THE STRUCTURE AND PROPERTIES OF CRYSTAL DEFECTS

MATERIALS SCIENCE MONOGRAPHS

Advisory Editor: C. LAIRD

Vol. 1 Dynamic Mechanical Analysis of Polymeric Material (Murayama)
Vol. 2 Laboratory Notes on Electrical and Galvanomagnetic Measurements (Wieder)
Vol. 3 Electrodeposition of Metal Powders (Călușaru)
Vol. 4 Sintering – New Developments (Ristić)
Vol. 5 Defects and Diffusion in Solids. An Introduction (Mrowec)
Vol. 6 Energy and Ceramics (Vincenzini)
Vol. 7 Fatigue of Metallic Materials (Klesnil and Lukáš)
Vol. 8 Synthetic Materials for Electronics (Jakowlew, Szymański and Włosiński)
Vol. 9 Mechanics of Aerospace Materials (Nica)
Vol. 10 Reactivity of Solids (Dyrek, Haber and Nowotny)
Vol. 11 Stone Decay and Conservation (Amoroso and Fassina)
Vol. 12 Metallurgy of Environmental Fracture (Briant)
Vol. 13 The Use of High–Intensity Ultrasonics (Puškár)
Vol. 14 Sintering – Theory and Practice (Kolar, Pejovnik and Ristić)
Vol. 15 Transport in Non–Stoichiometric Compounds (Nowotny)
Vol. 16 Ceramic Powders (Vincenzini)
Vol. 17 Ceramics in Surgery (Vincenzini)
Vol. 18 Intergranular Corrosion of Steels and Alloys (Čihal)
Vol. 19 Physics of Solid Dielectrics (Bunget and Popescu)
Vol. 20 The Structure and Properties of Crystal Defects (Paidar and Lejček)

MATERIALS SCIENCE MONOGRAPHS, 20

THE STRUCTURE AND PROPERTIES OF CRYSTAL DEFECTS

Proceedings of the Symposium on the Structure and Properties of Crystal Defects, Liblice, Czechoslovakia, June 13–17, 1983

Edited by

V. PAIDAR and L. LEJČEK

Institute of Physics, Czechoslovak Academy of Sciences, Prague, Czechoslovakia

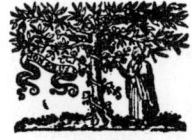

ELSEVIER
Amsterdam – Oxford – New York – Tokyo 1984

Distribution of this book is being handled
by the following publishers

for the U.S.A. and Canada
ELSEVIER SCIENCE PUBLISHING COMPANY, INC.
52 Vanderbilt Avenue, New York, N.Y. 10017

for the East European Countries, China,
Northern Korea, Cuba, Vietnam and Mongolia
SNTL – Publishers of Technical Literature
Spálená 51, 113 02 Praha 1, Czechoslovakia

for all remaining areas
ELSEVIER SCIENCE PUBLISHERS B.V.
Molenwerf 1
P.O.Box 211
1000 AE Amsterdam, The Netherlands

ISBN 0-444-99627-3 (Vol. 20)
ISBN 0-444-41685-4 (Series)

Copyright SNTL – Publishers of Technical Literature, Prague 1984
and The Society of Czechoslovak Mathematicians and Physicists

All rights reserved. No part of this publication may be reproduced, stored in a retrieval system or transmitted in any form or by any means, electronic, mechanical, photocopying, recording, or otherwise, without the prior written permission of the publisher.

Printed in Czechoslovakia

PREFACE

The aim of this symposium was to provide an appraisal of current knowledge of the structures of crystal defects and to elucidate the implications for various physical properties of crystals with defects. The scope of the symposium was restricted to dislocations, grain boundaries (internal interfaces) and, to a lesser extent, to more complex defects such as cracks. Point defects and external surfaces were excluded because they are considered in detail elsewhere; for example, International Surface Science Conferences (Warwick 1983) and European Conferences on Solid Surfaces (Gent 1982) are regularly organized. An emphasis was placed on defect structure at the atomic level and on mechanical properties of crystals with defects. The electrical properties of defects, and in particular defects in semiconductors, were not included since the specialized symposium on this subject was held in Hünfeld/Fulda in 1978 and a similar symposium was announced for this year.

Physicists, metallurgists and materials scientists from 13 countries participated in the symposium: 39 participants came from 9 western countries and 40 participants from 4 eastern countries.

Written contributions were presented in two ways at the symposium. The first consisted of 38 full-length papers which were presented orally. The second consisted of 44 short communications, which were presented in poster sessions, and only 3 of them were presented orally. The contribution are divided into 5 subject classifications:
1) The structure and properties of dislocations in metals and alloys with close-packed lattices
2) The structure and properties of dislocations in metals and alloys with a b.c.c. lattice
3) The structure and properties of defects in non-metallic materials
4) The structure and properties of grain boundaries
5) Collective behaviour and interaction of defects

This part of the symposium proceedings contains only the full-length papers. The short communications and abstracts of the full-length papers were published separately and made available only to the symposium participants.

June, 1983

V. Paidar
Symposium Secretary

Organizing Committee:

M. Bucki
J. Gemperlová
L. Lejček
V. Novák
V. Paidar
N. Zárubová

Program Committee:

J. Čadek
V. Dvořák
V. Karel
F. Kroupa
P. Lukáč
B. Šesták

Opening Address

It is my great pleasure to welcome you on behalf of the Institute of Physics, Czechoslovak Academy of Sciences here, in the Liblice castle, on the occasion of the international symposium on the Structure and Properties of Crystal Defects.

The physics of defects had been the favourite domain of physicists working in metallurgy for a long time even when the attention of most physicists was primarily paid to the perfect crystals. The defects proved to be very useful for the description of the plastic properties of materials at a submacroscopic level. Later, when the foundations of the concepts of the theory of defects, for example dislocations, had been convincingly established an interest in defects increased also in other branches of physics like liquid crystals, superconductivity, superfluidity and in research fields rather distant from the physics of metals like biology or geophysics.

Judging by the number of physicists interested in this Symposium it is apparent that the fundamental aspects of the physics of defect are still very attractive. The understanding of materials at the atomic level is essential to determine the microstructure and through this the macroscopic properties. Due to such experimental methods like high resolution techniques in electron microscopy and due to still increasing use of large high-speed computers for atomistic simulations our knowledge of defect structure has recently improved very substantially and it can be anticipated that this tendency will continue to the future.

In our Institute, the physics of defects has been traditionally studied in the Department of Physics of Metals but a growing interest in this subject is appearing also in other Departments. Problems of physics of metals such as cyclic plasticity, phase transformations associated with creep deformation, metallic glasses and surface layers are being investigated in our Department of Physics of Metals, and they are recognized as important up to date topics, where the crystal defects play a dominant role. All of them represent complex scientific tasks with significant technological implications. However, our Institute, which is the largest institute in the Czechoslovak Academy of Sciences, is not oriented only to the physics of metals. In fact larger capacities are devoted to the physics of semiconductors, magnetism, physics of low temperatures and even to the physics of elementary particles. The Institute of Physics participates also in the space materials research in the program Intercosmos, and we are also interested in solar energy materials and amorhpous materials.

I am sure that the recent results of the research of many famous laboratories from several continents, which will be presented at this Symposium, are undoubtedly contributing to the present development of the physics of materials.

It is the aim of this meeting to bring together a number of distinguished experts actively working in the field of crystal defects and to enhance the exchange of ideas among people studying various types of materials.

On behalf of the Institute of Physics and the symposium organizers I would like to thank all of you who have come to attend the Symposium and, in particular, those who have kindly prepared the contributed papers and short communications.

I wish you a pleasant stay, many interesting lectures and stimulating discussions.

Dr. A. Tříska
Deputy Director
Institute of Physics
Czechoslovak Academy of Sciences

CONTENTS

Preface v
Opening Address vii
Contents ix

Trends in the physics of dislocations and cracks . . . 1
    F. Kroupa

Section 1 : THE STRUCTURE AND PROPERTIES OF DISLOCATIONS IN METALS AND ALLOYS WITH CLOSE-PACKED LATTICES

Core structure of dislocations in f.c.c. base metals and alloys 19
    V. Paidar

The effects of dislocation core structure on flow in $L1_2$ ordered alloys 37
    D.P. Pope, V. Vitek

Dissociation of dislocations and plastic deformation modes in long period ordered alloys 53
    G. Vanderschaeve

Moving dislocations in aluminium-base alloys investigated by TEM and NMR techniques 75
    J. Th. M. De Hosson, O. Kanert

Temperature dependence of stacking fault energy 91
    T. Imura, H. Saka

Dislocation core structures in close-packed-hexagonal metals 102
    D.J. Bacon

Motion of dislocations in HCP metals 121
    P. Lukáč

Section 2 : THE STRUCTURE AND PROPERTIES OF DISLOCATIONS IN METALS AND ALLOYS WITH A BCC LATTICE

Dislocations in b.c.c. metals and ordered alloys and compounds with b.c.c.-based ordered structures . . . 131
    M. Yamaguchi, Y. Umakoshi

Kinked screw dislocations in the body-centred cubic lattice 148
    M.S. Duesbery

Application of tight binding techniques to crystal defect calculations 159
    D.M. Esterling

Motion of dislocations in b.c.c. metals at low temperatures 167
    S. Takeuchi, T. Hashimoto, K. Maeda

The low-temperature flow stress of high-purity α-iron single crystals 175
    D. Brunner, J. Diehl, A. Seeger

Selection of slip systems in low temperature deformation of niobium 184
    M. Meshii, Gun Woong Bang

Electron microscope studies of crystal dislocations . . 193
    L. P. Kubin

Theory of yield stress of dilute b.c.c. alloys 205
    H. Suzuki

The Snoek-Köster relaxation in body-centred cubic metals . 215
    M. Weller, M. Tietze, J. Diehl, A. Seeger

On the dislocation arrangement in Fe-3wt%Si single crystals after deformation in tension between 113 and 573 K . . . 223
    B. Šesták, M. Bucki

Dislocation mobility and overcoming of local barriers at low temperature as deduced from internal friction data . . 236
    V. I. Startsev, V. Ya. Platkov

Section 3 : THE STRUCTURE AND PROPERTIES OF DEFECTS IN
                NON-METALLIC MATERIALS

Defects in ionic crystals and oxides 251
    J. Philibert

Sessile dissociation and plastic deformation in $MgO.n.Al_2O_3$ spinels 266
    R. Duclos

The effects of OH^- ions on the dislocation mobility and the plastic deformation parameters of LiF crystals at low temperatures 275
    S.V. Lubenets, E.I. Ostapchuk, F. Appel, H.-J. Kaufmann

Dislocation in ionic crystals 282
    M. P. Puls

Disclinations in Sm C* liquid crystals 293
    L. Lejček

Section 4 : THE STRUCTURE AND PROPERTIES OF GRAIN BOUNDARIES

The structure of grain boundaries 301
    A. G. Crocker

Ideal and non-ideal coherent interfaces between f.c.c. and h.c.p. metallic crystals 318
    A. P. Sutton, J. W. Christian

Grain boundary sliding in metals and related phenomena . . 328
    I. Saxl, V. Skleničка, J. Čadek

Investigation of interphase interfaces by transmission
electron microscopy 338
    A. Gemperle

TEM and diffraction studies of the Mo-Mo_2C phase boundary . 350
    M. Florjancic, M. Rühle

Section 5 : COLLECTIVE BEHAVIOUR AND INTERACTION OF DEFECTS

Field theory of defects in Bravais crystals 357
    E. Kröner

Dislocation fields 370
    H. O. K. Kirchner

Simulation of kinks and jogs in dislocations using point
force arrays 384
    J.-P. J. Georges, C. S. Hartley

Interaction of dislocation with crystal surface and
emergence of dislocation on surface 397
    A. M. Kosevich, Yu. A. Kosevich

Continuum mechanics and collective behaviour
of dislocations 406
    B. Pegel

Disclination physics of plastic deformation 418
    A. E. Romanov, V. I. Vladimirov

Equilibrium configuration of dislocations around a crack
tip 427
    G. Michot, G. Champier

Electron microscope observation of crack propagation and
a dislocation model of fracture 438
    S. M. Ohr

Creep rate and microstructure of f.c.c. metals 447
    D. Caillard, J. L. Martin

Short communications presented at the symposium . . . 459

Acknowledgements 463

TRENDS IN THE PHYSICS OF DISLOCATIONS AND CRACKS
F. Kroupa
National Research Institute for Materials,
Opletalova 25, 113 12 Prague 1, Czechoslovakia

1. Introduction

In the early days of the physics of crystal defects, the general properties of defects were studied in the first approximation as independent of the details of their internal structure. However, it became soon evident that the defect properties are influenced by the crystal structure and by the type of interatomic forces which determine the defect structure and mobility. We shall discuss the development to a more atomistic approach in the theory of defects which play the main active role in plastic deformation and fracture, i.e. of dislocations and cracks.

While the theory of dislocations was developed mostly in physics, cracks were studied more in applied science. Our discussion of these two types of defects will be rather asymmetric: it will try to increase the interest of physicists in the problems of cracks. Some analogies between two very different types of line defects, dislocations and crack fronts, will be stressed.

2. Dislocations

2.1 Dislocations in crystals

After the introduction of the concept of a crystal dislocation in 1934, the theory of dislocations remained a hypothesis till the experimental proof of their existence in crystals and verification of their basic properties between 1950-1955. Since that time, theory of dislocations has developed into a set of facts on dislocations based both on theoretical and experimental investigation (see e.g. /1/).

It can be divided into three main regions:
i) Properties of individual dislocations in the crystal lattice, their mutual interactions and interactions with other crystal defects.
ii) Microscopic explanation of the plastic deformation of single crystals and of polycrystalline materials under different conditions (where dislocation motion plays the main active role).
iii) Influence of dislocations (or of plastic deformation) on other physical properties of crystalline solids, e.g. elastic, electrical, magnetic, thermal and optical properties, the role of dislocations in phase transformations, in crystal growth etc.

We shall concentrate on the properties of individual dislocations. Different models have been developed for a theoretical description of various dislocation properties.

2.2 Continuum models

Theory of dislocations in crystals found its first model ready in dislocations in continuum called also Volterra dislocations, introduced in the theory of elasticity already in 1907 (for a review see /2/) as a self-stress field in a doubly connected body.

The continuum model of a crystal dislocation, usually simplified for a singular dislocation line, had to be generalized for movable dislocations. A very useful new concept of force on a dislocation was introduced based on energy changes with a virtual or real displacement of a dislocation segment in the system: external forces - elastically stressed body - dislocation - other defects.

The continuum model gives good results for the problems where the long-range stress field of dislocations is important and surprisingly also sound results in some cases which are clearly beyond the scope of a continuum treatment, for example for properties of jogs and kinks on dislocations or for interaction of dislocations with point defect. The reason is that a lot of atomistic information and information on lattice geometry can be combined with the continuum model.

Different elastic properties of the continuum are assumed: linear isotropic, anisotropic or non-linear.

Let us mention, for illustration, the case of a screw dislocation in b.c.c. metals. In isotropic theory, it does not differ from dislocations in other lattices and its dilatation stress field is zero. Therefore, it should have only a weak interaction with point defects. However, it is known from experiments that interaction of interstitials such as carbon and nitrogen with screw dislocations in iron is as strong as with edge dislocations. This effect was explained within the isotropic theory when the main atomistic information was put in the point defect properties. The interstitials in b.c.c. metals produce tetragonal distorsions in the [100] directions and have a strong interaction even with the screw dislocation dilatation - free stress field.

The anisotropic theory leads to important corrections of the results of isotropic theory and has also discovered or explained some new phenomena, e.g. instability of dislocations in some directions in crystals with high anisotropy.

For screw dislocation in b.c.c. metals, the dilatation stress field is already non-zero, however weak - at least for iron.

Non-linear theory has been used practically only for explanation of special effects which do not follow from the linear theory, for example of the volume change due to a dislocation.

For a description of dislocation groups, theories of a continuous distribution of dislocations have been developed where the dislocation lines are smeared out into continuous functions of position. A continuous distribution of dislocations in a plane (which can be called a Somigliana dislocation) is used for description of planar dislocation groups, such as pile-ups and dislocation walls. A continuous distribution of dislocations in space has been developed especially by Kondo, Kröner, Bilby (see e.g. /1,2/) into a general theory of geometry of deformed continuum, of internal stresses and of plastic deformation. Nevertheless, the application to the collective behaviour of dislocations during plastic deformation has not yet reached the original expectations.

Disclinations or rotational dislocations (in contrast to translational dislocations called simply dislocations) were already introduced in continuum by Volterra. While disclinations are important elementary defects in liquid crystals and probably also in polymers, in crystals no disclinations exist as elementary line defects with a large Frank vector corresponding to the crystal rotational symmetry. Disclinations with irrational Frank vectors are used as a model for description of the stress fields of some dislocation groups in crystals.

2.3 Dislocation splitting

Dislocation splitting was introduced originally in 1952 as a dissociation of a perfect dislocation in the f.c.c. or h.c.p. lattice into two partials connected by a ribbon of stacking fault. Some more complicated dissociations were later observed, e.g. splitting of a dislocation in a plane into a larger number of partials in some non-metallic crystals with a complicated lattice.

To describe the three-fold symmetry of screw dislocations in b.c.c. metals, different splittings on three planes of the $\{110\}$ or $\{112\}$ type into four or three partials were proposed. These splittings are sessile and to move the screw dislocation in the slip plane, it must be transformed by external stress with the help of thermal activation into a glissile planar splitting. For small widths of splitting of the order of a few b, the splitting should be understood as a rough model of the core of a perfect dislocation.

In all these cases, the Burgers vectors of the partials and the type of stacking fault were chosen from simple crystallographic considerations. The concept of splitting was later generalized for the case where the stacking fault as an infinite planar defect is not stable, however, the ribbon in the split configuration can be stabilized by the decrease of the dislocation elastic energy. From the known dependence of the stacking fault energy on the relative displacement in the fault plane (the so called γ- surface) the Burgers vectors can be found /3/. The partials with irrational Burgers vectors (connected by non-equilibrium stacking faults) are called fractional dislocations.

In ordered metals, the structure of the superdislocation can be treated as splitting, where ordinary dislocations take the role of partials in the superlattice and the antiphase boundaries take the role of stacking faults. Besides, the ordinary dislocations can also be split into partials connected by stacking faults.

The concept of splitting has proved very fruitful for explanation of dislocation properties in some lattices. Its success is due to the fact that new additional information based on the properties of a special crystal lattice is added to the continuum model. Nevertheless, the splitting of dislocations does not seem to be a general phenomenon and has not been observed in some ionic crystals, nor in b.c.c. metals.

2.4 Atomistic models

There exists a wide class of problems which cannot be treated within the continuum model, the main being the Peierls-Nabarro stress due to the lattice periodicity, and generally the dislocation core structure, energy and properties.

Let us first mention two atomistic models of a rather historical importance, the Frenkel-Kontorova model and the Peierls-Nabarro model.

The Frenkel-Kontorova model treats one atomic row in a periodic potential, nevertheless, it was able to demonstrate the upper limit of the dislocation velocity and later also the influence of the form of the periodic potential on the Peierls-Nabarro stress.

The Peierls-Nabarro model forms a dislocation in a body consisting of two elastic half-spaces with forces between the surfaces depending periodically on the local relative displacement. The model could also be listed among the continuum models with one crystallographic information added - periodic interaction along the slip plane. The Peierls stress was first found using this model and its sensitivity to the chosen force law shown.

The PN model has been generalized for the dislocation core spread along three intersecting slip planes for description of a sessile screw dislocation in b.c.c. metals /4/. The corresponding distribution of the dislocation density $\rho(x) = db/dx$ calculated with the force law derived from a γ - surface for α-Fe on the $\{110\}$ planes is shown in Fig. 1. It can be roughly approximated by three fractional dislocations with Burgers vectors $b_1 = b_2 = b_3 = 0.272$ b at distances r = 2.5 b from the middle fractional dislocation with $b_4 = 0.184$ b. The stress necessary for a sessile-glissile transformation of the screw dislocation core has also been found.

The main disadvantage of the PN model is the treatment of the discrete core structure along the slip plane only, one of advantages is a clear graphic interpretation of the core which can be used for interpretation of more complicated three-dimensional atomistic models.

The attempts to describe a dislocation in a three-dimensional lattice already started in 1955 and became frequent after 1965 when computers enabled a numerical treatment of interaction of a large number of ions /5,6/. The central difficulty of the dislocation core simulation is no more connected with computation, but with the main physical information delivered to the model, i.e. the ion interaction, especially in the heavily distorted core-region. The detailed arrangement of the ions in the core, the core energy and the Peierls-Nabarro stress depend sensitively on the chosen forms of interionic potentials, which are not yet known with sufficient accuracy. Thus e.g. for α-Fe different potentials were used and only the features of the solution that did not depend on the exact form of the potentials were considered as valid /7/. High Peierls-Nabarro stress (at low temperatures) of screw dislocations due to the threefold core symmetry and predicted by the splitting models was confirmed by simulation.

For a rough quantitative treatment of plastic deformation in technical applications, surprisingly little theoretical information based on the continuum model is usually used. However, for a detailed description of plastic deformation in materials with special crystal structure, much more theoretical information is necessary, even from atomistic models. As an example, let us mention the b.c.c. metals, where the sessile structure of the screw dislocation core and the strong interaction of dislocations with interstitial impurities are responsible for a steep increase of the yield point with decreasing temperature. Another example are ordered alloys where mechanical properties are primarily given by the structure of superdislocations. One of the best explained processes is the high-temperature creep, where another type of atomistic information has been used, namely on diffusion which is the rate controlling process: though the creep deformation is mostly due to dislocation glide, its rate is controlled by climbing.

2.5 Outlook

Most of the basic properties of dislocations in crystals have been cleared up and the main attention has shifted to a quantitative treatment of the properties of individual dislocations and their different interaction and, especially, to applications in plastic deformation or generally in materials science.

Nevertheless, some basic problems remain still open, the most important being the structure of the dislocation core (the distribution of ions and also of electrons) and its behaviour under stress in different lattices with different bonds. Further development of the theory of crystal defects thus depends on further development of the electron theory of solids, which should deliver reliable interionic potentials or a self-consistent treatment of the distorted core region.

Some help may come from experiments, e.g. from microscopic experiments on the core structure using high-resolution TEM, however, also from macroscopic experiments. Some detailed theories of plastic deformation and of the influence of dislocations on other physical properties are based on certain assumptions on the dislocation core structure, and from the measurement of these macroscopic properties these assumptions may be checked.

There are also important open problems in the behaviour of large ensembles of dislocations, especially the explanation of instabilities of dislocation distributions in an external stress field and formation of non-homogeneous distributions of dislocations observed in deformed crystals.

3. Cracks

3.1 Elementary and complex cracks

A crack is a discontinuity in a body along a surface A bounded by a line s (which is closed or terminates on the body surface). It is, therefore, a planar (or generally a surface) defect formed by two free surfaces A^+, A^- bounded by a linear defect C called the crack front, crack root or crack tip.

If no other defect has been formed during the crack formation the crack will be called elementary (Fig. 2a). If the formation of the crack is accompanied with formation of other defects in its vicinity the crack will be called complex (Fig. 2b).

In contrast to dislocations, cracks have no self-stress field (complex cracks might have a stress field at the crack front due to other defects, especially to dislocations, however, it is usually a short-range field with respect to the crack dimensions).

The main elastic interaction of a crack with an external stress field is due to the change of the external field in the crack vicinity as some of the stress components have to be zero at surfaces A^+, A^-. The redistribution of the external stress field leads to a stress concentration at the crack tip.

Cracks are formed in two steps: crack nucleation and growth.

The crack nucleation is often an easy process (e.g. to get rid of microcracks in ceramics is as difficult as to get rid of dislocations in metals) and the main attention is paid to the growth of pre-existing cracks.

Fracture, i.e. the process of crack nucleation and growth, is usually classified according to the way of the crack growth.

From the point of view of microscopic mechanisms of the crack growth, we distinguish cleavage fracture, ductile fracture, fatigue fracture, high temperature creep fracture, etc. From the position of the crack path in polycrystalline materials, intergranular and transgranular fracture is distinguished. From the point of view of mechanics, the crack growth can be stable or unstable. Different modes of fracture can take place in the same material, depending on stress, temperature and environment.

The effective fracture energy γ_{ef} which must be delivered for formation of a unit crack area can be generally written as

$$(1) \quad \gamma_{ef} = 2\gamma_o + \gamma_H + \gamma_K + \gamma_D ,$$

where besides the surface energy term $2\gamma_o$ and internal energy of formed defects γ_D, the term γ_H is the energy transformed into heat (e.g. via dislocation motion at the crack tip) and γ_K the kinetic energy.

The effective surface energy ranges from $\gamma_{ef} \approx 2\gamma_o \approx 1$ J/m^2 for elementary cleavage cracks in ionic crystals or traditional ceramics to $\gamma_{ef} \approx 10^5$ J/m^2 for complex ductile cracks in metals.

Crack growth can be considered as a motion of a line defect - crack front. Different models have been developed to describe its properties.

3.2 Continuum models: fracture mechanics

The task of fracture mechanics - FM /8,9/ is to describe the properties of cracks in stressed bodies in order to be able to predict their behaviour. It assumes a pre-existing crack, i.e. is not interested in crack nucleation, and does not discuss the microscopic mechanisms of crack extension. All theoretical studies in FM use the methods of continuum mechanics and, therefore, FM can be called a continuum model of cracks or of crack fronts.

The following procedure is used in the theoretical approach of FM. A body of a given form and dimensions (characterized by data L) with a crack (data l) is stressed by external forces (data P) and the mechanical properties of the body are characterized within the continuum mechanics by data M (e.g. elastic, plastic, creep properties). The resistance to crack extension is not included in M.

The first step of FM is introduction of a scalar "driving parameter" X which should characterize the effect of the system stressed body + loading at the crack front and which can be calculated by the methods of continuum mechanics as

(2) $X = X(l, L, P, M)$.

In the linear fracture mechanics (LFM) the validity of the theory of elasticity in the body is assumed, in the nonlinear fracture mechanics (NLFM) plastic deformation (or other energy absorbing processes) is assumed in the whole body or at least in the zone in front of the crack tip (plastic zone).

FM postulates that the crack will not extend if the criterion of crack stability is satisfied,

(3) $X < X_c$,

where X_c, the critical value of the parameter X, is a new material constant (not included among M). For $X > X_c$ the loaded body with a crack loses stability and the crack quickly extends.

In some materials, e.g. in ceramics, or under special conditions, e.g. at high temperatures even in metals, a slow subcritical extension of cracks takes place for $X < X_c$. The crack velocity depends on the driving parameter X and is usually described as

(4) $v = dl/dt = A \ X^n$,

where A and n are further material constants of FM.

Within the phenomenological approach of FM, the condition of crack stability (3) and the velocity of subcritical crack growth (4) can be considered as postulates and their validity should be confirmed from experiments on bodies with cracks (especially the independence of (3) and (4) from the body and crack dimensions). Different parameters X are used in LFM and NLFM and, for some of them, attempts are made in FM to derive at least the criterion (3) from energy considerations.

Let us note that the material constants of FM (like X_c, A, n) depend not only on chemical composition, but very sensitively (more than the material constants M) also on microstructure, temperature and environment.

Three modes of deformation are usually assumed (Fig. 3) and are distinguished by indices I, II, III. For simplicity, tension mode I will be further assumed and index I left out.

Within the LFM, the calculated stress concentration at the front of a sharp crack tends to infinity. The tensile stress σ_{yy} in front of the crack (for $\varphi = 0$, $x = r \ll 1$) can be written as

(5) $\sigma_{yy} = K(l,L,P) \ (2\pi r)^{-\frac{1}{2}}$,

where K is called the stress intensity factor and is the main driving parameter X of the LFM. It can be calculated from the given form of the body with crack and given external forces. K is a measure of intensity of the stress concentration in front of the crack tip, and the crack stability criterion $K < K_c$ seems to be sound in the cases where the tensile stress governs the crack growth by cleavage without (or only with a small) plastic zone. The material constant K_c (i.e. the critical value of the stress intensity factor K) is called fracture toughness. An equation of type (4), $v = AK^n$, is used for subcritical crack growth.

Another pair of parameters is also used in LFM, the crack extension force G and its critical value G_c. G is defined as

(6) $G = - \partial(W-L_p) / \partial l$,

where W is the elastic energy of the body with a crack and L_p the work of external forces P, the derivative is taken with respect to the virtual displacement of the crack front. Therefore, G has the meaning of the force per unit length of the crack front or of energy which the body and loading system release when the unit crack front moves a unit distance (G can also be called the energy release rate).

However, G does not represent an independent parameter in LFM. From its definition a relation between G and K follows,

(7) $G = K^2(1 - \nu^2) / E$

for plain strain. The stability criterion $G < G_c$ is, therefore, equivalent to $K < K_c$ in the LFM, nevertheless, it brings an interesting interpretation: G_c has the meaning of energy necessary for extension of the crack over a unit surface and, therefore, it is equal to the effective fracture energy γ_{ef} from eq. (1). The criterion $G(l,L,P,M) < \gamma_{ef}$ is a direct generalization of the original Griffith criterion $\sigma < \sigma_{Gr} \approx \sqrt{E\gamma_{ef}/l}$ by taking into account the form and dimensions of the finite body and the position of the crack.

When a plastic zone develops at the crack tip the stress distribution changes and depends on materials constants such as yield point and work hardening coefficient which enter among constants M. Different driving parameters X are used for this case in the NLFM, especially the crack opening displacement δ and the Rice J-integral with the meaning close to the crack extension force. However, the NLFM fails when the plastic zone is large and when one driving parameter X need not be sufficient to describe the crack behaviour. To find the proper driving parameters, the investigation of the microscopic mechanisms of crack growth seems to be necessary.

A crack under stress in a body and the stress concentration can be modelled by a continuous planar distribution of virtual (so-called crack) dislocations and also the plastic zone ahead of the crack can be modelled by a continuum planar distribution of real dislocations /8/. This model has remarkable versatility and can be used either as a special formulation of FM (as a treatment of cracks in continuum profiting from the mathematical apparatus of the theory of dislocations) or in discussion of microscopic mechanisms of crack growth.

There are formal similarities between the treatment of the crack front in FM and the treatment of a dislocation in the continuum model. Thus e.g. the expression of the crack extension force G with the help of the stress intensity factor K is an analogy of the Peach-Koehler formula, i.e. the expression of the force on dislocation with the help of the local value of external stress.

However, the force action on dislocations is much better understood. The force component in the slip plane is due to shear stresses and leads to dislocation glide while the force perpendicular to the slip plane is due to normal stresses and leads to dislocation climb at high temperatures only. These two type of motion are usually independent and can be treated separately in a three-dimensional stress field.

The force action on the crack front seems to be well understood only in the simplest case, the growth of an elementary cleavage crack due to tensile stress across the crack plane. The combination of modes I, II, III leads to crack extension mechanisms which are not independent even for elementary cracks and, especially, for complex cracks. The effect of a three-dimensional stress on crack growth is, therefore, complicated and difficult to solve within the phenomenological approach of FM.

3.3 Microscopic mechanisms of crack growth

Fracture mechanism maps /10/ are diagrams showing the fields of dominance of a given mechanism of fracture in a given material in dependence on two variables: tensile stress - temperature. They can be constructed empirically by assembling the fracture data of a given material or theoretically via models for the individual fracture mechanisms. Their simplified examples for b.c.c. and f.c.c. metals (polycrystalline metals of technical purity) in Fig. 4 are divided into the following fields:

CL   - cleavage fracture with three subfields distinguished, CL_1 (growth from pre-existing cracks), CL_2 (cleavage crack nucleates during the preceding small plastic deformation by twinning or slip) and CL_3 (cleavage crack is formed after a considerable plastic deformation): in all these cases, the fracture path can be transgranular or intergranular;

LTD - low temperature ductile fracture (usually by nucleation of holes at inclusions and necking of regions between the holes by localized plastic deformation) leading usually to a transgranular, in some cases (with inclusions preferentially at boundaries) to intergranular crack path;

TC   - transgranular creep fracture (a high temperature analogy of LTD at relatively high stresses, not typical for usual creep conditions),

IC — intergranular creep fracture (by formation and coalescence of cavities along the grain boundaries under typical creep conditions-high temperatures and low stresses);

R — rupture (ductile fracture by macroscopic necking or shearing to zero cross section);

DYN — dynamic fracture at very high stresses (when the strain rate exceeds $\dot{\varepsilon} \approx 10^6 \text{ s}^{-1}$ and elastic and plastic waves become important).

Note that the concept of fracture-mechanism maps is very different from the concepts of fracture mechanics. Time-to-fracture is understood as a sum of the pre-nucleation period, time for nucleation and time of crack growth. It shows the field of dominant fracture mechanisms in coordinates σ - T which is sound if the crack nucleation is the main part of the time-to-fracture. However, if crack growth forms the main part of time-to-fracture, the average stress σ is not the proper parameter, the mechanism of the crack growth and its velocity are governed by some of the parameters X of fracture mechanics which also depend on specimen geometry and crack length.

Some attempts to construct the crack growth-mechanism maps for bodies with pre-existing cracks in other coordinates (e.g. K_I-T) have already been made, however, it again can be argued that, under different conditions, different X parameters are rate controlling.

Nevertheless, the fracture-mechanism maps show graphically, though only approximately, the sensitive dependence of mechanisms of crack growth (and partly also of crack nucleation) on the type of material and on external conditions, especially on loading and temperature.

Let us comment on the main difference between the fracture behaviour of b.c.c. and f.c.c. metals. The occurence of the cleavage cracks in b.c.c. metals at low temperature is a consequence of the steep increase of the yield stress with decreasing temperature in these metals, due mainly to the low mobility of screw dislocations and to the effect of interstitial impurities like carbon with tetragonally distorted neighbouring lattice leading to strong interaction with all dislocations (including screws). Therefore, an effective plastic zone cannot develop in b.c.c. metals at low temperatures.

There is no general mechanism of crack nucleation and growth which could be common to all crystalline materials under different conditions. The individual mechanisms depend on the type of bond, on the crystal structure and microstructure (e.g. grain size, distribution of dislocations, inclusions etc.), on physical conditions (the level and type of stress, temperature, environment) and even on geometrical conditions (the dimensions and form of body and crack).

The number of papers discussing different aspects of fracture mechanisms is so large that we shall not attempt to review them (see e.g. /8,11/) and shall only add a few comments.

The atomistic structure in the plane of an elementary crack has already been considered /8/ and the treatment of braking of bonds in the crack tip reminds the PN model of a dislocation. The crack loses stability when the crack opening displacement reaches a critical value. Modern atomistic models of elementary cracks /6/ are based on a crack tip computer simulation in a block of ions. The stressed configuration before the lost of stability can be found and it can be judged whether the crack tip will extend as a brittle crack or will be blunted by emission of dislocations. Similarly as in the atomistic models of dislocations, these models need more information on the ion interaction in the heavily distorted regions to reach quantitative results.

For complex cracks, the situation at the crack front is so complicated that usually only some aspects of the process leading to crack growth are discussed and only in a few cases the theory is able to predict the crack behaviour and the time-to-fracture.

We shall mention one example which is already well understood, namely the intergranular creep fracture.

Fracture in polycrystalline metals at high temperatures ($T/T_M > 0.4$) and small stresses ($\sigma/E < 10^{-3}$) leading to low creep deformation rates ($\dot{\varepsilon} < 10^{-6} s^{-1}$) has the following main features: the creep ductility is low, usually smaller then 1% (in materials which at the same temperature at higher stress have ductility between 10 and 50%) and fracture is intergranular.

The main mechanism of this special fracture is nucleation of cavities at the grain boundaries by grain boundary sliding and their subsequent growth mainly by vacancy diffusion along grain boundaries to the cavities. This process covers approximately 90% of the time-to-fracture, an intergranular crack is formed by coalescence of cavities and in the final stage of fracture the crack quickly extends along the cavitated grain boundaries (so that it reminds brittle fracture).

Detailed theories have been developed /12/ which made it possible to divide the IC field in fracture-mechanism maps into subfields with special dominating mechanism of cavity growth (simple diffusional growth, strain enhanced diffusive growth, constrained diffusive growth, etc.) leading to different dependences of the rate of cavity growth on σ and T.

The success of the theory of IC is due to good understanding of the main atomistic process involved, namely diffusion. Note that the IC of specimen without larger pre-existing cracks cannot be traeted by the methods of fracture mechanics as the process controlling the time-to-fracture is the crack nucleation.

However, another important problem is now in the centre of interest in high temperature failure, namely the subcritical growth of pre-existing cracks (formed e.g. as a technological defect or as a result of low cycle fatigue or thermal fatigue) under creep conditions. Both the microscopic approach and fracture mechanics are used /13/. The crack can grow as a result of two competing processes: (i) enhanced cavity growth in the stress concentration in front of the crack tip and coalescence of the cavities, (ii) relaxation of the stress concentration by creep deformation, plastic deformation and even by cavitation.

The microscopic theories have to consider the stress relaxation within the continuum mechanics and are able to derive for special materials and conditions the velocity of the crack growth $v = A X^n$ with the proper parameter X and the values of constants A,n following from the theory.

3.4 Outlook

Two approaches have been developed in the investigation of fracture.

The first - fracture mechanics - based on continuum treatment seems to be victorious in applications for the time being. It starts with a pre-existing crack and cannot, therefore, treat the cases where the crack nucleation is the rate controlling process (e.g. IC) or where the crack does not form at all (e.g. failure by rupture). Its main merit is the description of the crack stability and growth in the bodies with cracks of a given form and size, based on mechanics of continua. Its main disadvantage is the neglect of the microscopic mechanisms of fracture which leads to difficulties in describing crack growth in complicated cases (e.g. with a large plastic zone) and in some cases the fracture mechanics fails as a theory based on one driving parameter X.

The second approach - microscopic - is far from being a unified theory and is formed by a mosaic of individual cases. With respect to the variety of material properties and external conditions, it cannot develop into a unified theory. Nevertheless, in some cases the microscopic approach is already able not only to explain qualitatively the crack nucleation and growth but also to derive a quantitative description of the rate of these processes and predict the time-to-fracture. Until recently the main disadvantage of the microscopic approach was that it concentrated too much on the vicinity of the crack tip only and ignored the effect of the geometry of the whole body with the crack and the volume mechanical properties which have influence on the stress concentration near the crack tip.

Further understanding of fracture needs without doubt more experiments on recognition of the main microscopic mechanisms of crack nucleation and growth in different types of materials in different fields of conditions.

Another trend which has already started is bringing together the detailed microscopic approach and the formal general approach of fracture mechanics. The continuum treatment of fracture mechanics can clear out the conditions under which the microscopic investigation of the crack front is made. The results of experimental and theoretical investigation of microscopic mechanism of fracture should deliver to the fracture mechanics, for the given material and conditions, the identification of the governing driving parameters, the criterion of the crack stability and the laws of the subcritical crack growth.

4. Concluding remarks

Let us stress in conclusion that motion of line defects is generally more complicated than motion of point defects: line defects change during their motion their form, length, local character and properties. So for example edge dislocation may form parts of screw dislocations with completely different properties, the stress concentration at the crack front changes with the crack growth.

Dislocations and elementary crack fronts can be considered as elementary line defects.

There are only two types of motion of dislocations, gliding and climbing, with clear driving parameters, force $b\tau$ in the slip plane or $b\sigma$ on the extra half plane, and these two types of motion are, at least in first approximation, independent even in a three-dimensional stress field σ_{ij}.

For elementary cracks loaded by pure modes I, II, III, the proper driving parameters seem to be K_I, K_{II} and K_{III}. However, in a general stress field σ_{ij}, the mutual interaction of the modes and proper driving parameter or parameters are not yet known.

To describe a crack front of a complex crack as a line defect is an obvious simplification. It is a region of complicated processes of plastic deformation in a nonhomogeneous stress field in the proximity of free crack surfaces, processes of damage (for example microcracks) formation and interaction of these processes.

Nevertheless, for all three line defects - dislocations, elementary and complex crack fronts, the main problem seems to be common: to get more experimental information on their internal structure and to incorporate these facts into the theories of their motion.

References

/1/ Dislocations in crystals (Ed. F.R.N. Nabarro), Vol. 1-5,
North Holland Publ. Comp., Amsterdam 1979.

/2/ Teodosiu C.: Elastic models of crystal defects, Springer, Berlin 1982.

/3/ Vítek V., Kroupa F.: Phil. Mag. 19 (1969) 265.

/4/ Lejček L., Kroupa F.: Czech. J. Phys. B26 (1976) 528.

/5/ Interatomic Potentials and Simulation of Lattice Defects (Ed. P.C. Gehlen,
J.R. Beeler, R.I. Jaffee), Plenum Press, New York 1972.

/6/ Computer Simulation for Materials Applications (Ed. R.J. Arsenault,
J.R. Beeler, J.A. Simmons) Part 1,2, NBS, Gaithersburg 1979.

/7/ Vítek V.: Crystal Lattice Defects 5 (1974) 1.

/8/ Fracture (Ed. H. Liebowitz) Vol 1-7, Academic Press, New York 1968-1972.

/9/ Fracture Mechanics of Ceramics (Ed. R.C. Brandt, D.P. Hasselman,
F.F. Lange) Vol. 1-6, Plenum Press, New York 1974-1982.

/10/ Gandhi C., Ashby M.F.: Acta Met. 27 (1979) 1565.

/11/ Development in Fracture Mechanics (Ed. G.G. Chell) Vol. 2,
Applied Science Publ., London 1981.

/12/ Svensson L.E., Dunlop G.L.: Internat. Metals Rev. (1981) 109.

/13/ Sadananda K., Shahinian P.: Metal Science 15 (1981) 425.

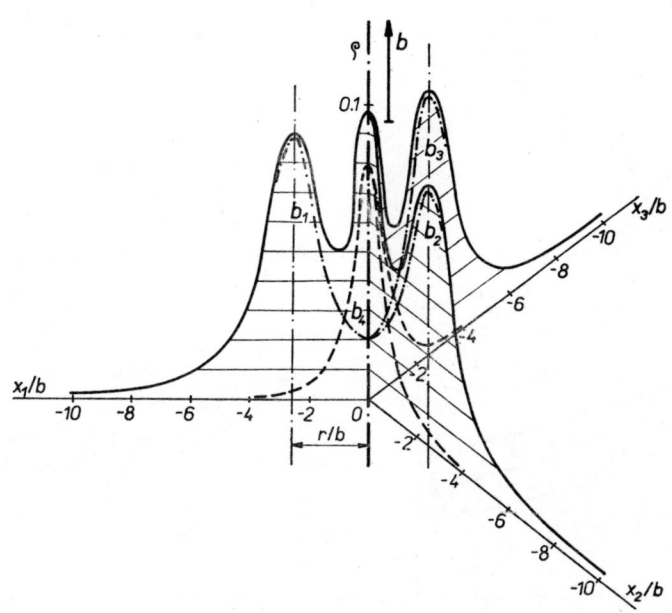

Fig. 1 Dislocation densities $\rho(x)$ in the dislocation core of a screw dislocation in α- Fe extended along three $\{110\}$ planes within a generalized PN model /4/.

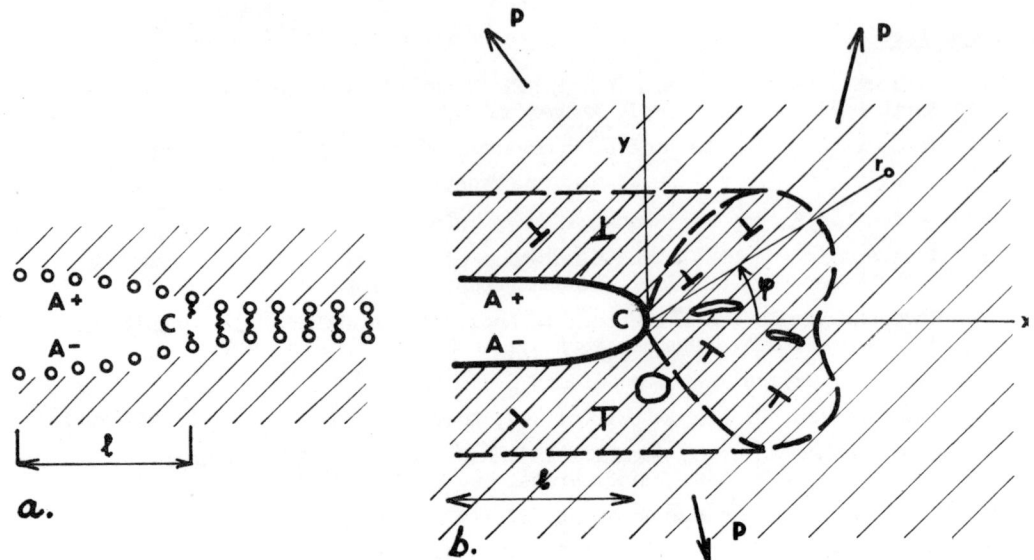

Fig. 2   a) Elementary crack, b) complex crack

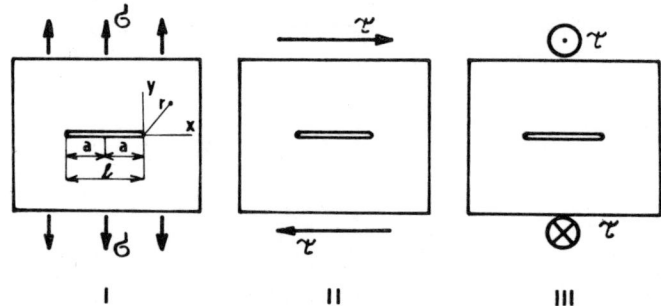

Fig. 3   Three modes of deformation near the crack

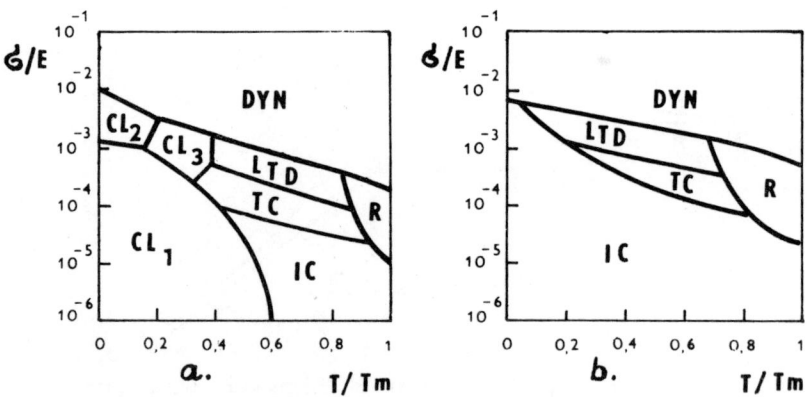

Fig. 4   Schematic fracture-mechanism maps for a) BCC metals, b) FCC metals /10/.

- 16 -

SECTION 1

THE STRUCTURE AND PROPERTIES OF
DISLOCATIONS IN METALS AND ALLOYS
WITH CLOSE-PACKED LATTICES

CORE STRUCTURE OF DISLOCATIONS IN F.C.C. BASE METALS AND ALLOYS
V. Paidar
Institute of Physics, Czechoslovak Academy of Sciences,
Na Slovance 2, 180 40 Prague 8, Czechoslovakia

1. Dislocations and stacking faults in f.c.c. metals

1.1 Dislocation dissociation into Shockley partials

Modelling of lattice defects on computers to study their atomic structure started more than two decades ago. The history of dislocation core simulations began with the two-dimensional model of a close-packed atomic structure /1,2/. The interatomic forces were described by central pairwise potentials considering only the interaction between nearest neighbours. Such a simplified model was assumed to correspond to a rather untypical crystal of solid argon. Two-body central potentials have considerable calculation advantages following from simplicity of their use in defect modelling. It has been shown later in various papers that some qualitative properties of defects which can be revealed by computer simulations are essentially independent of a particular potential form.

Classical papers on $1/2 \langle 110 \rangle$ dislocation core structure in f.c.c. metals by Cotterill and Doyama were published in the mid sixties /3,4/. The calculations for both edge and screw dislocations were carried out with a Morse potential in a three-dimensional model. It was demonstrated that the relaxed core configuration is dissociated into two Shockley partials with the $1/6 \langle 112 \rangle$ Burgers vectors as had been suggested much earlier from the existence of a stable stacking fault in the f.c.c. lattice (see Fig. 1). In spite of the fact that the nature of dislocation dissociation can be regarded as a consequence of the lattice type, the width of the dissociation critically depends on the interatomic forces.

When the two partial dislocations are sufficiently far apart and when the stacking fault between them is well defined (i.e. when the displacement vector characterizing the fault is constant over the fault ribbon and equal to $1/6 \langle 112 \rangle$) then the stacking fault energy can be determined by elasticity theory, because its use to calculate the partial separation is then adequately justified. However, for wide partial dislocation cores or for their small separations estimates of the stacking fault energy based on elasticity theory are not reliable and an atomistic approach must be employed /5-7/. The relaxed dislocation core is usually wider than the core deduced from the elastic displacements of a singular dislocation and possesses an internal structure that cannot be derived from the elastic continuum. In consequence, the separation of partials with singular cores obtained from elasticity theory is often different from the separation of relaxed cores.

A measurement of the stacking fault energy from the Shockley partial separation may lead for small separations to an incorrect result when a simplifying elasticity theory approach is used /7-10/. There is also an effect of the formation of dislocation images in the electron microscope /11/ since the image separation may differ from the actual partial separation. The difference of the stacking fault energy for copper deduced assuming anisotropic elasticity (about 40 mJm^{-2}) from the value obtained by the atomistic simulation of the core dissociation (70 mJm^{-2}) /7/ is considerable. For the same value of the stacking fault energy elasticity theory gives usually a narrower dislocation dissociation than the atomistic approach. The effect of the dislocation core structure on the partial separation was also studied using a Peierls model for the partial cores /9/. On the contrary to /7/, it was found that the partial separation should be smaller than the separation of the singular cores in the elasticity theory. Another model, in which the dislocation core was described by a continuous distribution of dislocations, was reported in /10/. It was shown that for the same separation of the partial dislocations a wide range of the stacking fault energies can be obtained assuming various dislocation distributions. In summary, various interatomic forces giving the same partial separation can lead to different values of the stacking fault energy because of a nonlinear character of those forces.

So far we have discussed the determination of the stacking fault energy from direct observations of the dissociated dislocations. However, there are several other methods use to experimentally determine the stacking fault energy /12/. Since the majority of them are indirect methods, a theoretical analysis must be employed to extract the fault energy from the experimental data. Due to inconsistences in applications of less than adequate relationships between experimental measurables and the fault energy, the spread in the reported fault energies is very wide /13/. A more recent review of the experimental measurements of the stacking fault energies including the energies of antiphase boundaries can be found in /14/, where the most reliable values are also picked out.

1.2 Calculations of the stacking fault energy

In the following we shall concentrate on theoretical evaluations of the fault energy. The number and spacings of the first and second neighbours in the f.c.c. lattice is the same as in the ideal h.c.p. lattice. Since the ideal non-relaxed stacking fault in the f.c.c. lattice represents a slice of the h.c.p. lattice its energy is entirely given by the interaction between more distant neighbours. On the other hand, the structure dependent part of the cohesive energy is largest for the nearest neighbours (first or second). Hence, when a reliable description of the interactomic forces is sufficiently accurate to determine the cohesive energy and the elastic constants, it need not necessarily yield the stacking fault energy with a similar accuracy.

For simple metals the stacking fault energy can be calculated using the pseudopotential theory /15-25/. The interatomic potentials derived from the pseudopotential theory are pairwise potentials oscillating for large atomic separations, r, as $\cos(2k_F r)/(2k_F r)^3$, where k_F is the Fermi wave number. Due to a long-range nature of the potential, the sum of the energy contributions of many interatomic bonds must be carefully estimated. Several summation methods have been proposed in the literature (for a review see /20/).

However, the theoretical estimates do not depend only on the method used for the summation of the atomic interactions, but are strongly affected by the atomic pseudopotential. It has been shown that reliable fault energies can be expected only for very accurate atomic pseudopotentials /19,20/.

Pseudopotential theory has been successfully applied to normal metals where d-electrons are essentially unimportant. For transition metals the calculation of stacking fault energy was carried out using a tight-binding description of the d band /26/. This method is capable of providing a qualitatively correct picture of the phase stability of the close-packed structures (f.c.c. and h.c.p.). However, because of simplifying assumptions (e.g. s-d mixing is neglected) only a right order of magnitude of the fault energies can be expected. In fact, all the theoretical estimates mentioned above should be compared with the stacking fault energy measured at 0 K, since the effect of temperature has not yet been theoretically considered. In spite of the uncertainty involved in the theory as well as in the experiments, our knowledge of the stacking faults in various close-packed metals and alloys has improved substantially and critically chosen estimates of the fault energies are fairly reliable.

1.3 Various core structures of 1/2 $\langle 110 \rangle$ dislocations

Besides the dissociation of the 1/2 $\langle 110 \rangle$ dislocations on $\{111\}$ plane there are indications that the 1/2 $\langle 110 \rangle$ dislocation might possess another core structures under certain circumstances. It has been reported in /27-31/ that slip on $\{110\}$ planes prevails at elevated temperatures in samples with the orientation of the deformation axis near to the $[001]$ direction. The plane with the maximum resolved shear stress then lies close to the (101) plane and the Schmidt factor is higher for this plane than for the (111) plane. Slip on $\{110\}$ planes is not confined only to materials with a large stacking fault energy on $\{111\}$ plane (as e.g. aluminium) but was observed in various other f.c.c. metals /28/. The occurrence of $\{110\}$ dislocation glide follows from slip pattern observations in an optical microscope /27-29/ and was deminstrated by electron microscopic study of "in-situ" deformation /30/ and by X-ray transmission topography /31/. It has been observed that $\{110\}$ slip is not composed of elementary glides on $\{111\}$ planes for the long dislocation segments moving on $\{110\}$ plane. The experiments mentioned above motivated theoretical papers where stacking faults and dislocation dissociations on $\{110\}$ plane were investigated /24,32/. In /32/ faults with displacement vectors 1/12 $\langle 110 \rangle$ and -1/12 $\langle 110 \rangle$ were proposed, but no stable stacking faults on $\{110\}$ planes were found for an aluminium potential at 0 K in /24/. However, when a lattice expansion was allowed a local minimum corresponding to the 1/4 $\langle 110 \rangle$ fault emerged and it was concluded that dislocation splitting on $\{110\}$ planes may be stabilized by a thermal expansion. Contrary to the dissociation on $\{111\}$ planes, which is entirely given by the lattice geometry, the dissociation on $\{110\}$ planes depends on the interatomic forces and therefore, is more complicated to be dealt with.

Another type of 1/2 $\langle 110 \rangle$ dislocation dissociation is into composite dislocations, which can glide on $\{100\}$ planes. They originate from a transformation of sessile Lomer-Cottrell dislocations. Recently the glide of composite dislocations has been systematically studied in /33-35/ using transmission microscopy methods (see also /30/). Since these dislocation segments are able to glide on $\{100\}$ planes, their core structure should be qualitatively different from sessile Lomer-Cottrell locks. The separation of $\{100\}$ atomic planes is the second largest (the most widely spaced planes are $\{111\}$ and the separation of the $\{110\}$ planes is the third largest in the f.c.c. lattice - see Fig. 1). A narrow core configuration which was dissociated on $\{100\}$ type plane was found in /36/ by computer simulations using an interatomic potential constructed for aluminium. Let us stress that the dissociation extending along certain crystallographic plane does not necessarily imply the existence of a stable stacking fault. Similar to b.c.c. metals /37/, dislocations may be split into fractional dislocations distributed along an appropriate plane even in the case when there is no stable stacking fault (the term partial dislocations is reserved for the splitting with a stable stacking fault).

2. Planar faults and dislocations in $L1_2$ ordered alloys

2.1 Stacking faults and antiphase boundaries

The number of general stacking faults, including the antiphase boundaries, in a superlattice is higher than in the basic lattice. Therefore, the core structure of superlattice dislocations is naturally more complex. In order to assess this problem it is necessary to study the stability of possible stacking faults and to evaluate their relative energies.

A superlattice of the $L1_2$ type is formed on the basic f.c.c. lattice where one sublattice (which is a simple cubic lattice) is occupied by B atoms while the remaining three sublattices are occupied by A atoms in the ordered structure of an A_3B alloy (see Fig. 2). If the position of the B sublattice in one part of the crystal is shifted with respect to its position in another part by a vector $1/2 \langle 110 \rangle$, such crystal regions are separated by an antiphase boundary (APB) /38/. The APB energy depends strongly on the orientation of the normal to the boundary plane. It was shown in /39/ on the basis of a simple model, where only the interaction between the nearest neighbours was taken into account, that the energy has a minimum for the $\{100\}$ plane. Besides the planar defects disturbing only long range order, there are defects deduced from the existence of the stacking fault on $\{111\}$ plane in the basic f.c.c. lattice. It is seen in Fig. 3 that three displacements $1/6 \langle 112 \rangle$ of the upper half-crystal with respect to the lower one (separated by the (111) plane) will set the atoms of the first atomic plane above the fault to the position exactly on the top of the atoms in the first atomic plane below the fault (e.g. the displacement $1/6 [\bar{1}\bar{1}2]$). Therefore, the energy of this hypothetical configuration will be very large and the configuration itself will be unstable. However, when the three displacements $1/6 \langle 112 \rangle$ are of the type $1/6 [\bar{2}11]$ (see Fig. 3), the stacking fault in the basic lattice is formed. Since the long range order is simultaneously disturbed the fault is called a complex stacking fault (CSF). Another stacking fault is formed when the "prohibited" displacement vector $1/6 [\bar{1}\bar{1}2]$ is extended to $1/3 [\bar{1}\bar{1}2]$. In this case there are no B-B nearest neighbours and the energy of the fault which is called a superlattice intrinsic stacking fault (SISF) can be expected to be relatively low. Notice that this fault had not been considered in the review paper /38/ and was employed in dislocation dissociations for the first time by Kear et al. /40/.

The stability of planar faults on $\{111\}$ and $\{100\}$ planes in the $L1_2$ structure was investigated in /41/ using a computer simulation technique introduced by Vitek /23/. A generalized stacking fault is characterized by an arbitrary displacement vector lying in the fault plane, and can be obtained by cutting the crystal along a crystallographic plane and displacing the two halves by the displacement vector. The fault energy as a function of the displacement vector can be represented by a so called γ-surface. Stable faults then correspond to the local minima in the γ-surface.

The stability of generalized stacking faults can be also revealed by symmetry considerations /42-43/. Since an intrinsic stacking fault represents a bicrystal with zero misorientation of the component crystals (the intrinsic stacking fault is fully specified by the plane normal and by the displacement vector), the symmetry properties of bicrystals /44/ can be applied to stacking faults.

For the displacements on the (111) plane it is sufficient to consider the displacements in $\langle 112 \rangle$ directions which conserve the mirror symmetry planes $\{110\}$ and colour reversing twofold rotations. Those are the displacements lying in $(\bar{1}01)$, $(0\bar{1}1)$, $(1\bar{1}0)$ planes designated in Fig. 3. Because the displacements zero, $1/3\,[\bar{1}\bar{1}2]$ and $1/3\,[\bar{2}11]$, lie at the intersection of three distinct $\{110\}$ mirror planes, these three points will correspond to the extrema on the γ-surface (the unfaulted crystal represents the absolute minimum, the $1/3\,[\bar{1}\bar{1}2]$ displacement represents an SISF and a maximum can be expected at $1/3\,[\bar{2}11]$). The existence of local minima at $1/6\,[\bar{2}11]$ (CSF) and $1/2\,[\bar{1}01]$ (APB) do not follow from the symmetry requirements and if such minima exist they need not be situated at $1/6\,[\bar{2}11]$ and $1/2\,[\bar{1}01]$ but their positions may be shifted along $[\bar{2}11]$ or $[1\bar{2}1]$ directions, respectively. However, the SISF displacement vector must be $1/3\,[\bar{1}\bar{1}2]$. A non-crystallographic generalized stacking fault vector is not limited only to the $L1_2$ structure, but was first reported for the DO_3 structure /45/. Notice that when an absolute minimum is found at $1/3\,[\bar{1}\bar{1}2]$ this implies that the $L1_2$ structure is unstable and a DO_{19} structure will possesses a lower energy. The most striking conclusion of the investigation of $\{111\}$ faults is that both CSF and APB may be unstable, meaning that the existence of $L1_2$ ordered alloys with just one stable stacking fault on $\{111\}$ planes (SISF) is theoretically permitted.

Analogous arguments can be applied to the faults on (010) and (101) planes (see Fig. 4 and 5, respectively). For the faults on (010) planes, there are three non-equivalent points of intersection of mirror planes, namely, the zero displacement, $1/2\,[\bar{1}01]$ and $1/2\,[001]$, which correspond to extrema on the γ-surface. The first point is the unfaulted crystal, the second represents the APB and at the third one, a maximum can be expected. Let us note that when the energy of the APB on the $\{100\}$ plane is very low, decreasing to zero value, the $L1_2$ structure will transform to the DO_{22} structure, a structure which can be manufactured from the $L1_2$ structure by a regular set of APB´s parallel to one of the $\langle 100 \rangle$ directions.

On the (101) plane, there are four non-equivalent points of intersection of symmetry planes, namely the zero displacement, $1/2\,[\bar{1}01]$, $1/2\,[\bar{1}11]$ and $1/2\,[010]$, where extrema of γ-surface required by the superlattice symmetry are located. The first two points correspond to the unfaulted crystal and APB, respectively.

The extrema at the remaining two points might be saddle points (if a maximum is assumed at 1/4 $[\bar{1}21]$), although the possibility that a local minimum may appear at these two points cannot be ruled out. In the case of the f.c.c. lattice, i.e. when the difference between A and B atoms (see Fig. 5) is ignored, the atomic plane lying in between the $(\bar{1}01)$ planes marked in Fig. 5 becomes a mirror symmetry plane and extrema of γ- surface will be at the zero displacement, 1/4 $[\bar{1}21]$, 1/2 $[010]$ and 1/4 $[\bar{1}01]$. The following types of extrema can be expected at these points: a minimum, maximum and two saddle points, respectively. However, as mentioned above, a local minimum was found at 1/4 $[\bar{1}01]$ under certain circumstances /24/. This implies that metastable stacking faults on $\{110\}$ planes with the displacement vectors 1/2 $[\bar{1}11]$ or 1/2 $[010]$ might exist in some $L1_2$ ordered alloys as well.

2.2 Dislocation dissociations

A superlattice dislocation with the Burgers vector $[\bar{1}01]$ can be dissociated on (111) planes into two 1/2 $[\bar{1}01]$ superpartials separated by an APB /46/ according to the reaction

$$[\bar{1}01] = 1/6\,[\bar{1}\bar{1}2] + 1/6\,[\bar{2}11] + 1/6\,[\bar{1}\bar{1}2] + 1/6\,[\bar{2}11] \qquad (1)$$

(each superpartial is further split into two Shockley partials). Another possibility was proposed in /40/ where 1/3 $\langle 211 \rangle$ superpartials coupled together by an SISF are dissociated according to the reaction

$$[\bar{1}01] = 1/6\,[\bar{1}\bar{1}2] + 1/6\,[\bar{2}11] + 1/6\,[\bar{1}2\bar{1}] + \\ + 1/6\,[\bar{1}2\bar{1}] + 1/6\,[\bar{1}\bar{1}2] + 1/6\,[\bar{2}11] \qquad (2)$$

(in this reaction all three faults on the (111) plane, CSF, APB and SISF, are involved). The dissociation with SISF will occur only when the APB energy is sufficiently high and the SISF energy is sufficiently low so that the reduction of the superpartial interaction energy will more than offset the higher self-energy of the 1/3 $\langle 211 \rangle$ superpartials compared with the 1/2 $\langle 110 \rangle$ superpartials /47-49/.

A detailed structure of dislocation cores can be revealed only by atomistic studies of the core configurations. It has been shown by computer simulation technique (for details of the method and model used see /50,51/) that the dissociation of a screw dislocation according to the first reaction describes well the actual atomistic structure. However, since the splitting of the superpartials may occur on two distinct $\{111\}$ planes (i.e. the Shockley partials lie in the (111) plane of the APB, as in the case of the first reaction, or are situated in the $(1\bar{1}1)$ plane), an alternative reaction may take place

$$[\bar{1}01] = 1/6\,[\bar{1}12] + 1/6\,[\bar{2}\bar{1}1] + 1/6\,[\bar{1}12] + 1/6\,[\bar{2}\bar{1}1] \qquad (3)$$

where the planes of splitting of both $1/2\,[\bar{1}01]$ superpartials are inclined 70.5° to the plane of the APB. Of course, there are two additional cases where the leading superpartial lies on the APB plane but the trailing does not, and the other way round. All four cases are schematically depicted in Fig. 6. Only the first type of dissociation (marked a in Fig. 6) is entirely glissile while the three remaining types are sessile.

In the case of the dissociation into $1/3\,\langle 211\rangle$ superpartials bounded by SISF, the core strcutures revealed by computer simulations are different from the core described by reaction (2). Three distinct core configurations were found for $1/3\,\langle 211\rangle$ superpartials (see schematic drawings in Fig. 7). The first core is narrow, spatially distributed (non-planar) and characterized by a shuffle displacement of one atomic row in the $[\bar{1}01]$ direction (i.e. along the dislocation line of the $[\bar{1}01]$ screw superdislocation). The second core is spread into two adjacent (111) planes. The screw component of the $1/3\,[\bar{2}11]$ dislocation is confined to the plane just above the SISF and is very similar to the dissociation of a $1/2\,[\bar{1}01]$ dislocation into $1/6\,[\bar{1}\bar{1}2]$ and $1/6\,[\bar{2}11]$ Shockley partials. The edge component is distributed in both the (111) planes, however, the $1/6\,[\bar{1}2\bar{1}]$ partial is located in the SISF plane just below the left $1/6\,[\bar{1}\bar{1}2]$ partial. Therefore, the structure of the second core may be interpreted as a dissociation into two overlapping $1/6\,[\bar{2}11]$ partials. The third core is distributed along the two $\{111\}$ planes of the $[\bar{1}01]$ zone, i.e. along the (111) SISF plane and along the $(1\bar{1}1)$ plane as well. The screw component is spread only onto the $(1\bar{1}1)$ plane and resembles a dissociation into $1/6\,[\bar{1}12]$ and $1/6\,[\bar{2}\bar{1}1]$ Shockley partials, while the edge component lies on the both $\{111\}$ planes. Since the $1/2\,[\bar{1}2\bar{1}]$ partial is located at the intersection of the $\{111\}$ planes together with the $1/6\,[\bar{2}11]$ partial, the structure of the third core may be interpreted as a dissociation

$$1/3\,[\bar{2}11] = 1/6\,[\bar{1}12] + 1/6\,[\bar{3}10]\,. \qquad (4)$$

It appears that only the second core is glissile whereas the first and third cores are sessile as has been shown in /51/. For the interatomic potentials used in /50,51/, the first core has the lowest energy and, moreover, the second configuration transforms to the first one at a relatively low stress level. Since the third core is stable only when the CSF is stable, it seems that the first configuration is the most important one, at least for $L1_2$ ordered alloys with high energy or unstable CSF. Nevertheless, it is not possible a priori to rule out the possibility that the second configuration is favoured over the first one in some systems. No core configuration in which all three planar faults on (111) plane are involved has been found by computer simulations in unstressed crystals. Only when a rather high external stress is applied to a crystal containing the first core does the core decomposes into a $1/2\ [\bar{1}01]$ dislocation split in the adjacent plane above the SISF plane and a $1/6\ [\bar{1}2\bar{1}]$ edge component which remains coupled with the atomic row forming a step between the APB and SISF planes. This dissociation in the stressed crystal is quite similar to that described by reaction (2), however, the plane of CSF and APB differs from the plane of the SISF and, moreover, there is a row of atoms parallel to $[\bar{1}01]$ displaced by about $1/4\ [\bar{1}01]$. To move such a core, a shuffling must occur which is presumably responsible for the sessile nature of this core. Let us emphasize that the dissociation

$$1/3\ [\bar{2}11] = 1/6\ [\bar{2}11] + 1/6\ [\bar{2}11] \qquad (5)$$

is "prohibited" in one plane, as there is a local maximum for the displacement $1/6\ [\bar{2}11]$ on the γ- surface, but this dissociation arises when the core structure is not confined just to one plane. Indeed, the dissociation according to reaction (5) appears in the second unstressed core, in an intermediate configuration of the stressed first core and in a glissile configuration of the stressed third core (at a high stress level) /51/. An essential difference between the first and second core is the atomic shuffling which takes place in the first but does not in the second. It is not yet clear under which circumstances the shuffling can occur. Providing that shuffling is difficult, the $[\bar{1}01]$ screw dislocations dissociated into $1/3\ \langle 211 \rangle$ superpartials are sessile, and a behaviour similar to the $1/2\ \langle 111 \rangle$ screw dislocations in b.c.c. metals /37/ may be expected. For instance, the stress necessary to move a dislocation will decrease with increasing temperature because motion involves the repeated release of sessile dislocation cores by thermal activation.

The $[\bar{1}01]$ dislocation on the (010) plane is dissociated into two 1/2 $[\bar{1}01]$ superpartials separated by APB because the APB is the only stable planar fault on the (010) plane. If the CSF is stable on the $\{111\}$ plane, the core structure of 1/2 $[\bar{1}01]$ superpartials on (010) is similar to the cores schematically shown in Fig. 6, i.e. core is spread either onto the (111) or the ($1\bar{1}1$) plane (Fig. 8). Thus the core configuration of superpartials can be represented by the dissociation 1/6 $[\bar{1}\bar{1}2]$ + 1/6 $[\bar{2}11]$ or 1/6 $[\bar{1}12]$ + 1/6 $[\bar{2}\bar{1}1]$, respectively. Different core configurations were found for unstable CSF /50/. In this case the core can be spread simultaneously onto both the (111) and ($1\bar{1}1$) planes. Since the splitting into one plane is more pronounced than into the other, there are again two core configurations, which are related by a mirror symmetry plane lying on the (010) or (101) plane. In both cases (stable or unstable CSF) the energy of the two configurations is the same, and thus we can call them energetically degenerate cores. No core of the 1/2 $[\bar{1}01]$ superpartial dissociated onto the (010) plane was found in /50/. Therefore, the 1/2 $[\bar{1}01]$ cores are sessile, regardless of the stability of CSF. This conclusion is in agreement with the experimental finding that there is a high Peierls stress for dislocation motion on $\{010\}$ planes /52/.

2.3 Relationship between the core configuration and the stability of $L1_2$ structure

Dislocation mobility is essentially affected by the dislocation core structure, planar cores are glissile, in contrast with spatially distributed cores, which are usually sessile. It was pointed out above that the type of dissociation is controlled by the energies (or stability) of planar faults, in particular APB and SISF. It is not easy to calculate these energies and when a dissociation for example with SISF is not favoured, the SISF energy cannot be determined experimentally because the fault does not occur. On the other hand a change of composition or temperature may cause an appropriate change of SISF energy and a dissociation with SISF becomes preferred. Alternation of the type of dissociation will manifest itself in a qualitative change of dislocation properties. Since the variation of fault energy is closely related to the phase stability, tendencies for changes in types of dissociation can be deduced from the occurence of certain crystal structures /49,53/.

When a change of composition leads to a phase transformation of the $L1_2$ structure into the DO_{19} - Cd_3Mg structure (or related structures DO_{24} - Ni_3Ti and Al_3Pu), the SISF energy will decrease to zero with such compositional variation. Cosequently, dissociation with SISF will be favoured and mechanical properties corresponding to the behaviour of $1/3 \langle 211 \rangle$ superpartials can be expected. For sessile cores, it means, for instance, that the flow stress will decrease with temperature in analogy with the b.c.c. metals. Indeed, this kind of behaviour has recently been observed for some $L1_2$ ordered alloys /54-58/.

Another type of instability of the $L1_2$ structure is associated with the phase transformation from $L1_2$ into DO_{22} - Al_3Ti structure (and related structures as DO_{23} - Al_3Zr). In this case the APB energy on $\{010\}$ planes is decreasing to zero with concentration changes which promote the occurence of the DO_{22} structure. Since the APB energy is anisotropic and is lowest on $\{010\}$ plane /39/, a dislocation can lower its energy by cross-slipping from the $\{111\}$ octahedral slip plane onto the $\{010\}$ cube plane. However, the dislocation is immobilized on the $\{010\}$ plane because of the non-planar nature of the $1/2 \langle 101 \rangle$ superpartial cores as stated earlier. Immobilization of $1/2 \langle 101 \rangle$ screw dislocations by cross-slip onto $\{010\}$ plane was proposed in /59/ as a reason for the anomalous increase of flow stress with rising temperature in $L1_2$ ordered alloys. The cross-slip process will not be discussed here since it is described in detail in /60/. Let us only note that when the APB energy on $\{010\}$ is decreasing, the cross-slip driving force is increasing and a more pronounced increase of the flow stress can be expected.

It has been illustrated in the above two examples how information about structural phases can be useful to assess the variation of the fault energies with compositional changes, thus make it possible to predict changes in dislocation core structures and, consequently, trends in mechanical properties.

3. Conclusions

In the present review of the dislocation core structure in f.c.c. metals and in ordered alloys with the $L1_2$ structure, emphasis has been placed on the role the planar faults play in determining the basic features of the core dissociation. The problems encountered in stacking fault calculations are surveyed and various possibilities of dislocation dissociations in f.c.c. metals are briefly discussed. Planar faults in $L1_2$ superlattice are investigated on the basis of symmetry conservation rules and potential displacement vectors are found for the faults on $\{111\}$, $\{010\}$ and $\{101\}$ planes. The core configurations of the $[\bar{1}01]$ superlattice screw dislocation are summarized and it is shown how the occurence of crystal structure variants is correlated with mechanical properties controlled by dislocation cores.

References

/1/ Englert A., Tompa H.: J. Phys. Chem. Solids 21 (1961) 306.
/2/ Englert A., Tompa H.: J. Phys. Chem. Solids 24 (1963) 1145.
/3/ Cotterill R.M.J., Doyama M.: Phys. Rev. 145 (1966) 465.
/4/ Doyama M., Cotterill R.M.J.: Phys. Rev. 150 (1966) 448.
/5/ Perrin R.C., Englert A., Bullough R.: Interatomic Potentials and Simulation of Lattice Defects, eds. P.C. Gehlen, J.R. Beeler, R.I. Jaffee, Plenum Press, N.Y. 1972, p. 509.
/6/ Basinski Z.S., Duesbery M.S., Taylor R.: Interatomic Potentials and Simulation of Lattice Defects, eds. P.C. Gehlen, J.R. Beeler, R.I. Jaffee, Plenum Press, N.Y. 1972, p. 525.
/7/ Norgett, Perrin R.C., Savino E.J.: J. Phys. F 2 (1972) L73.
/8/ Perrin R.C., Savino E.J.: J. Microscopy 98 (1973) 214.
/9/ Seeger A., Schöck G.: Acta Metall. 1 (1953) 519.
/10/ Cockayne D.J.H., Vitek V.: phys. stat. sol. (b) 65 (1974) 751.
/11/ Cockayne D.J.H., Ray I.L.F., Whelan M.J.: Phil. Mag. 20 (1969) 1265.
/12/ Symposium on the Measurement of Stacking Fault Energy, Pittsburgh, 1969. The papers from the Symposium are published in Met. Trans. 1 (1970) 2366-2486.
/13/ Gallagher P.C.J.: Met. Trans. 1 (1970) 2429.
/14/ Coulomb P.: J. Microscopie et Spectroscopie Electronique 3 (1978) 295.
/15/ Harrison W.A.: Pseudopotentials in the Theory of Metals, Benjamin, New York 1966, p. 207.
/16/ Hodges C.H.: Phil. Mag. 15 (1967) 371.
/17/ Devlin J.F.: J. Phys. F 4 (1974) 1865.
/18/ Blandin A., Friedel J., Saada G.: J. Physique Coll. 27 (1966) C3 - 128.
/19/ Beissner R.E.: Phys. Rev. B 8 (1973) 5432.
/20/ Simon J.P.: J. Phys. F 9 (1979) 425.
/21/ Harrison E.A.: phys. stat. sol. (a) 19 (1973) 487.
/22/ Harrison E.A.: Acta Metall. 20 (1972) 1397.
/23/ Vitek V.: Phil Mag. 18 (1968) 773.

/24/ Vitek V.: Scripta Met. 9 (1975) 611.
/25/ Rao P.V.S.: J. Phys. F 5 (1975) 611.
/26/ Papon A.M., Simon J.P., Guyot P.: Phil. Mag. 39 (1979) 301.
/27/ Le Hazif R., Poirier J.D.: Scripta Met. 6 (1972) 367.
/28/ Le Hazif R., Dorizzi P., Poirier J.D.: Acta Metall. 21 (1973) 903.
/29/ Le Hazif R., Poirier J.D.: Acta Metall. 23 (1975) 865.
/30/ Caillard D.: Thesis, University of Toulouse (1976).
/31/ Pichaud B., Minari F.: Scripta Met. 14 (1980) 1171.
/32/ Edelin G.: Scripta Met. 6 (1972) 1185.
/33/ Karnthaler H.P.: Phil. Mag. A 38 (1978) 141.
/34/ Korner A., Karnthaler H.P.: Phil. Mag. A 42 (1980) 753.
/35/ Korner A., Karnthaler H.P.: Phil. Mag. A 44 (1981) 275.
/36/ Esterling D.M.: Acta Metall. 28 (1980) 1287.
/37/ Vitek V.: Crystal Lattice Defects 5 (1974) 1.
/38/ Marcinkowski M.J.: Electron Microscopy and Strength of Crystals, eds. G. Thomas, J. Washburn, Interscience, N.Y. 1963, p. 333.
/39/ Flinn P.A.: Trans. AIME 218 (1960) 145.
/40/ Kear B.H., Giamei A.F., Silcock J.M., Ham R.K.: Scripta Met. 2 (1968) 287.
/41/ Yamaguchi M., Vitek V., Pope D.P.: Phil. Mag. A 43 (1981) 1027.
/42/ Yamaguchi M., Pope D.P., Vitek V., Ukamoshi Y.: Phil. Mag. A 43 (1981) 1265.
/43/ Umakoshi Y., Yamaguchi M.: phys. stat. sol. (a) 68 (1981) 457.
/44/ Pond R.C., Bollmann W.: Phil. Trans. Roy. Soc. London 292 (1979) 449.
/45/ Paidar V.: Czech. J. Phys. B 26 (1976) 865.
/46/ Marcinkowski M.J., Brown N., Fisher R.M.: Acta Metall. 9 (1961) 129.
/47/ Kear B.H. Oblak J.M., Giamei A.F.: Met. Trans. 1 (1970) 2477.
/48/ Suzuki K., Ichihara M., Takeuchi S.: Acta Metall. 27 (1979) 193.
/49/ Paidar V., Pope D.P., Yamaguchi M.: Scripta Met. 15 (1981) 1029.
/50/ Yamaguchi M., Paidar V., Pope D.P., Vitek V.: Phil. Mag. A 45 (1982) 867.
/51/ Paidar V., Yamaguchi M., Pope D.P., Vitek V.: Phil. Mag. A 45 (1982) 883.
/52/ Copley S.M., Kear B.H.: Trans. AIME 239 (1967) 977.
/53/ Paidar V.: Kovové materiály 21 (1983) 169.
/54/ Wee D.M., Suzuki T.: Trans. Japan Inst. Metals 20 (1979) 634.
/55/ Wee D.M., Noguchi O., Oya Y., Suzuki T.: Trans. Japan Inst. Metals 21 (1980) 237.
/56/ Pope D.P., Russell J., Harris D.: J. Metals 32 (1980) No.12,61.
/57/ Suzuki T., Oya Y., Wee D.M.: Acta Metall. 28 (1980) 301.
/58/ Suzuki T., Oya Y.: J. Mater. Sci. 16 (1981) 2737.
/59/ Kear B.H., Wilsdorf H.G.F.: Trans. AIME 224 (1962) 382.
/60/ Pope D.P., Vitek V.: following paper in this volume.

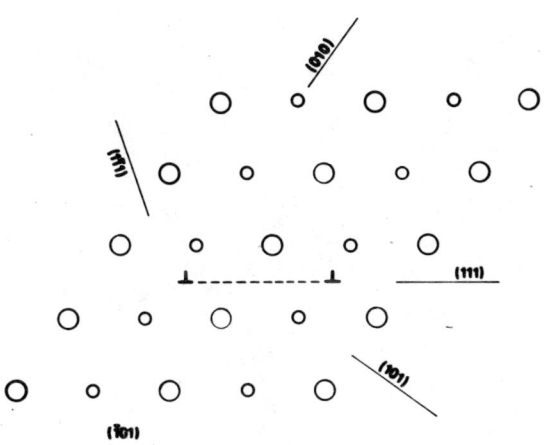

Fig. 1 Schematic view of a 1/2 $[\bar{1}01]$ dislocation dissociated on the (111) plane into Shockley partials, 1/6 $[\bar{1}\bar{1}2]$ and 1/6 $[\bar{2}11]$. Two alternating $(\bar{1}01)$ atomic planes are distinguished by large and small circles.

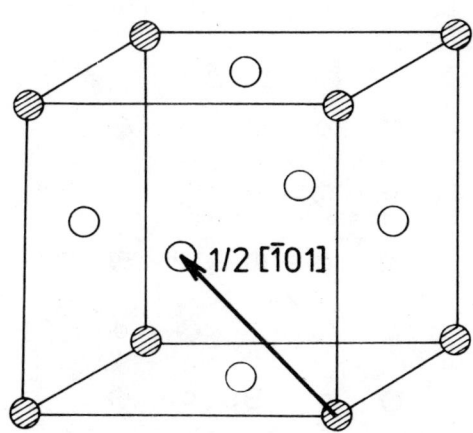

Fig. 2 The elementary cell of the $L1_2$ ordered structure of an A_3B alloy (atoms B are distinguished by hatching).

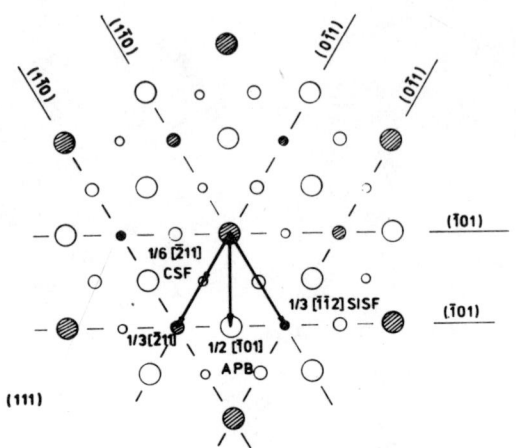

Fig. 3 Crystallographic displacement vectors of generalized stacking faults on the (111) plane: $1/6\,[\bar{2}11]$ for complex stacking fault, $1/2\,[\bar{1}01]$ for antiphase boundary and $1/3\,[\bar{1}\bar{1}2]$ for superlattice intrinsic stacking fault. Three different atomic layers are distinguished by large, medium and small circles; open circles represent A atoms and hatched circles represent B atoms in an A_3B alloy with the $L1_2$ structure.

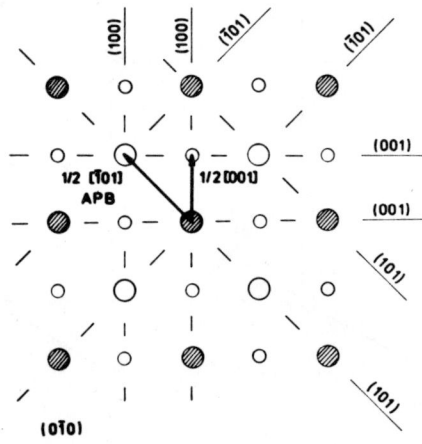

Fig. 4 Symmetry of the intrinsic generalized stacking faults on the (010) plane in the $L1_2$ structure. Two alternating atomic planes are distinguished by large and small circles

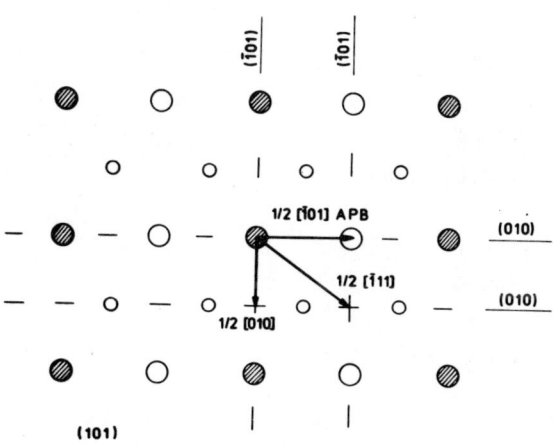

Fig. 5 Symmetry of stacking faults on the (101) plane in the L1$_2$ structure.

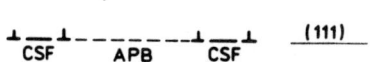

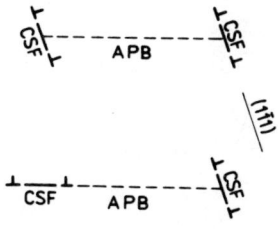

Fig. 6 Four different dissociations of the $[\bar{1}01]$ dislocation when the $1/2[\bar{1}01]$ super-partials are bounded by APB.

- 35 -

Fig. 7 Three distinct core structures of $1/3[\bar{2}11]$ superpartials. Core configurations designated as 2) and 3) correspond to the reactions (5) and (4), respectively.

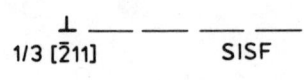
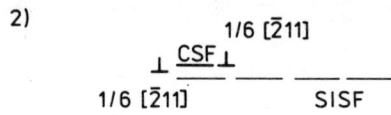
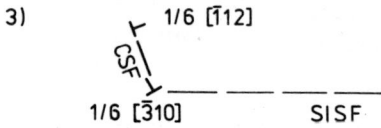

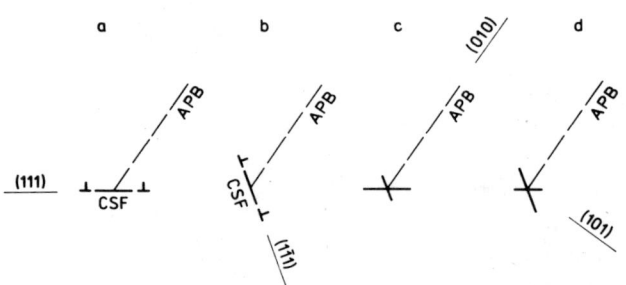

Fig. 8 Dislocation dissociation on the (010) plane. Only the structure of one $1/2[\bar{1}01]$ superpartial is schematically shown. In a and b the CSF is stable and it is unstable in c and d.

THE EFFECTS OF DISLOCATION CORE STRUCTURE ON
FLOW IN L1$_2$ ORDERED ALLOYS

D. P. Pope and V. Vitek

Department of Materials Science and Engineering,
University of Pennsylvania, Philadelphia, PA 19104, USA

I. Introduction

The flow stress of a number of AB$_3$ ordered alloys having the L1$_2$ structure is anomalous in a number of ways. Since the L1$_2$ structure is based on the fcc structure, with the majority atoms on the face centered positions and the minority atoms on the corners, these anomalies appear, at first glance, to be all the more strange. In this paper we will first describe these anomalies, then show how these anomalies can be related to the configurations of dislocation cores in these materials (as described by Paidar in the preceeding paper in this volume [1]), and finally, the results of recent experiments will be described which are in remarkably good agreement with the predictions of the model.

The flow stress of a large number of alloys having the L1$_2$ structure increases with increasing temperature as first shown by Flinn, Fig. 1 [2]. These data, obtained on polycrystalline Ni$_3$Al, show that the flow stress is rather insensitive to temperature changes at low temperatures, then dramatically increases with increasing temperature until a peak is reached, after which the flow stress drops sharply. Flinn proposed that deformation of this material occurs by motion of pairs of 1/2[$\bar{1}$01](111) dislocations separated by antiphase boundary (APB) on (111) planes, and that the increased flow stress with increasing temperature is due to diffusion-controlled changes of the dislocation configuration, Fig. 2. Flinn proposed that dislocations are dissociated on (111) planes at low temperatures as shown in Fig. 2(a), but as the temperature is raised, diffusive mechanisms allow climb of one dislocation so that the pair is now separated by low energy APB on the (010) plane, Fig. 2(b), and is therefore immobilized. APB's on (010) planes are expected to have a low energy since there are no nearest neighbor violations across such faults. Stoloff and Davies [3] showed that such a diffusion-controlled mechanism does not operate since the flow stress is only very slightly strain rate-dependent.

Other mechanisms involving intrinsic lattice effects [3,4,5] and changes in long range order [6] were also proposed, but it has been subsequently shown that variations of the Flinn model are most capable of explaining the experimental results.

In addition to the anomolous increase of the flow stress, later experiments on several different $L1_2$ ordered alloys have shown the following: (i) In the temperature regime where the flow stress increases with increasing temperature, i.e., below the peak temperature, slip occurs mostly on the $[\bar{1}01](111)$ system but above the peak temperature slip occurs mostly on $(001)[\bar{1}10]$ [7] (for samples oriented in the standard $[001]$-$[011]$-$[1\bar{1}1]$ unit triangle). (ii) The dislocation structure in samples deformed below the peak temperature consists mostly of long straight screw dislocations [8], indicating that screw dislocations are less mobile than edge and mixed dislocations. (iii) The amount of the increase of the critical resolved shear stress (CRSS) with increasing temperature depends on the offset strain used in the flow stress measurement. The CRSS measured at an offset strain of 10^{-3} shows the anomalous increase, but the CRSS measured at an offset strain of 10^{-5} to 10^{-6} is almost constant below the peak temperature [9,10]. (iv) At temperatures below the peak temperature the CRSS for $(111)[\bar{1}01]$ slip, as measured in compression, is highest for samples with the highest RSS on the $(010)[\bar{1}01]$ cube cross slip system and lowest for samples with the lowest RSS on that system [11], i.e., there is a breakdown of Schmid's law. (v) The CRSS depends on the sense of the applied uniaxial stress. For samples oriented near [001] the tensile CRSS exceeds the compressive and the opposite occurs on the $[011]$-$[1\bar{1}1]$ side of the unit triangle [12].

The first model to successfully explain observations (i)-(iv) above (but not (v)), was proposed by Takeuchi and Kuramoto [11]. This model is based on the Flinn calculations of the difference in the APB energy on (010) and (111) [2], the Kear-Wilsdorf cross-slip mechanism [13], and the proposal by Thornton et al [9] that the Kear-Wilsdorf mechanism is applicable to the flow stress increase. The Flinn calculation of the anisotropy of the APB energy, based on nearest neighbor interactions, showed that the APB energy on (010) is much lower than on (111). Kear and Wilsdorf [13] suggested that a screw dislocation with a $[\bar{1}01]$ Burgers vector, dissociated into two dislocations with

1/2[$\bar{1}$01] Burgers vector (which may themselves be dissociated) separated by APB, can minimize its energy by cross slipping from (111), where it is mobile, to (010), where it is immobile, Fig. 3. The driving force for cross slip is the difference in APB energy on the two planes. Takeuchi and Kuramoto combined the above qualitative ideas into a quantitative theory in the following way. They proposed that short segments of 1/2[$\bar{1}$01](111) screw dislocations cross slip to (010) and provide localized pinning points around which the segments remaining on the (111) plane must bow in order to continue motion. The frequency of formation of these cross slipped segments per unit length of dislocation, $f(T, \tau_{cb})$, was assumed to be given by the following,

$$f(T, \tau_{cb}) = A \exp\left[\frac{-H + \tau_{cb} V}{kT}\right] \quad (1)$$

where T is the temperature, τ_{cb} is the resolved shear stress on the [$\bar{1}$01](010) system, H is the activation energy, V the activation volume and k is Boltzmann's constant. Equation (1) says that the formation of a cross slipped segment is a thermally activated process, the activation energy of which is reduced by the RSS on the [$\bar{1}$01](010) cross slip system, the component of the applied stress tensor which promotes cross slip. After making additional assumptions about the nature of the dislocation motion on (111) planes, Takeuchi and Kuramoto showed that the increase of the CRSS for [$\bar{1}$01](111) slip over the low temperature value, $\Delta\tau_{pb}$, is given by

$$\Delta\tau_{pb} = B \exp\left[\frac{-H + \tau_{cb} V}{3kT}\right] \quad (2)$$

where B is a constant. If a Schmid factor ratio N is defined such that $\tau_{cb} = N\tau_{pb}$, then the variation of N with position in the unit triangle is as shown in Fig. 4(a). Note that N increases (and therefore τ_{cb} increases) with increasing distance from [001]. Since τ_{cb} depends on the orientation of the uniaxial stress axis, equation (2) predicts a breakdown of Schmid's law, and that the breakdown should occur as described in (iv) above. The results of compressive flow stress measurements on Ni$_3$Ga [11], Ni$_3$Ge [14], and Ni$_3$Al [15-17] were shown to be in agreement with this model.

However the results of later experiments by Lall et al [18] on Ni_3Al indicated that the Takeuchi and Kuramoto model is incomplete. Lall et al measured the compressive flow stress of a number of differently oriented samples, studying more orientations than were tested by previous investigators, and found significant deviations from the orientation dependence predicted by the model. Lall et al suggested that the difference is due to the fact that an additional stress component is required in equation (2). This stress component, τ_{pe}, acts on the edge components of the Shockley partials which comprise the $1/2[\bar{1}01]$ (111) superpartial dislocations. Since these edge components have equal magnitude and opposite signs, τ_{pe} acts to extend or constrict these partials on the (111) plane. τ_{pe} is taken to be positive if it reduces the width and negative if it increases the width of splitting. The ratio of τ_{pe}/τ_{pb}, defined as Q, is shown in Fig. 4, plotted for the case of tension. Note that Q is negative near [001] (cross slip is aided) and is positive on the other side of the triangle. Lall et al proposed a modified form of equation (2),

$$\Delta \tau_{pb} = B \exp\left[\frac{-H + \tau_{cb}V_1 + \tau_{pe}V_2}{3kT}\right]. \qquad (3)$$

Since τ_{pe} changes sign when the sense of the applied stress is changed from compression to tension, equation (3) predicts that the tensile CRSS should exceed the compressive for Q<0 and the opposite should occur for Q>0.

The predictions of equation (3) were confirmed by Ezz et al [12], Fig. 5, with one important lack of agreement: the CRSS measured in tension and compression are not equal for Q=0 in Fig. 4, and it appears that the orientation at which they are equal is considerably to the left of the Q=0 line. These differences are related to details of the dislocation core configuration that were understood only after results of simulation experiments were completed by Yamaguchi et al [19] and Paidar et al [20], as discussed by Paidar [1] in the paper immediately preceeding this one.

II. Effects of Dislocation Core Structure on Flow: APB Splitting.

It was found in [19,20] that when the superpartials dissociate on (111) according to,

$$[\bar{1}01] = 1/2[\bar{1}01] + 1/2[\bar{1}01] \qquad (4)$$

such that the superpartials are separated by APB, then the cores of the 1/2[$\bar{1}$01](111) dislocations dissociate into a planar configuration, similar to Shockley partials, see Fig. 6(a). However if the leading superpartial cross slips onto the (010) plane, then its core dissociates onto either the (111) plane, 6(b), the (1$\bar{1}$1) plane, 6(c), or both planes simultaneously 6(d). This implies that as soon as a 1/2[$\bar{1}$01] screw dislocation cross slips onto the (010) plane, its core redissociates onto the (111) or (1$\bar{1}$1) plane, thereby immobilizing the dislocation on the (010) plane. The dislocation only moves a distance of b/2 on the (010) plane before it can redissociate on the (1$\bar{1}$1) plane, where b = 1/2[$\bar{1}$01]. Consequently, the dislocation does not bow out onto the (010) plane, rather, cross slip occurs by the production of a double kink on the line as shown in Fig. 7. This cross slip process was treated in detail by Paidar et al [21] in the following manner.

Since the dislocation segment cross slips only a distance w=b/2 on the (010) plane before it can be immobilized, Paidar et al [21] assumed that cross slip occurs by the simultaneous formation of a constriction on the dislocation on the (111) plane, a shift of the core by a distance equal to an integral number times b/2 on (010), and a redissociation on (1$\bar{1}$1). That is, it was assumed, as did Friedel [22], that redissociation of the cross slipped dislocation occurs as soon as it is formed. The only difference here is that the core of the cross slipped segment shifts by b/2 on (010) during this process. Such a cross slip event will be favorable whenever $\gamma_0 > \sqrt{3}\gamma_1$, where γ_0 and γ_1 are the APB energies on (111) and (010), respectively. The activation enthalpy for a segment of critical length cross slipping a distance b/2 on (010) is given by:

$$H_c = 2W + b \left\{ C - [(\gamma_1/\sqrt{3} - \gamma_0 + \tau_{cb} b) \mu b^3/8\pi]^{\frac{1}{2}} \right\}, \quad (5)$$

where W is the sum of the energies of constrictions on the (111) and (1$\bar{1}$1) planes, C is the self energy of the kink per unit length, and μ is the shear modulus. Successive additional jumps as well as jumps of longer length are possible, leading to the various configurations shown in Fig. 8, but Paidar et al [21] showed that the initial jump of length b/2 is rate controlling. If equation (5) is expanded in a Taylor series, and if only the terms linear in τ_{cb} are retained, then equation (5) reduces to the form of equation (2).

The core configuration has thus far entered into the analysis by limiting the distance of the jump onto the (010) plane. However, in addition, the core width before and after the jump controls the magnitude of W, as was shown by Escaig [23] for cross slip in fcc metals. W is given by

$$W = W_0 \left[1 + \beta_1 \tau_{pe} - \beta_2 \tau_{se} \right] \quad (6)$$

where τ_{se} is the resolved shear stress on the edge components of the Shockley partials on the $(1\bar{1}1)$ plane, W_o is the energy when both τ_{pe} and τ_{se} are zero and β_1 and β_2 are constants which depend on the width of the unstressed superpartials. Both τ_{pe} and τ_{se} are taken to be positive when the applied stress increases the width of the partials. The signs of the two stresses change with changes in the sense and orientation of the applied stress. Consequently, equation (6) predicts an orientation dependent tension/compression asymmetry of the flow stress. If equation (6) is inserted into equation (5), the dependence of H_c on temperature, orientation, and sense of the applied uniaxial stress is obtained. Following Takeuchi and Kuramato [11], the CRSS for $[\bar{1}01](111)$ slip is therefore:

$$\Delta \tau_{pb} = B \exp \left[-H_c / 3kT \right]. \quad (7)$$

Reasonable values of the parameters in equations (5) and (6) were estimated from the experiments of Ezz et al [12] and the results were used to make the predictions shown in Fig. 9. The model predicts that: (i) The CRSS for $(111)[\bar{1}01]$ slip measured in tension should exceed that in compression for orientation near [001]. (ii) For orientations somewhere between [001] and the $[012]-[\bar{1}13]$ great circle the tensile and compressive results should be equal, and (iii) on the other side of this great circle the compressive CRSS should exceed the tensile. (iv) For orientations near [011] the compressive CRSS should greatly exceed the tensile. Umakoshi et al [24] performed flow stress experiments on Ni_3Al single crystals to check these predictions, and the results are shown in Fig. 10. Note that predictions (i)-(iv) above are all confirmed. To our knowledge, only a core width change of the type discussed here can give rise to the kinds of asymmetries shown in Fig. 10.

Finally, we ask which is the more important mechanism leading to the anomalous flow stress increase with temperature, the "cross slip" effect controlled by τ_{cb} in equation (5) or the "core width" effect controlled by τ_{pe} and τ_{se} in equation (6)? Consider the schematic diagrams shown in Fig. 11. If several samples are oriented along the [001]-x line in Fig. 11(a), then the "cross slip" effect should always lead to a flow stress increase as the tensile or compressive axis is moved away from [001] as shown in Fig. 11(b), since τ_{cb} always promotes cross slip and τ_{cb} increases with angular deviation from [001]. The "core width" effect changes as shown in Fig. 11(c). The observed flow stress is the sum of the two effects and the results of Ezz et al [12] and Umakoshi et al [24] show trends as shown in Fig. 11(d). Note that the compressive flow stress increases with deviation of the axis from [001], but the tensile flow stress initially decreases. This initial decrease for the tensile test suggests that the "core width" effect is more important. It further suggests that the good agreement between the Takeuchi and Kuramoto model (which does not include the core width effect) and the results of compressive flow stress measurements on Ni_3Ga [11], Ni_3Ge [14] and Ni_3Al [15-17] may have been fortuitous.

III. Effects of Core Structure on Flow: SISF Splitting

The dislocation core simulations of Yamaguchi et al [19] and Paidar et al [20] also showed that when the ratio of the APB energy on (111) to the superlattice intrinsic stacking fault (SISF) energy on (111) is sufficiently high, then dislocations dissociate on (111) planes according to

$$[\bar{1}01] = 1/3\,[\bar{2}11] + 1/3\,[\bar{1}\bar{1}2] \qquad (8)$$

In this case the superpartials are separated by SISF and the cores may be highly nonplanar. These dislocations were found to have a very high Peierls stress, and therefore the flow stress of such a material is expected to increase sharply with decreasing temperature at low temperature. Wee et al [25] have recently discovered a number of Pt-based $L1_2$ alloys, the flow stress of which indeed behaves like this. More recent experiments on single crystalline Pt_3Al by Wee et al [26] have shown that both (111)[$\bar{1}01$] and (001)[$\bar{1}10$] slip occur in samples oriented in the standard triangle, and the slip system activated depends on the orientation of the compression axis, Fig. 12. Note that the CRSS for both slip systems increases sharply at low temperatures. The CRSS for $(111)[\bar{1}01]$ slip is expected to increase for the reasons stated above. The CRSS for $(001)[\bar{1}10]$ slip increases since dislocation cores in L1$_2$ materials never dissociate on cube planes. The data in Fig. 12 are not conclusive, however, since we do not yet have direct evidence confirming that SISF splitting does, indeed, occur in Pt$_3$Al.

IV. Summary

Our current level of understanding of the flow processes in L1$_2$ ordered alloys could not have been obtained without a knowledge of the possible dislocation core configurations in these alloys. For alloys which show an anomalous increase of the flow stress with increasing temperature, a knowledge of the core structure provided the critical insight which suggested the application of the Friedel/Escaig cross slip model. This led to the prediction and confirmation of an orientation dependent tension/compression asymmetry, and a more detailed understanding of the cross slip process. In the case of L1$_2$ alloys which show an increasing flow stress with decreasing temperature, the interpretation based on a nonplanar dislocation core appears most promising, but more evidence is required before this interpretation can be considered to be confirmed.

V. References

1. Paidar, V., Preceeding paper in this volume.
2. Flinn, P.A., Trans TMS-AIME, 218 (1960) 145.
3. Davies, R.G. and Stoloff, N.S., Trans TMS-AIME, 233 (1965) 714.
4. Johnston, T.L., McEvily, A.J. and Tetelman, A.S., in High Strength Materials, (V.F. Zackay, ed.) pp. 363-381, Wiley, New York, 1965.
5. Copley, S.M. and Kear, B.H., Trans. TMS-AIME, 239 (1967) 977.
6. Pope, D.P., Phil. Mag., 25 (1972) 917.
7. Staton-Bevan, A.E. and Rawlings, R.D., Phys. Stat. Solidi (a), 29 (1975) 613.
8. Kear, B.H. and Hornbecker, M.F., Trans. ASM, 59 (1966) 155.
9. Thornton, P.H., Davies, R.G. and Johnston, T.L., Met. Trans. 1A (1970) 207.
10. Mulford, R.A. and Pope, D.P., Acta Met., 21 (1973) 1375.

11. Takeuchi, S. and Kuramoto, E., Acta Met., 21 (1973) 45.
12. Ezz, Salah S., Pope, D.P. and Paidar, V., Acta Met., 30 (1982) 921.
13. Kear, B.H. and Wilsdorf, H.G.F., Trans. TMS-AIME, 224 (1962) 382.
14. Pak, H.R., Saburi, T. and Nenno, S., Trans. Jap. Inst. Metals, 18 (1977) 617.
15. Saburi, T., Hamona, T., Nenno, S. and Pak, H-R., Jap. J. Appl. Phys., 16 (1977) 267.
16. Kuramoto, E. and Pope, D.P., Acta Met., 26 (1978) 207.
17. Aoki, K. and Izumi, O., Acta Met., 26 (1978) 1257.
18. Lall, C., Chin, S. and Pope, D.P., Met. Trans. 10A (1979) 1323.
19. Yamaguchi, M., Paidar, V., Pope, D.P. and Vitek, V., Phil. Mag., 45 (1982) 867.
20. Paidar, V., Yamaguchi, M., Pope, D. P. and Vitek, V., Phil. Mag. 45 (1982) 883.
21. Paidar, V., Pope, D.P. and Vitek, V., to be published.
22. Friedel, J. in Dislocations and Mechanical Properties of Crystals, (J.C. Fisher, W.G. Johnston, R. Thomson and T. Vreeland, Jr., ed.) pp. 330-32, John Wiley, New York (1957).
23. Escaig, B. in Dislocation Dynamics, (A.R. Rosenfield, G.T. Hahn, A.L. Bemet, Jr. and R.I. Jaffee, ed.) pp. 655-77, McGraw-Hill, New York (1968).
24. Umakoshi, Y., Pope, D.P. and Vitek, V., to be published.
25. Wee, D.M., Noguchi, O., Oya, Y. and Suzuki, T., Trans. JIM, 21 (1980) 237.
26. Wee, D.M., Pope, D.P. and Vitek, V., to be published.

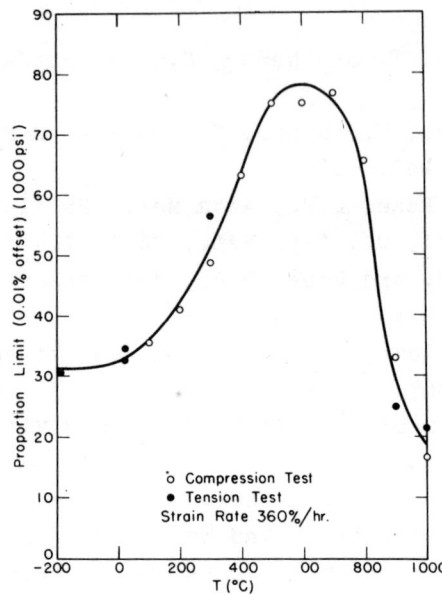

Fig.1 The flow stress of polycrystalline Ni_3Al as a function of test temperature as measured by Flinn [2].

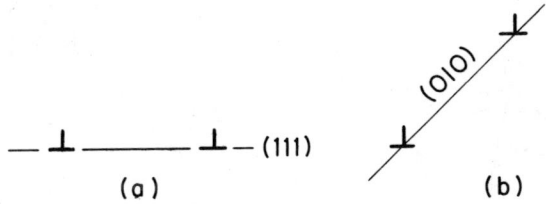

Fig.2: (a) The configuration of a $[\bar{1}01]$ superdislocation dissociated into two $1/2\,[\bar{1}01]$ partial dislocations separated by APB on (111) at low temperatures.
(b) The configuration after diffusive rearrangement at elevated temperatures leading to immobilization [2].

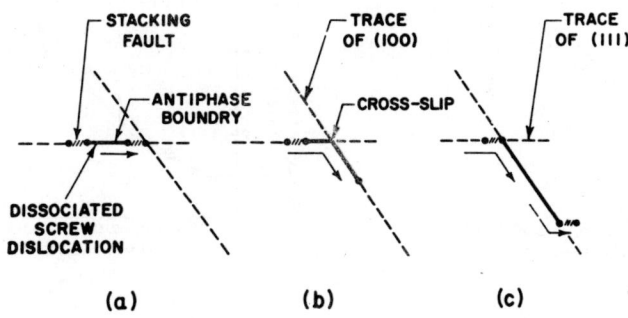

Fig.3: The mechanism of cross-slip from (111) to (010) planes leading to dislocation pinning as proposed by Kear and Wilsdorf [13].

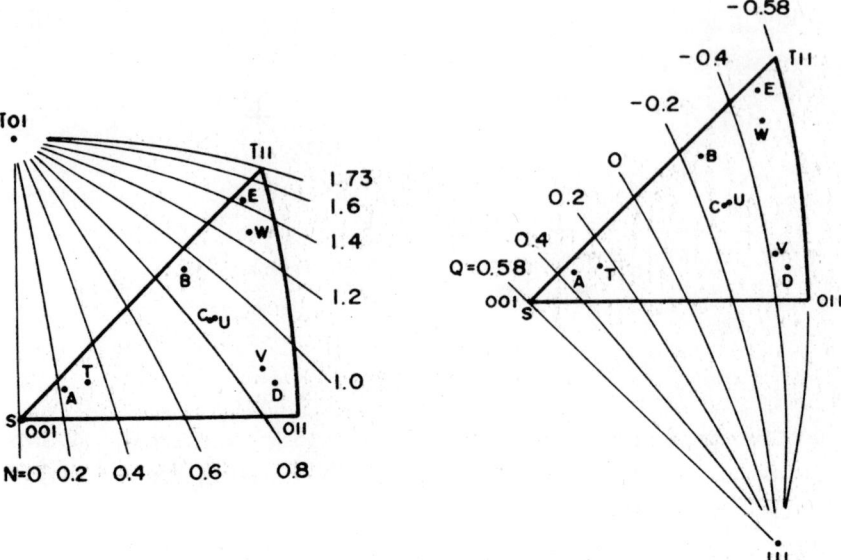

Fig.4: Plots of N and Q as a function of position in the unit triangle.

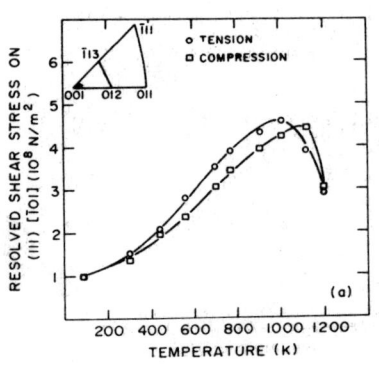

(a)

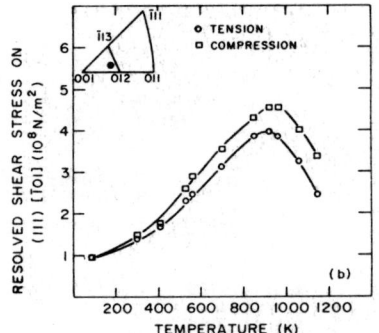

(b)

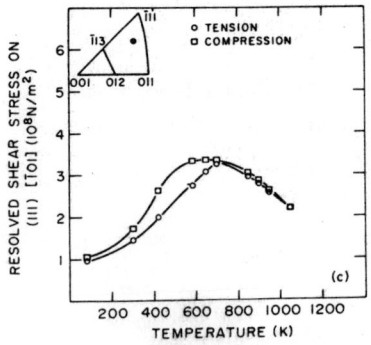

(c)

Fig.5: The CRSS for (111) $[\bar{1}01]$ slip of Ni_3(Al, Nb) as a function of temperature, orientation and sense of the applied stress [12].

- 48 -

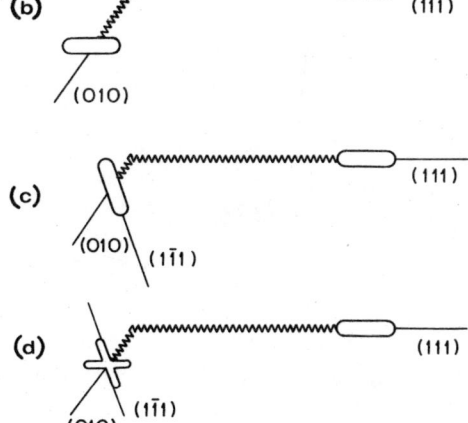

Fig.6: (a) A pair of 1/2[$\bar{1}$01] screw superpartials with planar cores separated by APB on (111).
(b) The configuration in (a) after cross slip of the leading partial onto (010) and redissociation on (111). (c) As (b), but with redissociation on (1$\bar{1}$1). (d) As in (b) but with simultaneous redissociation on (111) and (1$\bar{1}$1) [19,20].

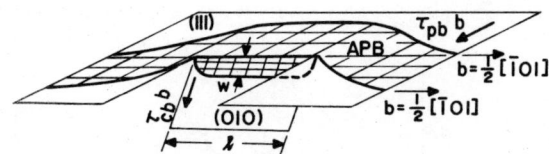

Fig.7: Cross slip of a 1/2 [$\bar{1}$01] screw dislocation from the (111) to the (010) plane by the formation of a pair of double kinks.

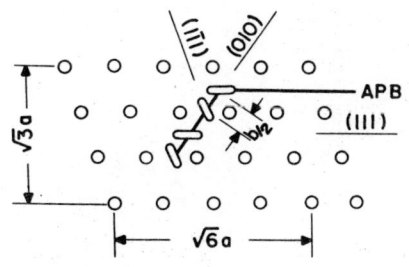

Fig.8: Possible core configurations after jumps of various lengths onto the (010) plane.

- 49 -

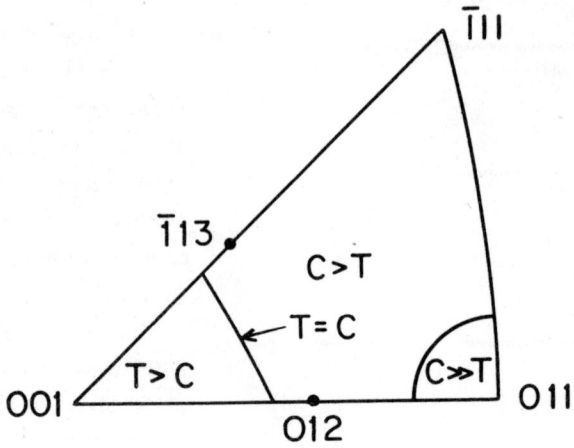

Fig.9: The predictions of the Paidar et al [21] model for the orientation dependence of the tension/compression flow stress asymmetry of Ni_3Al.

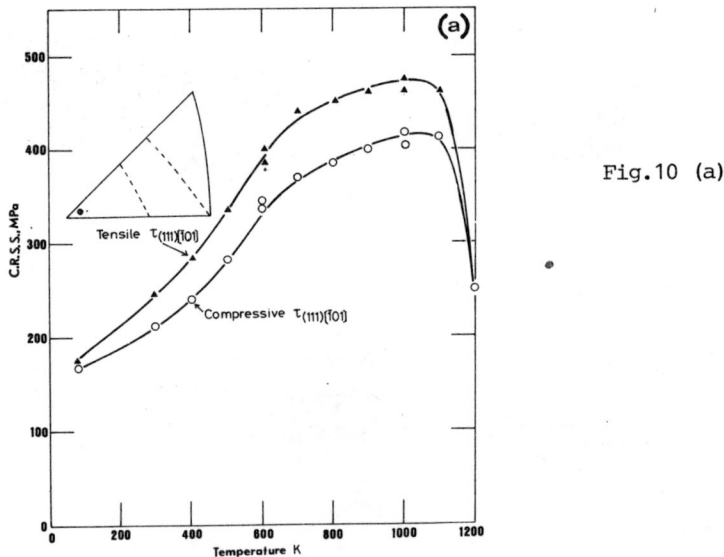

Fig.10 (a)

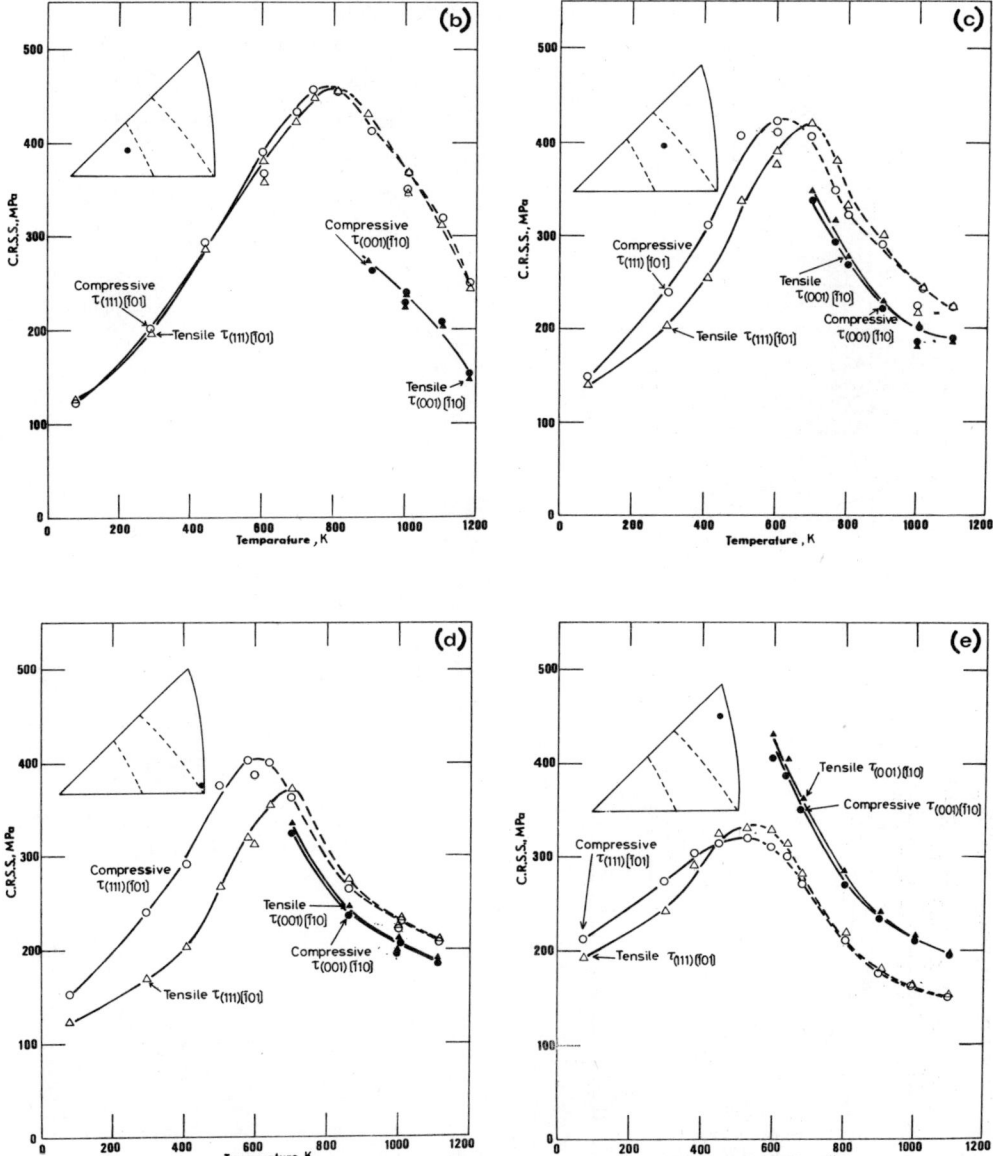

Fig.10: (a)-(e) The flow stress measurements of Umakoshi et al [24] performed on Ni_3Al to check the predictions of the Paidar et al [21] model as shown in Fig.9.

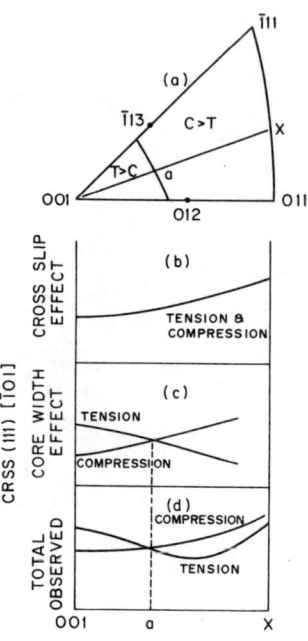

Fig.11: (a) The trends predicted by the Paidar et al [21] model for the (111) [$\bar{1}$01] CRSS for orientations along [001] -x. (b) The trends of the "cross slip effect". (c) The trends of the "core width effect". (d) The trends actually observed by Ezz et al [12] and Umakoshi et al [24].

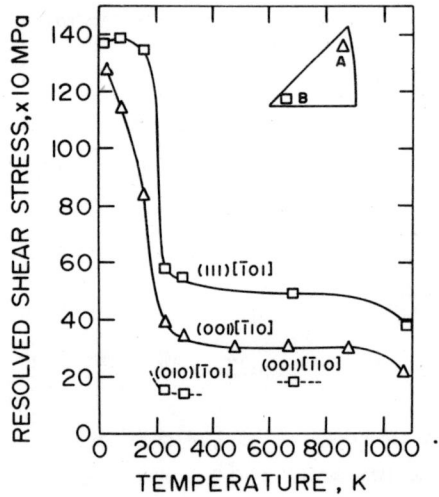

Fig.12: The CRSS for (111) [$\bar{1}$01] and (001) [$\bar{1}$10] slip as a function of temperature in Pt$_3$Al [26].

DISSOCIATION OF DISLOCATIONS AND PLASTIC DEFORMATION MODES IN LONG PERIOD
ORDERED ALLOYS

G. Vanderschaeve

Laboratoire de Structure et Propriétés de l'Etat Solide (LA C.N.R.S. n° 234),
Université des Sciences et Techniques de Lille, 59655 Villeneuve d'Ascq Cedex,
France.

Abstract

Deformation modes in long period ordered alloys (with periodic antiphase boundaries every M cube planes) are analyzed using transmission electron microscopy.

Depending on the relative energies of the geometrical stacking fault and the order fault left behind by a dislocation pair, two different deformation modes are observed

(i) When M is small (Ni_3V, M=1 ; $Ag_3 Mg$, M≃2), plastic deformation proceeds in extending numerous geometrical stacking fault ribbons, resulting in a profuse twinning of the crystal. Some peculiarities of twins propagation across the ordering structure as well as their implications on the mechanical properties of these alloys are discussed.

(ii) In $Cu_3 Pd$ (M≃8), deformation is carried out by dislocations pairs. Mechanical properties of this alloy are analyzed by comparing the long period ordered structure with a small domain Ll_2 alloy.

1 - Introduction

The structure of long period ordered alloys can be thought as derived from the Ll_2 structure by regular step shifts repeating in the cube plane at each M unit cell distance (fig. 1). Since the long period can adopt with equal probability any one out of the three cube directions of the parent phase, a domain structure results, consisting of order twins with coherent {110} twin planes [1,2] (fig. 2). Thus when dislocations are moved through the crystal, they continually cross the domain boundaries and mechanical properties of these alloys are affected by conditions governing the propagation of dislocations through these boundaries.

The present paper reports electron microscope observations on deformed long period ordered alloys Ni_3V (M=1), $Ag_3 Mg$ (M≃2) and $Cu_3 Pd$ (M≃8), with special attention to the dissociation of dislocations and its influence on the domain boundary crossing. When the average separation M of periodic antiphase boundaries is large enough, the deformation is carried out by slip of paired dislocations. When M is small, providing the geometrical stacking fault energy is sufficiently low, the predominant deformation mechanism is microtwinning.

2 - Structural aspects of stacking and order faults and propagation of dislocations in long period ordered alloys

2.1 - Dislocations and stacking faults

The ordering pattern and the stacking sequence of {111} close packed planes are described hereafter. Let the composition of the alloy be A_3B. In the {111} plane of the $L1_2$ structure, the B atoms form a triangular lattice. The unit cell in this plane has twice the lattice parameter of the disordered phase. The effect of the periodic half diagonal shift is to transform triangles into rectangles. Therefore, the ordering pattern of B atoms in close-packed planes consists of (M-1) strips of triangles alternating with one strip of rectangles (fig. 3). In view of the tetragonal symmetry the <110> directions are no longer equivalent.

The stacking sequence involves 3 × 2M {111} planes and can be written as :

$$\ldots A_{2M} \ B_{2M} \ C_{2M} \ A_1 \ B_1 \ C_1 \ A_2 \ B_2 \ C_2 \ \ldots$$

Notice that the perfect stacking does not involve B-B atomic pairs.

Table 1

Shortest Burgers vectors of partial dislocations bounding a geometrical stacking fault in the (d) ≡ (111) plane.

domain	[100]	[010]	[001]
1°/ M odd	2δB	2δA	2δC
	4Aδ	4Bδ	4Aδ
	4Cδ	4Cδ	4Bδ
	(3M-2)Bδ	(3M-2)Aδ	(3M-2)Cδ
M = 1	Bδ	Aδ	Cδ
	4Bδ	4Aδ	4Cδ
2°/ M even	2δB	2δA	2δC
	4Aδ	4Bδ	4Aδ
	4Cδ	4Cδ	4Bδ
	(3M-2)Bδ±AC	(3M-2)Aδ±BC	(3M-2)Cδ±AB
M = 2	4Bδ±AC	4Aδ±BC	4Cδ±AB

A geometrical stacking fault (i.e. a stacking fault without any wrong first neighbour bond) is made by shifting the B_1 plane into the C_{2M} position, resulting in the following stacking sequence :

$$\ldots A_{2M}\ B_{2M}\ C_{2M}\ A_1\ +\ C_{2M}\ A_1\ B_1\ C_1\ A_2\ B_2\ C_2\ \ldots$$

Such an intrinsic stacking fault is formed by a thin lamella of two extra planes. Its energy per unit area will be termed γ_G. The Burgers vectors of partial dislocations bounding a geometrical stacking fault on the right are listed in Table 1 for the three possible orientations of the superperiod $|3|$, using Thompson's notations $|4|$. In the $Ni_3 V$ alloy such partials are particular simple Shockley partials ; partials like $4A\delta$ can propagate through all domains without disturbing chemical order.

2.2 - Domain boundaries crossing and propagation of dislocations

Let us consider now the propagation of dislocations through domains. On crossing a domain boundary the Burgers vectors of dislocations are conserved[*]; however since the structure has a different orientation on both sides of the interface, the relative orientation of Burgers vector and structure is different. This causes a perfect dislocation in a domain (i.e. a dislocation pair) to introduce in the new domain an order fault with a certain number of uncorrect atomic bonds.

In the (111) plane of a [001] domain, the shortest lattice translation is 2BA ; the passage of one CA dislocation restores the geometrical order, but leaves an order fault, characterized by one uncorrect B-B bond per atom, as represented in fig. 4a. The energy per unit area associated with such a defect (so-called antiphase boundary) is termed γ_o. A second CA dislocation in the same glide plane and following the first one, restores both geometrical and chemical order, except in the neighbourhood of rectangles (fig. 4b) : the intersection of the glide dislocation pair and periodic antiphase structure causes the development of new segments of antiphase boundaries in the slip plane, equivalent to a "step" on periodic antiphase boundary (fig. 4c). Therefore, the 2CA superdislocation, perfect in the [100] domain leaves when entering in a [001] domain an order fault characterized by 1/M uncorrect bonds per atom ; as far as we consider only first neighbours interactions the energy per unit area of such a defect is γ_o/M.

---

[*] The lattice deformation occuring at the disorder-order transformation is so small that the parallelism of the {111} planes in two different domains is sufficient to allow glide dislocations to propagate across the order twin boundary.

Since the moving dislocations frequently cross periodic antiphase boundaries, the surface of the order fault step grows as the number of dislocation pairs increases. Dislocations propagate in so-called planes with disturbed long range order |5-7|, where parts of antiphase surface alternate with those in which long range order is preserved. The M value in the alloys studied being not higher than 10, planes with disturbed long range order must arise in the initial stage of deformation. The passage of M paired dislocations leaves an antiphase boundary in the whole slip plane (fig. 5). However, as subsequent dislocation pairs move, the extent of the portion of antiphase boundary in the slip plane diminishes, whereas propagation of a unit dislocation leaves an antiphase boundary in the whole slip plane, so that deformation must be carried out by slip of paired dislocations. If the shear becomes equal to the periodic antiphase boundary separation, there should be a complete recovery of the ordered structure. We present in the following some electron microscopy experiments which indicates that deformation in the Cu - 20,3 at % Pd alloy (M = 7,6) is due to slip of paired dislocations (see paragraph 3.3).

During their movement dislocations can split in Shockley partials according to $CA \rightarrow \delta A + C\delta$. The propagation in the [001] domain of the leading $C\delta$ partial is accompanied by the creation in the slip plane of a complex (stacking + order) fault with energy $\gamma_G + \gamma_o (1 - \frac{1}{M})$ (*), since correct B-B pairs are preserved only in the neighbourhood of rectangles (fig. 6a). The trailing δA partial leaves an antiphase boundary (with energy γ_o), so that the effective surface tension acting on it is $\gamma_G - \gamma_o/M$. Extended stacking fault is expected to be observed if the surface tension is low. Dissociation mode of the subsequent CA dislocation should be very different : The leading $C\delta$ partial leaves in the slip plane a complex fault with energy $\gamma_G + \gamma_o$ (fig. 6b) and the δA partial is bounding an order fault with energy γ_o/M. The effective stacking fault energy is $\gamma_G + \gamma_o (1 - \frac{1}{M})$, higher than the previous one, so that the corresponding splitting of the CA dislocation would likely not be observed.

Let n superdislocations have passed in the slip plane. The effective surface tension acting on the trailing δA partial of the subsequent CA dislocation is $\Gamma_n = \gamma_G - \frac{n+1}{M} \gamma_o$. If Γ_n is low, a larger dissociation of the CA dislocation occurs, whereas the subsequent CA dislocation experiences an effective stacking fault energy $\gamma_G + \gamma_o (1 - \frac{n+1}{M})$ and does not dissociate. Such a complex configuration of dislocations, consisting of dislocation pairs followed by an alternation of extended stacking faults and unsplit dislocations has been observed in

---

(*) When M = 1 (Ni_3V) the $C\delta$ partial is leading a geometrical stacking fault (see table 1).

Cu 20 at % Pd alloy |7|. If Γ_n becomes negative, a complete dissociation of the unit dislocation occurs, and partial dislocations lie along the domain boundaries. Notice that the stacking fault cannot extend in another domain, for the propagation of the δA partial would create a different complex fault.

To sum up, according to this model, deformation is achieved by paired dislocations. Depending on the relative values of γ_G and γ_o/M, complete dissociation of single dislocations is possible.

Now, a second domain boundary crossing mode is discussed |3,8| ; in this case splitting of dislocations leads to the formation of a geometrical fault.

Let us consider a 2BC superdislocation, perfect in a [010] domain, stopped at the boundary with a [001] domain. As discussed above it leaves when entering the new domain an order fault with energy γ_o/M. If this energy is too high (for example for small M), the superdislocation dissociates according to 2BC → 2Bδ + 2δC. The 2δC partial is leading in the slip plane a geometrical fault (see table 1). In contrast the 2δA partial is stopped at the boundary, for it would have to trail behind a high energy order fault. Notice that a 2δC partial cannot enter a new domain, either [100] or [010], without creating a high energy complex fault.

This domain boundary crossing scheme should hold in any long period ordered alloy with a low geometrical stacking fault energy and accounts for the occurence of numerous stacking faults limited at domain boundaries, as observed in Ag_3 Mg |9|. It has been observed in Ni_3V by in situ straining experiments in a high voltage electron microscope (fig. 7). During deformation, some perfect dislocations dissociate when crossing a domain boundary ; the leading partial propagate in the new domain and is stopped at the next domain boundary.

2.3 - Splitting of dislocations

The preceeding discussion emphasizes that the predominant physical parameters controlling the propagation of dislocations in long period ordered alloys are the relative energies per unit area of the geometrical stacking fault (γ_G) and the order fault (γ_o), as well as the separation M of periodic antiphase boundaries. The analysis of dissociated dislocation configurations allows to estimate the energy of these defects.

In the Cu_3 Pd alloy, dislocation pairs lying in a domain where they are not perfect are frequently observed. Perfect superdislocations 2BA and 2DC in a [001] domain should be out of contrast when a $[00\bar{2}]^*$ reflection is operating, whereas the observed dislocation pairs in fig. 8 are in contrast with this reflection, indicating they are not perfect in this domain. From these observations, we conclude that $\gamma_o/M < \gamma_G$ in this alloy.

In Ag 22 at % Mg (M = 2) eightfold dissociated superdislocations are observed (fig. 9a) ; 8CA is a lattice translation in a [001] domain. Of special interest is the large dissociation seen at the third unit dislocation, as compared with others. This is an evidence that the geometrical stacking fault energy γ_G is lower than the various order fault energies, since in this case the leading partial leaves a geometrical stacking fault. Splitting could occur for the other unit dislocations also, but the complex fault formed in that case involves uncorrect Mg - Mg bonds, with a higher energy and correspondingly a narrower dissociation width |9|.

In this alloy a perfect superdislocation 2BA consists of two unit BA dislocations joined by an antiphase boundary (fig. 9b).

Referring to the previous paragraph, two different order faults are possible, due to the particular value of M (M = 2), namely type I and type II. Type I order fault, left behind by a unit dislocation, is characterized by one wrong Mg - Mg bond per atom ; type II order fault due to a 2CA shear involves on an average 1/2 uncorrect Mg - Mg bond per atom.

The measurement of peak separations on electron microscope images gives estimates of the fault energies. Taking for the shear modulus and Poisson's ratio the values $\mu = 3.4 \cdot 10^{10}$ Pa and $\nu = 0.354$ |10| known for pure silver as a substitute for the unknown elastic constants of Ag_3 Mg, one evaluates :

$$90 \text{ mJ/m}^2 \leq \gamma_o^I \leq 120 \text{ mJ/m}^2$$
$$70 \text{ mJ/m}^2 \leq \gamma_o^{II} \leq 90 \text{ mJ/m}^2$$
$$50 \text{ mJ/m}^2 \leq \gamma_G \leq 70 \text{ mJ/m}^2$$

Three remarks are made about these experimental results :

(i) The geometrical stacking fault energy γ_G is lower than the order fault energies γ_o^I and γ_o^{II}. So it is expected that domain boundary crossing leads to the formation of a geometrical stacking fault in the new domain.

(ii) When only first neighbours interactions have been taken into account, one should have $\gamma_o^{II} = \gamma_o^I/2$. The experimental results, which disagree with this assumption, suggest that interactions between second, and even third neighbours atoms are not negligible. This confirms previous results indicating that the ordering energies V_i for the first three coordination spheres are comparable to one another in value ($V_2/V_1 \simeq -1$; $V_3/V_1 \simeq -0,5$) |11|. Such high V_i/V_1 ratios have not previously been observed for ordering alloy (for Cu_3 Au $V_2/V_1 \simeq -0,2$; $V_3/V_1 \simeq 0$). The V_1 value has been determined from either X ray diffusion |11| or calorimetry |12| experiments as being $\simeq 6.10^{-21}$ J/atome ($V_1 \simeq 0,7$ kT_c). Taking into account the first two coordination spheres gives calculated order fault energies in correct agreement with experimental results

(iii) In some Ll_2 alloys, a 2BA superdislocation can dissociate according to $2BA \rightarrow 2B\delta + 2\delta A$; 1/3 <112> dislocations are coupled together by a geometrical stacking fault |13|. In the Ag_3 Mg alloy, the same dissociation scheme would induce the formation of a type II complex fault |9|, with energy $\gamma_o^{II} + \gamma_C > \gamma_o^{I}$. So dissociation according to $2BA \rightarrow BA + BA$, as observed fig. 9b, where unit dislocations are joined by a type I order fault (or antiphase boundary) will be prefered owing to the lower energy of the configuration.

In Ni_3V (M = 1), dissociation of perfect 2AB superdislocations in a [001] domain into unit dislocations connected by an order fault area has never been observed on electron micrographs, indicating that the corresponding order fault energy γ_o is probably higher than 250 mJ/m^2 |14|.

Due to the rectangular ordering of V atoms in close-packed {111} planes (fig. 3), $3C\delta$ dislocations are perfect dislocations. They are dissociated into three $C\delta$ partials (fig. 10 a) bounding a geometrical intrinsic-extrinsic stacking fault pair |15|. $3C\delta$ dislocations are probably formed during order annealing by recombination of CA and CB dislocations gliding on the same, or neighbouring, plane. Although they repel each other elastically, the recombination reaction is still favourable because it reduces the width of the high energy order fault area they leave behind, so that $3C\delta$ dislocations should be at least as numerous as 2AB superdislocations. All the observed $3C\delta$ dislocations are found to be screw in the undeformed material. It has been shown that this configuration is a minimum in the total energy of the CA and CB dislocations |15|.

The probable core structure of partial dislocations in the undeformed material is drawn on fig. 10 b. It is expected that the perfect $3C\delta$ dislocation would dissociate into two partials separated by a geometrical intrinsic stacking fault, according to the reaction $3C\delta \rightarrow 2C\delta + C\delta$. $C\delta$ dislocation is leading a geometrical fault in the [001] domain (see table 1). Finally, a more stable configuration is obtained by developping a $C\delta$ loop in the adjacent plane. For the long range elastic field of the ($2C\delta$, δC) doublet is equivalent to the one of a single $C\delta$ partial at a distance of a few lattice parameters and beyond, so that a triple $C\delta$ ribbon is produced, bounding an intrinsic - extrinsic fault pair.

A further stabilization of the extreme partial core ($2C\delta$, δC) is expected when the dislocation line is parallel to CB (or CA) directions. For the CB part can be exchanged by cross slipping on either ($1\bar{1}1$) $\equiv$ (a) or (010) planes, from the $2C\delta$ partial ($2C\delta \rightarrow \delta A + CB$, with $\delta A \perp CB$, thus only weakly interacting) to the attractive δC partial ($\delta C + CB = \delta B$), resulting in the configuration schematized on fig. 10 d. This configuration has been observed in slightly deformed material (fig. 10 c) : the narrower ribbon is extrinsic, as determined by dark field imaging |16|. Notice the straight character of the trailing partial, parallel to the direction [$10\bar{1}$] = BC, at the edge of the extrinsic fault, in agreement with the above model.

We never observe intrinsic-extrinsic stacking fault pairs bounded by either Aδ or Bδ partials in a [001] domain. This is a strong support for the mechanism described here, i.e. the dissociation of dislocations involves only a geometrical stacking fault, without any uncorrect first neighbour atomic bond.

The estimated energies are relatively low :

$$19 \text{ mJ/m}^2 \leq \gamma_G^i \leq 24 \text{ mJ/m}^2$$
$$36 \text{ mJ/m}^2 \leq \gamma_G^e \leq 45 \text{ mJ/m}^2$$

where γ_G^i and γ_G^e are the geometrical intrinsic and extrinsic stacking fault energies, respectively.

These low values, as compared to the stacking fault energy of pure nickel $\simeq 125 \text{ mJ/m}^2$ |17|, are in good agreement with previously reported results indicating that adding vanadium strongly reduces the stacking fault energy |18|.

2.4 - Propagation of geometrical stacking fault through domains

In Ni_3V and Ag_3Mg alloys, the geometrical stacking fault energy is lower than the order fault energies. In these alloys deformation should be carried out by propagation of partial dislocations leaving behind a geometrical stacking fault.

We consider now the propagation of geometrical stacking faults through domains. As shown in paragraph 2.2, a 2δC dislocation trailing a geometrical stacking fault in a [001] domain cannot enter another domain, either [100] or [010], without creating a complex fault. It happens however that 4Aδ dislocations bound a geometrical stacking fault in two different domains, and even in three different domains in Ni_3V (see table 1). In the third one (3M-2) Aδ or (3M-2) Aδ ± BC dislocations, depending on the evenness of M, bound such a defect. So it can be shown, from a geometrical point of view, that deformation in these alloys should proceeds as follows |3| : A packet of 2/3 <112> dislocations has to glide together on M adjacent layers. On crossing some domain boundaries, atomic rearrangement in the form of multipole nucleation is needed within the slip lamella in order to keep unperturbated chemical order. Of course dislocations leave their multipole at the exit boundary. Notice that 4Aδ dislocations are easily nucleated either by a pole mechanism, or by recombination of 2δC dislocation (trailing a geometrical stacking fault in a [001] domain) and perfect 2AB superdislocation |8|.

It is therefore expected that, in these alloys, plastic deformation proceeds in extending numerous stacking fault ribbons, resulting in a profuse twinning of the crystal. Such microtwins do preserve correct atomic bonding.

3 - Deformation modes in long period ordered alloys

In order to specify the influence of the various dissociation schemes on plastic deformation modes in long period ordered alloys, compression tests have been performed on Ni_3V (M=1), Ag 26,5 at % Mg (M = 5/3) and Cu 20,3 at % Pd (M = 7,6) alloys. The microstructure of deformed samples is analyzed using transmission electron microscopy.

3.1. - Effect of domain size on the mechanical properties of Ni_3V |14,19|

Very large domain sizes can be developed in this alloy by appropriate annealing treatments |1| ; the domain size in a polycrystal may reach a size as large as the grain size itself (0.1 mm) after annealing during six days at 950°C. Referring to the above discussion, simple Shockley partials like $C\delta$ could be slip dislocations in large domain crystals, while four fold Shockley partials like $4A\delta$ should be needed in small domain crystals, in order to propagate through domains without introducing uncorrect V-V atomic bonds.

Fig. 11 reports stress strain curves for single ($[\bar{1}13]$ compression axis) and polycrystals deformed at room temperature. Experimental determinations of yield stresses and workhardening rates are listed in Table 2.

Table 2
Yield stress and workhardening rate in Ni_3V alloy

	polycrystal		single crystal	
	small domains	large domains	small domains	large domains
Yield stress (M Pa)	1320	720	520	350
Workhardening (M Pa)	4800	12300	1850	2300

The ratio between yield stresses for small domain crystals and large domain ones is 1.8 for polycrystals and 1.5 for single crystals, respectively. When comparing nominal stresses for polycrystals to resolved shear stresses for single crystals, some value of the Taylor factor has to be introduced. Thus small domain samples behave consistently either as single or polycrystals : their yield stress ratio is 2.5 and the workhardening rates ratio is 2.6. In contrast large domain samples exhibit a surprisingly high polycrystalline workhardening rate, since the corresponding ratio is 5.3, to be compared to the yield stress ratio : 2.1. This will be discussed below in connection with the nature of slip dislocations which is proposed to be 1/6 <112> in large domain crystals, while being 2/3 <112> in small domain ones.

Electron microscopy observations of deformed samples show conclusively that deformation is carried out by propagation of widely extended stacking faults resulting in a profuse twinning throughout the crystal. In small domain crystals, twins propagate across the three possible domains (fig. 12a), while dark field experiments proove that long range chemical order is still preserved within the microtwin |20|. This provides a clear experimental evidence that in this case deformation is carried out by 2/3 <112> dislocations, since only these ones can trail a geometrical stacking fault in any domain, whatever the direction of the superperiod be. Deformation microstructures observed in large domain alloy are quite similar. As in small domain crystal, microtwinning is the predominant deformation mode. Fig. 12 b shows that microtwinning results from the propagation of Cδ Shockley partial dislocations on successive {111} layers in a [001] domain.

It is sometimes observed (fig. 12c) that twin bands change direction at domain boundary |21|. Such a zigzag propagation across the ordering structure is due to cross slip of partials via the stair rod mode |22|, in order to preserve correct atomic bonds.

From the above observations, it is assumed that the difference reported on small and large domain samples originates from the difference in Burgers vector length of the corresponding slip dislocations, the latter increasing from 1/6 <112> to 2/3 <112>, respectively. Detailed calculations of the propagation stress through a dislocation forest have been done following Fontaine's analysis |23| for Cδ and 4Aδ, 4Bδ or 4Cδ cutting through the same forest. They give the expected flow stresses in a ratio lying in between 1.5 and 1.9, depending on the particular averaging procedures used |19| ; such computed ratios are in good agreement with the experimental values reported above.

The second point of interest is the workhardening rates. As pointed out above large domain polycrystals workharden roughly twice as much than single crystals. This can be qualitatively related to the peculiarities of 1/6 <112> glide, which gives only four independent slip systems available (only one vector 1/6 <112> is allowed for each {111} plane in a single domain). Therefore as far as 2/3 <112> slips are not activated, deformation from neighbouring grains cannot be accomodated in the polycrystal (according to the well known Von Mises conditions), resulting in a higher workhardening rate. Single crystals cannot behave in the same way, for the deformation in neighbouring domains are not independent from each other, but are connected through orientation symmetries : the general state of deformation in the crystal depends on less than five parameters and can be accomodated more easily.

3.2 - Deformation microstructures in Ag 26,5 at % Mg (M = 5/3)

Electron microscope observations on deformed samples show that again deformation is carried out by propagation of widely extended stacking faults stopped at domain boundaries and by microtwinning extending through several domains |14|. From careful electron diffraction experiments, it is evidenced that twins do preserve the chemical order. So there is a strong reason to conclude that deformation twins are created by propagation of 2/3 <112> dislocations. Microtwins extending over the three possible domains have not yet been observed, probably because of the high stress level required to nucleate multipole at the third domain boundary$^{(*)}$. It should be noticed however that domains within the crystal are not distributed at random, since an alternation of two domain types (e.g. [100] and [010], with the third [001] direction common to the two domains) is sufficient to minimize or even cancel the elastic strains associated with the slight quadratic deformation due to ordering.

The yield stress of ordered alloy is about 2.4 times larger than the disordered alloy, in good agreement with previously reported results |12|. As in Ni_3V, the increase in flow stress is attributed to an increase of the stress required for mobile dislocations to move across the attractive forest dislocations.

3.3 - Deformation modes in Cu 20,3 at % Pd alloy (M = 7,6)

The yield stress of the ordered alloy is only 1.2 times larger than the disordered alloy, as previously reported by Buynova et al. |6|.

Fig. 13 shows a typical exemple of dislocation configurations in deformed alloys. Deformation is mainly due to paired dislocations, which are not dissociated into Shockley partials. We observe on the micrographs a weak fringe contrast, parallel to the intersections of slip planes with sample surface. This striped contrast is attributed by Buynova et al. |5-7| to planes with disturbed

---

(*) As shown recently |24| long period Ag_3 Mg in an exemple of "irregular arrangement with uniform mixing" structure in Fujiwara's terminology |25|. For M = 5/3 the corresponding giant unit cell is built with 10 $L1_2$ cubes, so that twin lamella involves simultaneous slip of five 2/3 <112> dislocations |14|.

long range order ; it results probably from the break of regular coupling between atoms of the slip plane and those of the neighbour plane : in this alloy thermal antiphase boundaries, when imaged with fundamental reflections, exhibits similar weak α-fringe contrast |2|.

It can be seen from fig. 14 that weak fringe contrast vanishes within some domains ; in these domains, long range order is not disturbed by slip of dislocations. This prooves that deformation is carried out by propagation of paired dislocations, which are perfect for this superperiod orientation, but not by slip of independent single dislocations.

Further confirmation is given by dark field imaging of slip induced order defects. It is well known that in long period ordered alloys, the occurence of periodic antiphase boundaries along (001) planes, for example, causes those $[hk\ell]^*$ $L1_2$ superstructure reflections to be split into so-called satellite $[hk\ell \pm 1/2M]^*$ ones, only when $h+k$ is odd |26|. The slip induced order defects are observed when imaging with a satellite reflection (Fig. 15a) ; they are out of contrast when imaging with a $L1_2$ structure reflection (Fig. 15b). That means that the corresponding fault vector is a $L1_2$ lattice translation, i.e. shear displacement is due to propagation of dislocations pairs. This is obviously related to the nature of the order fault left behind by a dislocation pair, when moving across periodic antiphase structure. As emphasized in paragraph 2.2, such an order fault involves only 1/M uncorrect atomic bonds, so its energy should be very low for high M.

After the passage of 2M superdislocations, there is a complete recovery of the ordered structure, so that propagation of dislocations in the same plane becomes more difficult. Dislocation sources operate in new planes, resulting in a very homogeneous deformation microstructure (Fig. 13). Evidence that a large number of slip planes is involved in plastic deformation of this alloy is also provided by the development of very fine, uniformely distributed slip traces on sample surfaces |27|.

In the course of their study on mechanical properties of $Cu_3 Pd$ alloys, Buynova et al. |5-7| come to the conclusion that plastic deformation involves intensive formation of stacking faults limited at domain boundaries, arising as a result of the motion of a single Shockley partial in planes with disturbed long range order |28|. It is expected that the apparent discrepancy between their observations and ours originates in a different degree of order in corresponding alloys. As shown in paragraph 2.2 a complete dissociation of unit dislocations should occur if the energy $\Gamma_n = \gamma_G - \frac{n+1}{M} \gamma_o$ becomes negative. Depending on the degree of order, the order fault energy γ_o (proportionnal to the square of long range order parameter) might be higher in Buynova's alloys than in ours, resulting in a negative value of Γ_n and consequently a large dissociation of

single dislocations. Notice that the ordered state is established in their
alloys by cooling over 4 months from 500°C to 270°C, at the rate of 2°C/day,
while the alloys used in our own experiments were held for 7 days at 455°C,
resulting possibly in a lower degree of order.

4 - Conclusion

Electron microscope study of deformed long period ordered alloys shows
that the main factors governing the plasticity of these alloys are the relative
values of γ_G and γ_o/M. When the average separation M of periodic antiphase
boundaries is large, deformation is carried out by slip of paired dislocations.
Dissociation of single dislocations can generate complex faults limited by
domain boundaries. When M is small, providing γ_G is sufficiently low, the predominant deformation mechanism is "ordered" microtwinning.

Acknowledgements

The author would like to thank B. Escaig for continuous encouragement and
stimulating discussions in the course of this work.

References

/1/ Tanner L.E. : Phys. Stat. Sol. 30 (1968) 685.
/2/ Vanderschaeve G. : Electron microscopy 1 (1980) 270.
/3/ Vanderschaeve G. : J. Physique 35 (1974) C7-47.
/4/ Thompson N. : Proc. Phys. Soc. 66B (1953) 481.
/5/ Buynova L.N., Syutkina V.I., Shashkov O.D., Yakovleva E.S. : Fiz. Metal.
    Metalloved. 29 (1970) 1221.
/6/ Buynova L.N., Syutkina V.I., Shashkov O.D., Yakovleva E.S. : Fiz. Metal.
    Metalloved. 33 (1972) 1195.
/7/ Buynova L.N., Syutkina V.I., Shashkov O.D., Yakovleva E.S. : Fiz. Metal.
    Metalloved. 34 (1972) 561.
/8/ Vanderschaeve G., Escaig B. : Phys. Stat. Sol. (a) 20 (1973) 309.
/9/ Vanderschaeve G., Coulon G., Escaig B. : Phys. Stat. Sol. (a) 9 (1972) 541.
/10/ Hirth J.P., Lothe J. : Theory of Dislocations, Mc Graw-Hill, New York
     (1970) p. 762.
/11/ Grayevskaia Ya. I., Iveronova V.I., Katsnel'son A.A., Popova I.I. :
     Fiz. Metal. Metalloved. 40 (1975) 195.
/12/ Gangulee A., Bever M.B. : Trans. A.I.M.E. 242 (1968) 278.
/13/ Kear B.H., Giamei A.F., Silcock J.M., Ham R.K. : Scripta Met. 2 (1968) 287.
/14/ Vanderschaeve G., Escaig B. : Strength of Metals and Alloys (I.C.S.M.A. 5
     Proceedings), P. Haasen, V. Gerold, G. Kostorz editors, Pergamon Press
     (1979), p. 83.

/15/ Vanderschaeve G., Escaig B. : J. Physique Lettres 39 (1978) L 74.
/16/ Gevers R., Art A., Amelinckx S. : Phys. Stat. Sol. 3 (1963) 1563.
/17/ Carter C.B., Holmes S.M. : Phil. Mag. 35 (1977) 1161.
/18/ Delehouzée L., Deruyttere A. : Acta Met. 15 (1967) 727.
/19/ Vanderschaeve G., Sarrazin T., Escaig B. : Acta Met. 27 (1979) 1251.
/20/ Vanderschaeve G., Sarrazin T. : Phys. Stat. Sol. (a) 43 (1977) 454.
/21/ Vanderschaeve G., Escaig B. : Phil. Mag. (1983), to be published.
/22/ Fleischer R.L. : Acta Met. 7 (1959) 134.
/23/ Fontaine G. : J. Physique 27 (1966) 323.
/24/ Guymont M., Gratias D. : Acta Cryst. 35 A (1979) 181.
/25/ Fujiwara K. : J. Phys. Soc. Japan 12 (1957) 7.
/26/ Sato H., Toth R.S. : Alloying Behavior and Effects in Concentrated Solid Solutions, T.B. Massalski editor, Gordon-Breach (1965) p. 295.
/27/ Syutkina V.I., Yakovleva E.S. : Fiz. Tverd. Tela 8 (1967) 2688.
/28/ Buynova L.M., Syutkina V.I., Shashkov O.D. : Fiz. Metal. Metalloved. 40 (1975) 180.

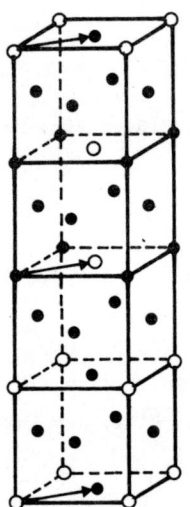

Fig.1 Example of long period ordered structure:

Ag_3 Mg (M = 2).

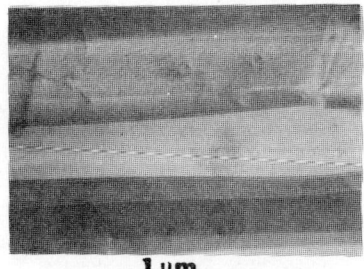

Fig.2 Domain boundaries in Cu$_3$Pd.

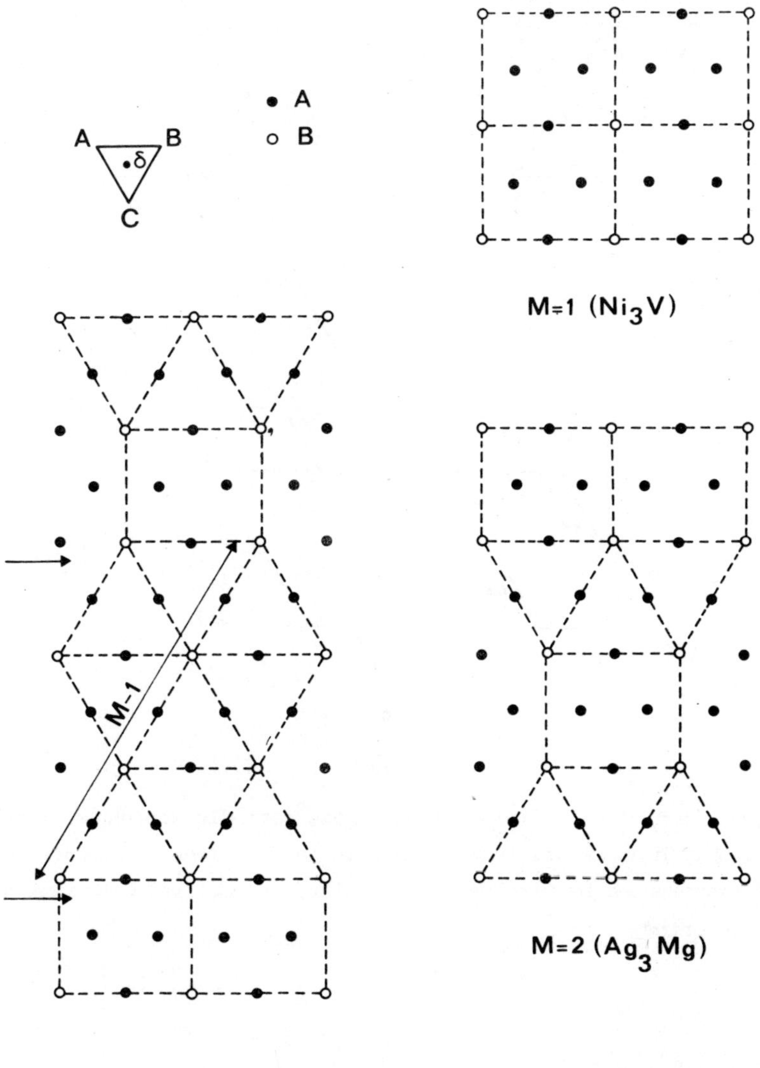

M=1 (Ni$_3$V)

M=2 (Ag$_3$Mg)

Fig.3 Atomic ordering in close-packed planes of long period ordered structures.

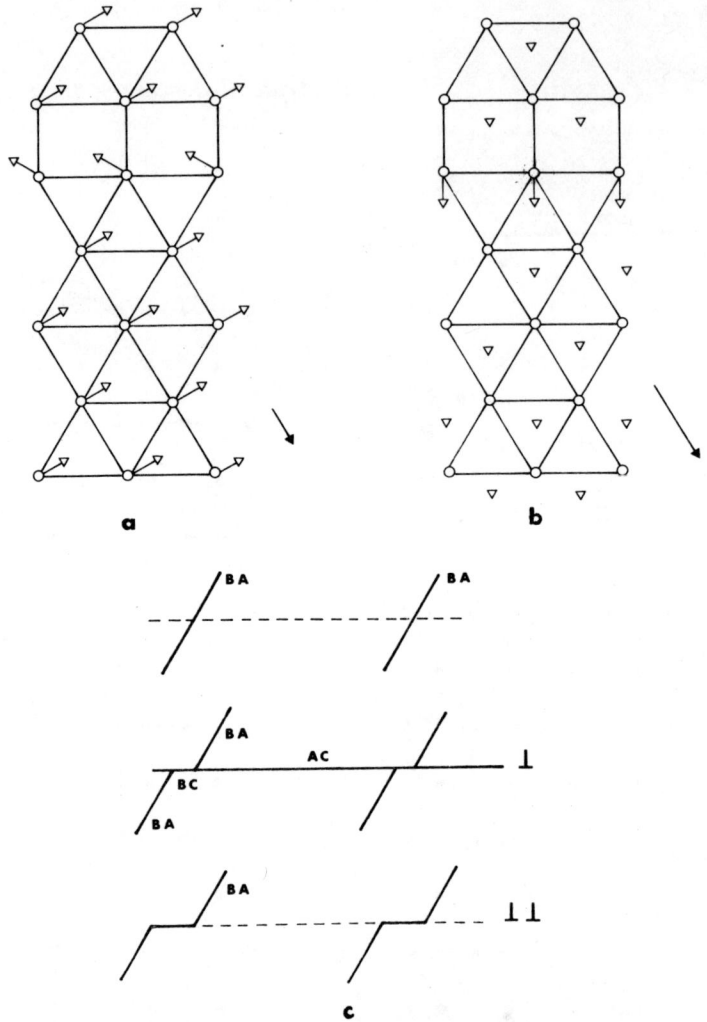

Fig.4 Propagation of unit dislocations across periodic antiphase boundary structure. Only B atoms are drawn. Atoms in the A_1 plane and in the adjacent plane are represented by circles and tringles, respectively. Uncorrect atomic bonds are reported.

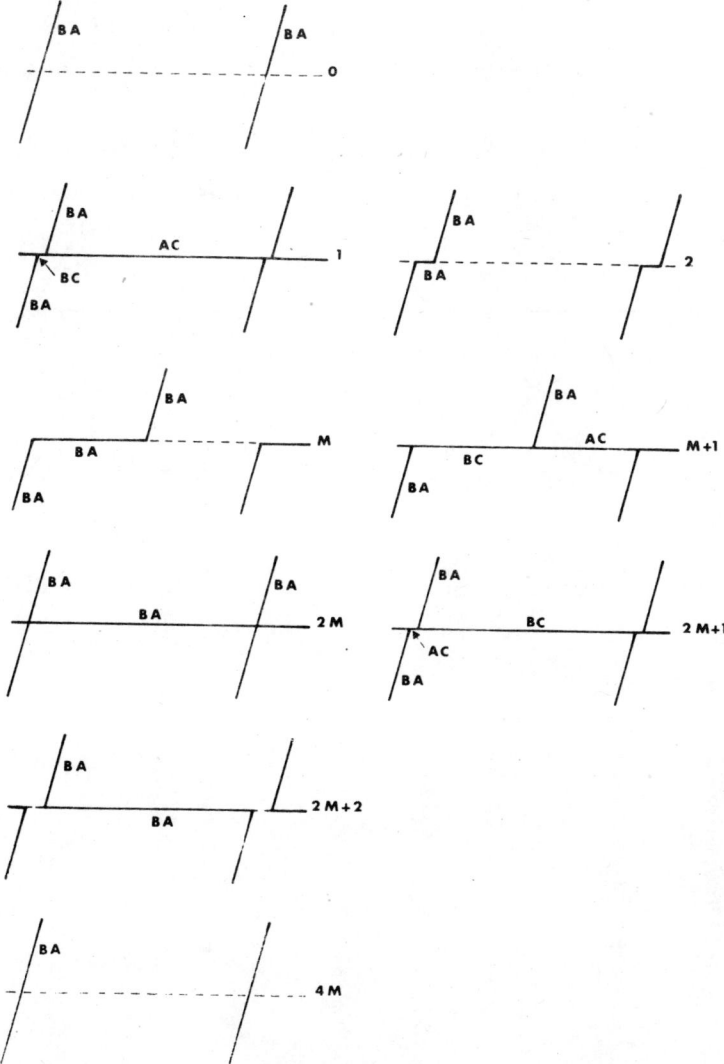

Fig. 5 Order faults area created by propagation of 1,2,...4M unit dislocations across periodic antiphase boundary structure.

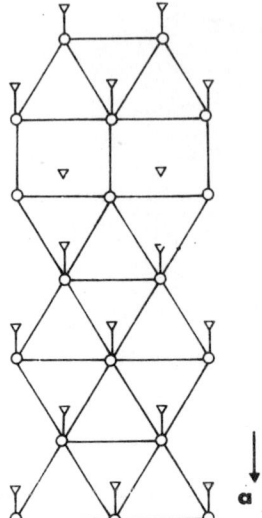 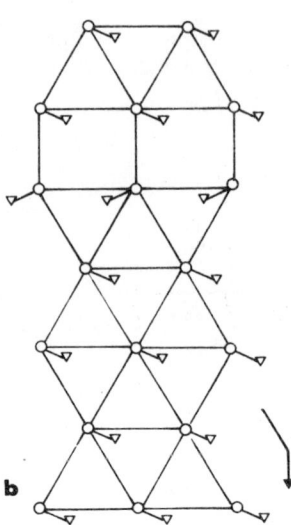

Fig.6 Nature of complex faults generated by splitting of unit dislocations.

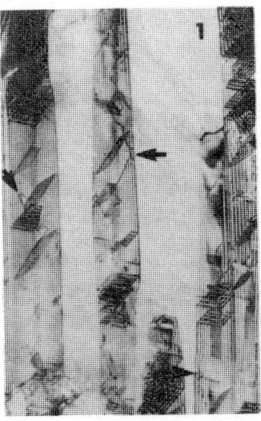 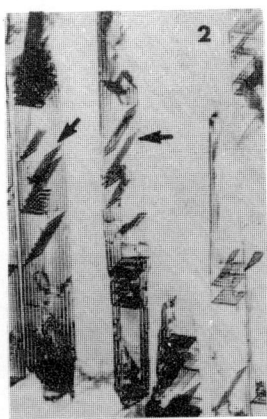 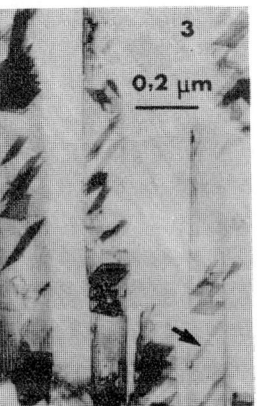

Fig.7 Dissociation of dislocations and propagation of geometrical stacking faults during in situ straining experiments in a Ni_3V alloy

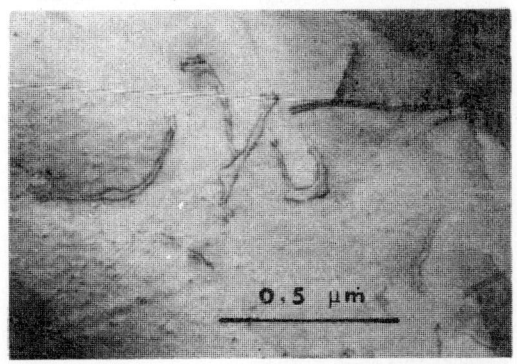

Fig.8 Dislocation pairs in Cu_3 Pd; their total Burgers vector is not a perfect lattice translations

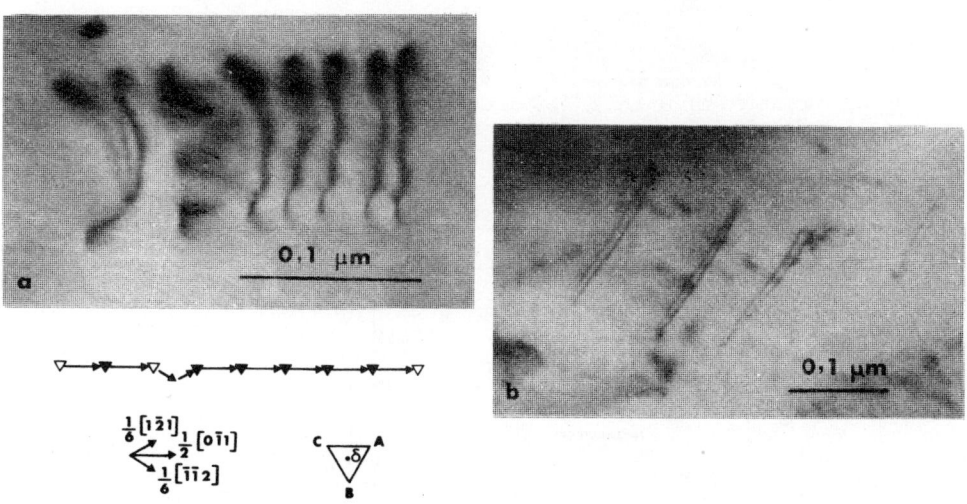

Fig.9a) Dissociation of a 4 110 superdislocation in Ag_3 Mg.
9b) Dislocation pairs in Ag_3 Mg.

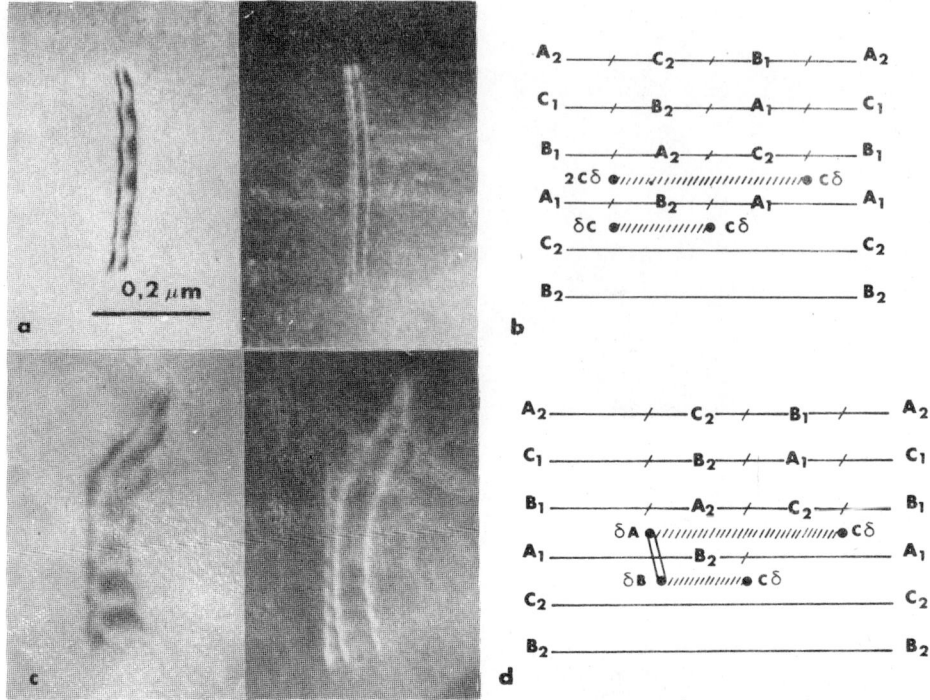

Fig.10 Dissociation of a 1/2 ⟨112⟩ dislocation in Ni_3V; a,b) undeformed material; c,d) slightly deformed material.

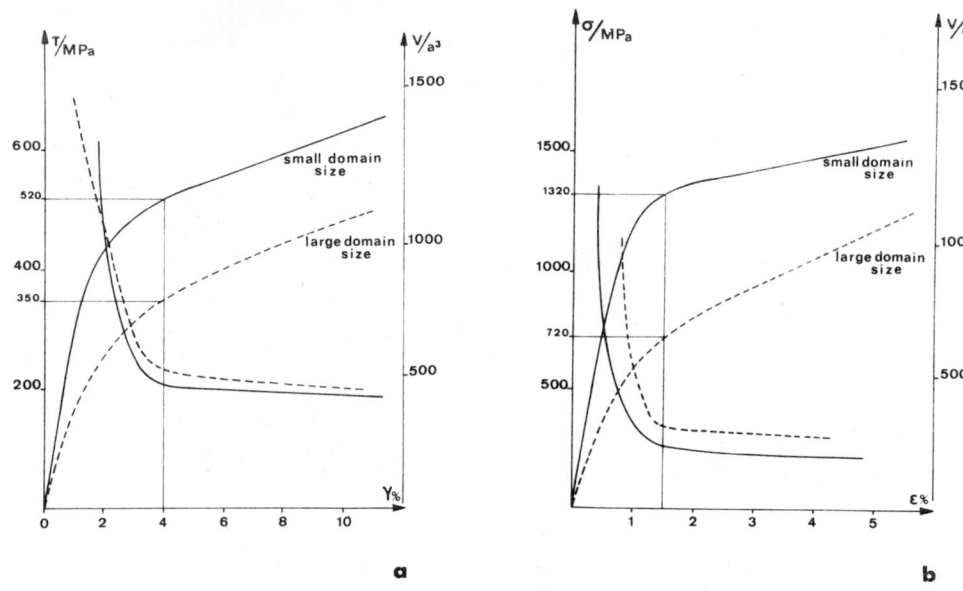

Fig.11 Stress strain curves for Ni_3V alloys a) single crystal; b) polycrystal.

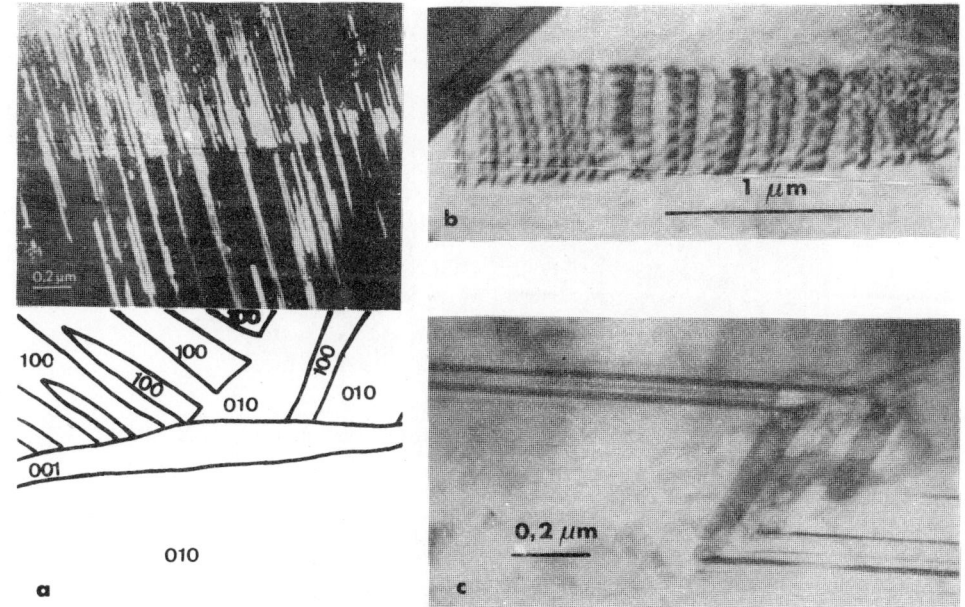

Fig.12 Microtwinning in Ni_3V a) small domain alloy; b) large domain alloy; c) zigzag propagation of microtwins.

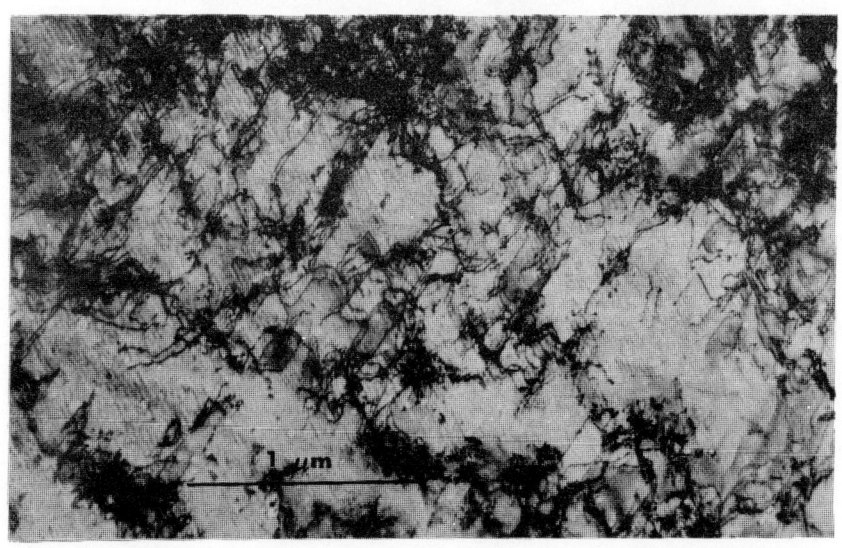

Fig.13 Typical deformation microstructure in Cu_3Pd.

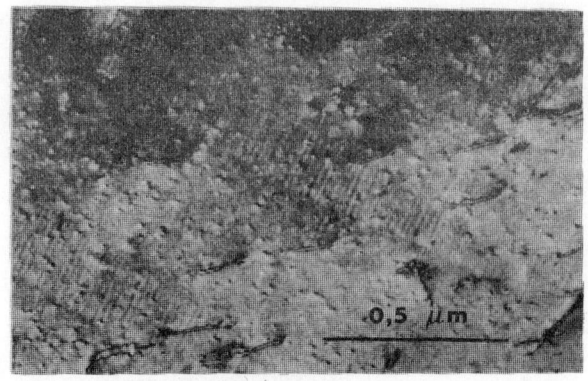

Fig.14 Vanishing of weak fringe contrast inside some domains ($Cu_3 Pd$).

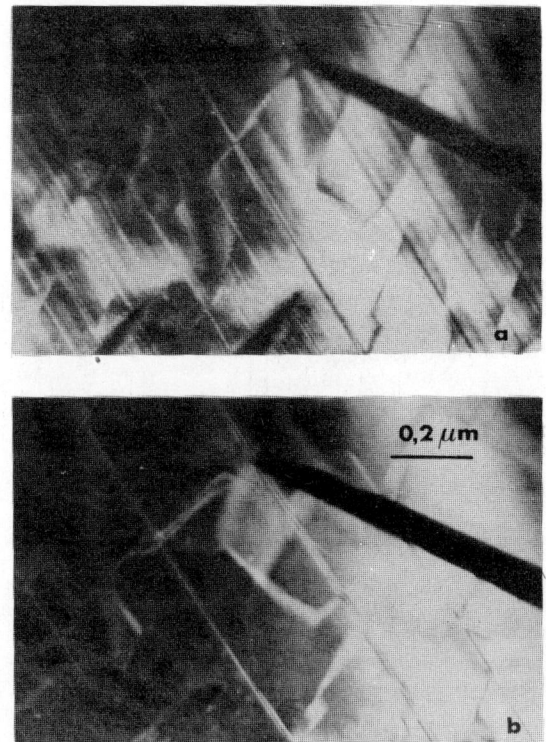

Fig.15 Dark field analysis of slip induced order defects in $Cu_3 Pd$
a) satellite reflection; b) $L1_2$ reflection.

MOVING DISLOCATIONS IN ALUMINIUM-BASE ALLOYS INVESTIGATED BY TEM AND NMR TECHNIQUES

J. Th. M. De Hosson
Department of Applied Physics, Materials Science Centre
University of Groningen, Nijenborgh 18
9747 AG Groningen, The Netherlands

O. Kanert
Institute of Physics, University of Dortmund
46 Dortmund 50, FRG

Abstract

Dislocation dynamics has been investigated by TEM/NMR in Al-Cu alloys containing plate-like precipitates (θ') and in Al-Li alloys containing spherical precipitates (δ'). The spin lattice relaxation rate in the rotating frame, $T_{1\rho}^{-1}$, of ^{27}Al has been measured as a function of the plastic strain rate $\dot{\varepsilon}$ at 77 K. From $T_{1\rho}$-measurements which were performed on pure Al, Al-1 at% Cu containing θ' plates and Al-2.2 wt% Li containing δ' precipitates, the mean jump distance of mobile dislocations is found. The mean jump distance has been determined as a function of strain. The precipitation hardening in the Aluminium-base alloys could be evaluated in terms of these NMR and TEM data.

Introduction

The startling increase in yield stress upon precipitation from solid solution, has lead to a great interest in precipitation hardening mechanisms in alloys. For example, the addition of lithium to aluminium results in a reduction of density and an increased modulus of elasticity compared with conventional aluminium alloys. Consequently, the development of aluminium-lithium alloys is highly desirable for structural applications especially in aerospace industry [1]. The basic strengthening mechanism of aluminium-lithium alloys is due to the formation of coherent δ' precipitates (ordered $L1_2$ phase Al_3Li)[2]. Another example is Al-Cu alloys containing non-deforming plate-like precipitates. The interplate spacing in the slip direction sets an upper limit for the slip distance, i.e. the actual distance traversed before a dislocation gets stuck. As a result the flow stress increases with decreasing interplate spacing.

To understand the strengthening mechanism and the increase in yield stress one must investigate the way in which moving dislocations interact with precipitate particles of a second phase. In this paper, a combined nuclear magnetic resonance and transmission electron microscopic study of the mechanism of dislocation motion in Al-2.2 wt% Li alloys and Al-1 at% Cu is presented. The *static* transmission electron microscopic observations of the instantaneous dislocation configuration and of the microstructure of the material are related to *in situ* nuclear spin relaxation measurements. Combining the evaluation of the two sets of data leads to detailed information about the effective mean jump distance L of mobile dislocations.

The NMR method of determining characteristics of dislocations is essentially based on the interaction between nuclear electric quadrupole moments and electric field gradients at the nucleus. If the nuclear environment is cubically symmetric there does not exist any static field gradient at the nucleus and interaction does not appear. However, around a dislocation that symmetry is destroyed and interactions between nuclear electric field gradients arise. As a matter of course, in order to apply the NMR technique to studies on dislocations, it is essential to have atomic nuclei with non-zero quadrupole moments; that requirement limits the choice of materials to be studied.

In the following we will focus mainly on plastic deformation experiments with a constant strain rate $\dot{\varepsilon}$. This type of experiment is governed by Orowan's equation [3]:

$$\dot{\varepsilon} = \phi \, b \, \rho_m \frac{L}{\tau_w} \, , \tag{1}$$

assuming a thermally activated, jerky motion of mobile dislocations of density

ρ_m. The motion may be considered to be jerky-like if the actual jump time τ_j is small compared to the mean time of stay τ_w at an obstacle. In Eq. (1), ϕ denotes a geometrical factor, b symbolizes the magnitude of the Burgers vector and L is the mean jump distance between obstacles which are considered to be uniform.

Theoretical Background

In the past we have shown that nuclear magnetic resonance is a useful tool for in situ investigations of dislocation motion in Al and in Al-Cu alloys. For detailed information of this technique reference is made to [4][5][6][7]. Only a concise review will be given here.

While deforming a sample with a constant strain rate $\dot{\varepsilon}$ the spin-lattice relaxation rate in a weak rotating field H_1 ("locking field"), $1/T_{1\rho}$, of the resonant nuclei in the sample is enhanced due to the motion of dislocations. The resulting total relaxation rate may be decomposed into a background relaxation rate $(1/T_{1\rho})_0$ and the contribution $(1/T_{1\rho})_D$ which is governed by the mechanism of dislocation motion, i.e. by Eq. (1):

$$\frac{1}{T_{1\rho}} = \left(\frac{1}{T_{1\rho}}\right)_0 + \left(\frac{1}{T_{1\rho}}\right)_D . \qquad (2)$$

In metallic systems, $(1/T_{1\rho})_0$ is due to fluctuations in the conduction electron-nucleus interaction. Whenever a dislocation changes its position in the crystal, the surrounding atoms have also to move, thus causing time fluctuations both of the quadrupolar and dipolar spin Hamiltonian for spins with $I > \frac{1}{2}$. However, the dipolar effects on the nuclear spin relaxation due to dislocation motion is negligible, and quadrupolar interactions dominate the relaxation behaviour.

The resulting expression for the relaxation rate induced by dislocation motion is given by:

$$\left(\frac{1}{T_{1\rho}}\right)_D = \frac{A_Q}{H_1^2 + H_{L\rho}^2} \frac{1}{\phi b} \cdot g_Q \cdot \frac{1}{L} \cdot \dot{\varepsilon} . \qquad (3)$$

Hence, for a given plastic deformation rate $\dot{\varepsilon}$ the nuclear spin relaxation rate is proportional to the inverse mean jump distance L. This relationship is used in the experiments to determine L. $H_{L\rho}$ is the mean local field in the rotating frame determined by the local dipolar field $H_{D\rho}$ and the local quadrupolar field $H_{Q\rho}$. The quadrupolar geometry factor g_Q in Eq. (3) which depends on the mean jump distance L approaches to one if L is of the order of 0.1 µm or higher. For ^{27}Al in aluminium, the quadrupolar coupling constant δ_Q has the value $2.85 \cdot 10^{-25}$ G² dyne^{-1}cm^4. The mean-squared electric field gradient $<V^2>$ of a dislocation of unit length in aluminium can be derived experimentally from an analysis of the line shape of the NMR signal which is quadrupole distorted by a known number of dislocations and $\delta_Q <V^2>$ appeared to be $3 \cdot 10^{-10}$ G² cm² (= A_Q).

Experimental Details

Sample preparation and transmission electron microscopic measurements

Polycrystalline samples with a grain size of the order of 100-200 μm were used. To avoid skin effect distortion of the NMR signal the NMR experiments were carried out on rectangular foils of size 27 mm x 12 mm x 40 μm.

The starting material for the Al-Cu alloys was 5N Al-1 at% Cu. After a homogenizing procedure at 550 °C for 2.5 days the material was rolled out to the thin foils with a thickness of about 40 μm and has then been cut by spark erosion to the sample size given above. The ultrapure aluminium samples were annealed a second time at 290 °C for 1 hour.

In order to get samples of solid solution the foils were annealed at 550 °C for 2.5 hrs and then quenched to 20 °C. Some of these samples were exposed to a third heat treatment (200 °C for 1 day) in order to produce plate-like precipitates of copper in these samples (θ'-phase in the Al:Cu phase diagram). The starting material for the Al-Li samples was Al-2.5 wt% Li. After a homogenizing procedure at 580 °C for 1 hr the material was rolled out to the thin foils with a thickness of about 40 μm and has then been cut by spark erosion to the sample size given above. Afterwards, the samples were annealed a second time at 580 °C for 7 min and quenched in water. In order to produce δ' precipitates of different sizes the samples were exposed to a third heat treatment (either 1 hr at 215 °C or 115 hrs at 245 °C). After the heat treatments, the Li content was measured by means of a Perkin Elmer spectrophotometer and appeared to be equal to 2.2 wt%. Transmission electron micrographs were taken by using a JEM 200 CX operating between 120 keV - 160 keV.

NMR measurements and deformation experiments

In the NMR experiment, the sample under investigation is plastically deformed by a servo-hydraulic tensile machine (ZONIC Technical Lab. Inc. Cincinnati) of which the exciter head XCI TE 1105 moves a driving rod with a constant velocity. The movement is controlled by a digital function generator which serves the Master controller of the exciter head. While the specimen was deforming, ^{27}Al nuclear spin measurements were carried out by means of a BRUKER pulse spectrometer SXP 4-100 operating at 15.7 MHz corresponding to a magnetic field of 1.4 T controlled by an NMR stabilizer (BRUKER B-SN 15). The NMR head of the spectrometer and the frame in which the rod moves formed a unit which was inserted between the pole pieces of the electromagnet of the spectrometer. The unit could be temperature-controlled between 77 K and 550 K. The spectrometer was triggered by the electronic control of the tensile machine. The trigger starts the nuclear spin relaxation experiment at a definite time during deformation. The general set-up of the whole tensile testing system is shown in the block diagram of Fig. 1. The NMR measurements discussed here were carried out at 77 K. At such a low temperature nuclear spin relaxation effects due to diffusive atomic motions are negligible. Calculations of the correlation times for Al, Cu, Li show that in fact Al, Cu and Li are immobile at 77 K. Therefore, an observable contribution of diffusive atomic motion to the measured relaxation rates does not occur.

The local fields $H_{L\rho}$ (Eq. 3) in Al-Cu and Al-Li were determined from ^{27}Al spin echo signal measurements [4] and were found to be 4.4 G and 3.75 G, respectively.

Figure 2 exhibits deformation curves of some of the Al-Cu samples measured at 77 K. In particular, the data demonstrate the different plastic behaviour of the Al-0.1 at% Cu (solid solution) sample and of Al-1 at% Cu (θ' - phase). The increase of the yield stress of the Al-1 at% Cu sample compared to Al-0.1 at% Cu and pure aluminium is about 70 MPa.

In figure 3 deformation curves of some of the samples at 77 K are depicted. In particular, the data demonstrate the different plastic behaviour of the Al-2.2 wt% Li alloys compared to ultrapure Al. The increase of the yield stress of the samples aged at 215 °C and aged at 245 °C, compared to ultrapure Al, is 92 MPa and 41 MPa, respectively.

Results and Discussion

Mean jump distance of moving dislocations in Al

In Figure 4 the mean jump distance measured by NMR in pure Al is illustrated as a function of strain. The mean jump distance L measured by NMR in Al has to be interpreted with care in terms of mean slip distance and statistical slip length (Λ_{st}). As commonly found in annealed f.c.c. metals, a cell structure is formed in Al after deformation at 77 K. As a result, the mean slip distance of dislocations is mainly determined by the cell size when the cell structure is well developed. The statistical slip length Λ_{st} will be of the same order of magnitude as the cell size ($\simeq$ 1-2 µm), i.e. much larger than the mean jump distance measured by NMR ($\simeq$ 0.1 µm for $\varepsilon \gtrsim$ 7%). A plausible explanation for this difference is that all moving dislocations, present both in the cell boundary and in the interior region of the cell, affect the spin lattice relaxation rate. The mean jump distance of dislocations measured by NMR is possibly related to the spacing of the dislocation tangles near the cell boundary ranging from 0.01 µm to 0.1 µm.

Assuming two different sets of corresponding mobile dislocation densities: ρ_1 in the interior of the cell and ρ_2 inside the cell wall the total spin lattice relaxation rate can be written as:

$$\left(\frac{1}{T_{1\rho}}\right)_D = \left(\frac{1}{T_{1\rho}}\right)_D^{(1)} + \left(\frac{1}{T_{1\rho}}\right)_D^{(2)} \quad . \tag{4}$$

Further, since $L_1 \gg L_2$ and $g_Q(L_1) \simeq 1$ and $g_Q(L_2) \simeq 0.6$ the total spin lattice relaxation rate measured by NMR is largely determined by the distance between forest dislocations inside the cell wall: $(T_{1\rho}^{-1})_D \simeq (T_{1\rho}^{-1})_D^{(2)}$.

Mean jump distance of dislocations in Al-1 at% Cu (θ')

In figure 4 the NMR results are displayed in the case of Al-1 at% Cu (θ'-phase). Figure 5 shows an electron micrograph of Al-1 at% Cu. The typical microstructure shows plate-like θ' precipitates. According to Russell and Ashby [8] the interplate spacing in the slip direction (Λ_p) sets an upper limit for the slip distance, i.e. the actual distance traversed before a dislocation gets stuck.

The mean jump distance of the dislocations measured by NMR can be associated with the effective interparticle spacing obtained from the transmission electron micrographs. The precipitates have a definitive angle with the glide plane (54° 44'). In the glide plane, their mean length of the obstacles D' is $(\pi/4)D$ and their mean thickness d' is $d\sqrt{3/2}$ [9][10]. The mean centre-to-centre spacing is then given by:

$$\lambda' = \sqrt{\frac{D' d'}{f}} \quad , \tag{5}$$

where f is the volume fraction of the precipitates. Following Foreman et al.[11] a distribution of linear parallel obstacles of length $S = D' - d'$ will give a hardening that is $1 + S/\lambda'$ times greater than for the associated distribution of point obstacles. The latter applies to aligned, line obstacles only. If we take into account the finite thickness of plate shaped particles the effective separation between the precipitates is

$$\Lambda_p = \frac{\lambda'}{1+S/\lambda'} - d' \quad . \tag{6}$$

From the transmission electronmicroscopic observations follows: $D = 0.36$ μm, $d = 0.005$ μm and $f = 0.03$. Substituting the values for D' and d' into Eq. (5) and Eq. (6) leads to $\Lambda_p = 0.11$ μm. The effective particle spacing obtained from the transmission electronmicroscopic observations is in good agreement with the mean jump distance of dislocations measured by NMR ($L_{NMR}=0.12$ μm, figure 4). The hardening is thus controlled by the microstructure at the beginning of deformation. It should be noted at this point that Λ_p, defined by Ashby [12] as a constant, is independent of the shear strain a. Thompson et al. [13] proposed a modification to the Ashby view point where Λ_p sets an upper limit to Λ_{st} and $\Lambda_{st} \simeq \Lambda_p$ at yield. Then at small strain the slip distance is $\simeq \Lambda_p$ and at large strain the slip distance is $\simeq \Lambda_{st}$. This situation was found in our experiments at the beginning of deformation $L_{NMR} \simeq \Lambda_p$. At larger strains the mean distance between the statistical dislocations is about 0.03 µm (figure 4).

For a theoretical evaluation of the yield stress, which is based on the NMR data, and for comparison with the deformation experiment the following theoretical expression of the yield stress is assumed:

$$\sigma = \sigma_0 + \frac{k_1 k_2}{2\pi\lambda} \mu b \ln\left(\frac{\lambda}{b}\right), \qquad (7)$$

where λ is the mean end-to-end spacing of the precipitates in the glide plane, k_1 is a statistical factor and k_2 is a factor depending on the character of the dislocation. σ_0 is considered to be the contribution to flow stress due to the residual solid solution ($\simeq$ 0.09 at% Cu). Eq. (7) is similar to the expression proposed by Ashby [16]. If in the case of Orowan by-passing the bowed-out dislocation between the θ' obstacles are not much affected by dipole interactions, the constant k_2 can be calculated on the basis of a line tension approximation [9] [10]. The maximum value thus obtained is 1.5 and the minimum value of k_2 is 1. Substituting the values in Eq. (7) and taking for $\lambda = L_{NMR} = 0.12$ µm, $\mu = 2.8 * 10^{11}$ dyn/cm² and $k_1 = 0.85$ [10] we found that the minimum of the Orowan stress is 54.5 MPa and the maximum value is found to be 81.8 MPa. It means that the yield stress due to the hardening effect of the precipitates lies in the range of 54.5 MPa to 81.8 MPa. From Eq. (7) it follows that this hardening effect has to be added to the contribution to flow stress due to the residual solid solution ($\simeq$ 0.09 at% Cu). This is in good agreement with the experimental stress-strain curves (Fig. 2): the increase of the yield stress of Al-1 at% Cu samples compared to Al-0.1 at% Cu in solid solution is about 70 MPa.

Mean jump distance of moving dislocations in Al-2.2 wt% Li aged at 215 °C (1 hr)

The results of the strain dependence of L measured by NMR are depicted in Fig.6. The spin-lattice relaxation rate was determined at a constant strain rate $\dot{\varepsilon} = 1.6$ s^{-1}. The shape of the L vs ε curve is quite similar to the curve obtained for ultrapure Al (Fig. 4). Apparently at the beginning of deformation the storage dislocation follows strictly geometrical or statistical rules which are not considerably influenced by temperature and strain rate. Assuming that the mean jump distance L is proportional to the statistical slip length Λ_{st} and that Λ_{st} is proportional to the slip line length Λ_L which decreases with increasing strain in pure f.c.c. metals, it means that

$$\frac{1}{L} \approx \varepsilon \ . \tag{8}$$

From Fig. 6 we find indeed that the inverse of the mean jump distance varies linearly with strain according to equation (8).

Two electron micrographs illustrating the microstructure of deformed Al-Li at 5% and 15% (fracture) are shown in Fig. 7 and Fig. 8, respectively. In Fig. 7 dislocation contrast has been used ($\vec{g} = [\bar{2}00]$) and in Fig. 8 δ' superlattice reflections have been used for imaging the Al_3Li precipitates. From the micrograph depicted in **Fig. 8** it is very difficult to conclude whether the precipitates are sheared or not. Therefore, we will base our arguments on the NMR and TEM results concerning the occurrence of either order hardening or Orowan hardening. When a dislocation passes through the ordered Al_3Li precipitate, an antiphase boundary is formed, of surface energy γ_{APB} per unit area. A complication which commonly arises in alloys containing ordered precipitates is that the dislocations travel in pairs, the second dislocation removing the disorder created by the first. In Fig. 7 such a superlattice dislocation ($\frac{1}{2}[101] \, (\bar{1}11)$) has been imaged. The mean separation is about r = 93 nm. Stereo electron micrographs revealed that the volume fraction f is 3.1 % and the mean diameter of the precipitates is $2\bar{R}$ = 15.2 nm. Taking μ = 0.3 10^5 MPa in the following equation

$$f \, \gamma_{APB} = \frac{\mu b^2}{2\pi r} \ , \tag{9}$$

leads to γ_{APB} = 135 mJ/m². This value should be regarded as the upper limit since any internal or friction stress should be subtracted. Obviously, residual stresses are present on the dislocations shown in Fig. 7. Brown and Ham [14] have calculated that when the first dislocation of a superlattice dislocation pair meets the Friedel condition, the second dislocation is pulled forward by the antiphase domain boundary remaining in the particles which it intersects. As the flow stress τ is increased from zero, the first dislocation bends forward more, while the second dislocation straightens out. The forward stress on the first dislocation is considerably increased by the interaction of the second dislocation with disordered particles. This is actually illustrated in Fig. 7. The Friedel spacing as well as the mean square spacing (0.076 μm and 0.062 μm, respectively) appear to be close to the mean jump distance L measured by NMR (see Fig. 6). Since the first dislocation meets the Friedel condition is this case ([14] $\pi T f/4\gamma < \bar{R}_s < T/\gamma$) and the second dislocation is nearly straight, the applied flow stress required for cutting the precipitates is given by:

$$\tau_a = \frac{\gamma}{2b} \, [(\frac{4\gamma \bar{R}_s \, f}{\pi T})^{\frac{1}{2}} - f \,] \tag{10}$$

Taking the experimental values mentioned before τ_a is found to be 31 MPa (line tension $T \simeq \frac{1}{2} \mu b^2$, $\bar{R}_s = \sqrt{\frac{2}{3}} \bar{R}$). This is in close agreement with the increase of the applied stress ($\tau_a \simeq \sigma_a/3$) compared to ultrapure Al (Fig. 3). As a matter of course, this increase should be compared with the as-quenched sample value. However, we could not obtain reproducible results for those samples as far as σ_Y (12 MPa - 28 MPa) is concerned. The onset of looping occurs when $\tau_a = \frac{1}{2} \tau_0$. The Orowan stress τ_0 is calculated to be 101 MPa. It means that as long as $\gamma_{APB} <$ 172 mJ/m² shearing of the precipitates will take place.

Mean jump distance of moving dislocations in Al-2.2 wt% Li aged at 245 °C (115 hrs)

The NMR results (L vs ε) are displayed in Fig. 6. Fig. 9 shows an electron micrograph of Al-2.2 wt% Li deformed until fracture strain. In this case the microstructure as well as the NMR results look very different compared to those treated in the previous section. From transmission electron micrographs the mean diameter appeared to be $2R = 0.129$ µm and the volume fraction $f = 5.7\%$. The average gap [15] between the particles is then given by 0.29 µm. This value is very close to the mean jump distance determined by NMR at low ε, indicating that in contrast to the previous section, Orowan hardening might be the predominant hardening-mechanism. Furthermore, Fig. 9 clearly shows that looping occurred during plastic deformation. The interparticle spacing in the slip direction sets an upper limit for the slip distance, i.e. the actual distance traversed before a dislocation gets stuck. The hardening is expected to be controlled by the microstructure at the beginning of deformation. In this case $\bar{R}_s > T/\gamma$ and we expect that the flow stress for cutting is given by [14]

$$\tau = (\frac{\gamma}{2b}) [(\frac{4f}{\pi})^{\frac{1}{2}} - f] . \qquad (11)$$

The cutting stress for the first dislocation approaches $\tau_1 = 2\tau + (\gamma/b)f$. At this stage the dislocation becomes sufficiently bent to loop around the particles by the Orowan process instead of cutting through them. The critical stress for looping is calculated to be $\tau_0 = 27.4$ MPa using the NMR data for the effective distance between the precipitates. Since the applied stress required for cutting (Eq. 11) is calculated to be 50.1 MPa, i.e. larger than $\tau_0/2$, the first dislocation reaches the looping stage. As a matter of course, as soon as looping occurs, two dislocations in equilibrium cannot be supported by a row of particles and the dislocation pair tends to spread apart. So, no "super lattice" dislocation pairs are observed (Fig. 9).

At higher strain values the mean jump distance is decreasing gradually from 0.2 µm at $\varepsilon = 5\%$ to 0.08 µm. The reasons for this decrease starting at $\varepsilon = 10\%$ are twofold. First of all 'statistically stored' dislocations, i.e. those that would accumulate during simple tension, will diminish the mean jump distance substantially. As can be deduced from Fig. 9, the mean distance between the statistical dislocations is certainly much smaller than the mean separation of the δ' precipitates. Secondly, since it is unlikely that each particle is to be intersected by only one slip plane, loops are expected to form vertical stacks. Any movement of dislocations lying on these particles (internal interactions, cross slip, etc.) affect the spin lattice relaxation rate. According to equation 4, the distance between the stacked loops is much smaller than the distance between the precipitates. Consequently, spin-lattice relaxation rate $(1/T_{1\rho})_D$ is more determined by the dislocation motion around the precipitates. As a result the mean jump distance measured by NMR is smaller than the actual mean particle spacing.

Conclusions

The conclusion may be drawn that pulsed nuclear magnetic resonance is a complementary new technique for the study of dislocations in metallic systems. Since the process of dislocation motion is made up of atomic movements nuclear magnetic resonance technique offers a possibility to determine the manner in which dislocations progress through the crystal as a function of time utilising nuclear spin relaxation as a tool.

It turned out that from the pulsed nuclear magnetic resonance experiments on Al and Al-Cu alloys the mean jump distance of moving dislocations can be deduced and subsequently the hardening effect due to precipitates in Al-1 at% Cu (θ') can be predicted. Also in Al-Li alloys the different hardening mechanisms could be evaluated by this approach. Nevertheless, it should be emphasized that Al-Li alloy is not an alloy system that exhibits only one type of hardening: i.e. either order hardening or Orowan hardening. In alloys like Al-Li there is actually a distribution of particle sizes which are used in the equations of the previous section. Plastic deformation is a local process and depends on the local characteristics of the microstructure. Therefore, some precipitates can also be shearable in the alloy system, mentioned in the latter section, and Orowan looping can take place in an alloy system treated as mentioned in the previous section as well. Nevertheless, spin-lattice relaxation measurements clearly indicate that the fluctuations in the quadrupolar field due to moving dislocations in these two alloys are quite different, from which a difference in dislocation dynamics may be concluded.

Acknowledgements

Thanks are due to Dr. L. Katgerman (Technological University - Delft) for providing us with the raw Al-Li material.

This work is part of the research program of the Foundation for Fundamental Research on Matter (F. O. M. - Utrecht) and has been made possible by financial support from the Netherlands Organization for the Advancement of Pure Research (Z. W. O. - The Hague) and the Deutsche Forschungsgemeinschaft, FRG.

References

[1] Aluminium-Lithium Alloys, Eds.:T.H. Sanders and E. A. Starke, Conference Proceedings AIME, 1981.
[2] Sanders, T. H. and Starke, E. A., Acta Metall. 30 (1982) 927.
[3] Orowan, E., Z. Phys. 89 (1934) 634.
[4] Tamler, H., Kanert, O., Alsem, W. H. M. and De Hosson, J. Th. M., Acta Metall. 30 (1982) 1523.
[5] Hackelöer, H. J., Kanert, O., Tamler, H. and De Hosson, J. Th. M., Rev. Sci. Instruments 54 (1983) 341.
[6] De Hosson, J. Th. M., Alsem, W. H. M., Tamler, H. and Kanert, O., in: Defects, Fracture and Fatigue (Eds.: G. C. Sih and J. W. Provan), Nijhoff - The Hague, p. 23 (1983).
[7] Tamler, H., Hackelöer, H. J., Kanert, O., Alsem, W. H. M. and De Hosson, J. Th. M., in: Nuclear and Electron Resonance Spectroscopies Applied to Materials Science (Eds.: E. N. Kaufmann and G. K. Shenoy), North Holland Amsterdam, p. 421 (1981).
[8] Russell, K. C. and Ashby, M. F., Acta Met. 18 (1970) 891.
[9] Merle, P., Fouquet, F., Merlin, J., Mat. Sci. & Engin. 50 (1981) 215.
[10] Kelly, P. M., Scripta Met. 6 (1972) 647.
[11] Foreman, A. J. E., Hirsch, P. B., Humphreys, F. J., NBS Spec. Publ. 317 Vol. 2 (1970) 1083.
[12] Ashby, M. F., Phil. Mag. 21 (1970) 399.
[13] Thompson, A. W., Baskes, M. I., Flanagan, W. F., Acta Met. 25 (1973) 1017.
[14] Brown, L. M. and Ham, R. K., in: Strengthening Methods in Crystals (eds.: A. Kelly, R. B. Nicholson), Applied Science Publ.-London, p. 12 (1971).
[15] Hazzledine, P. H. and Hirsch, P. B., Phil. Mag. 30 (1974) 1331.
[16] Ashby, M. F., Acta Metall. 14 (1966) 679.

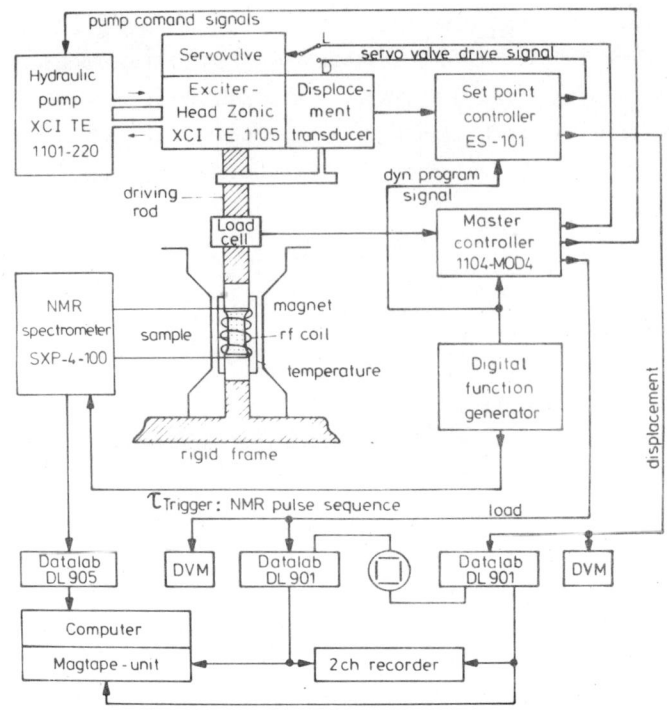

Fig.1: Scheme of the experimental set-up.

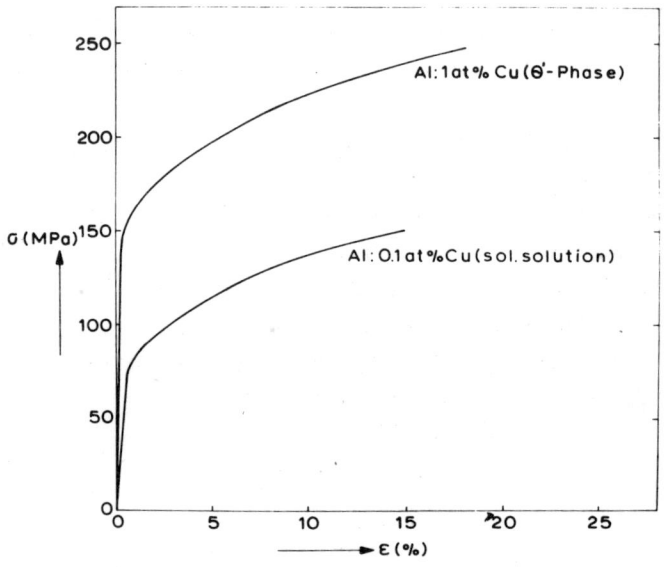

Fig.2: Experimental stress-strain curves at 77 K.

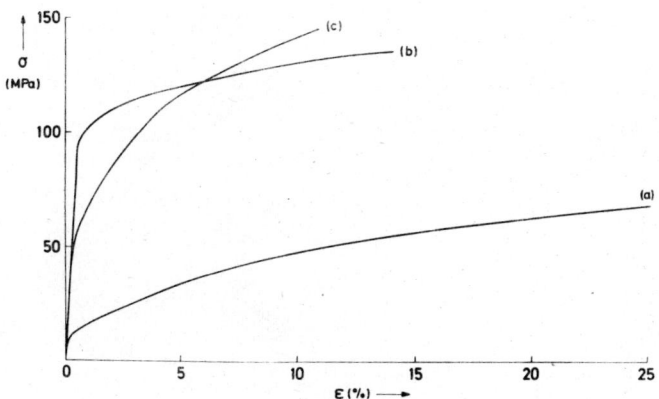

Fig.3: Experimental stress-strain curves of *some* of the foils meaured at 77 K.
(a) 5N Al; (b) Al-2.2 wt%Li aged at 215°C (1hr); (c) Al-2.2 wt% Li aged at 245°C (115 hrs).

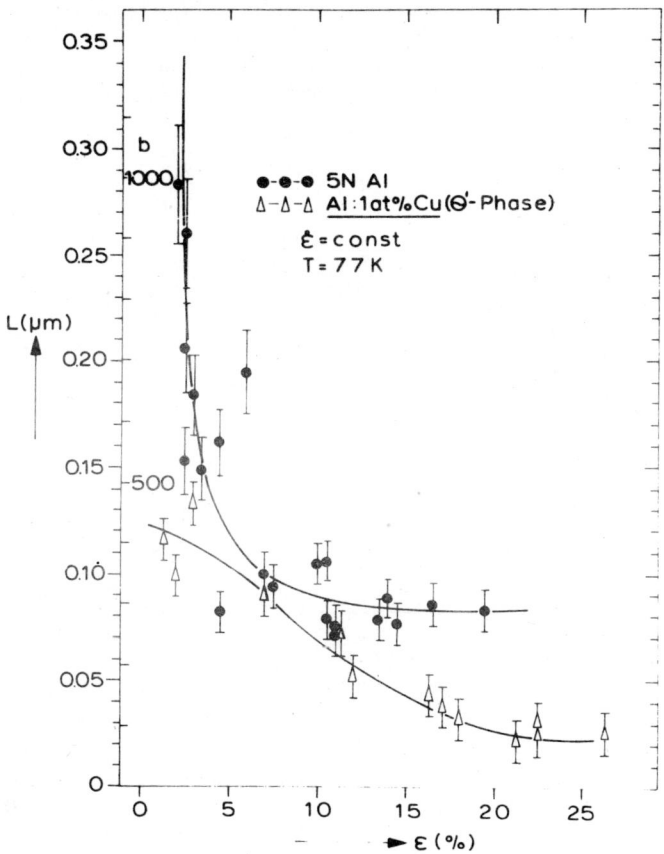

Fig.4: The mean jump distance measured by NMR as a function of strain ε in Al and in Al-1 at% Cu.

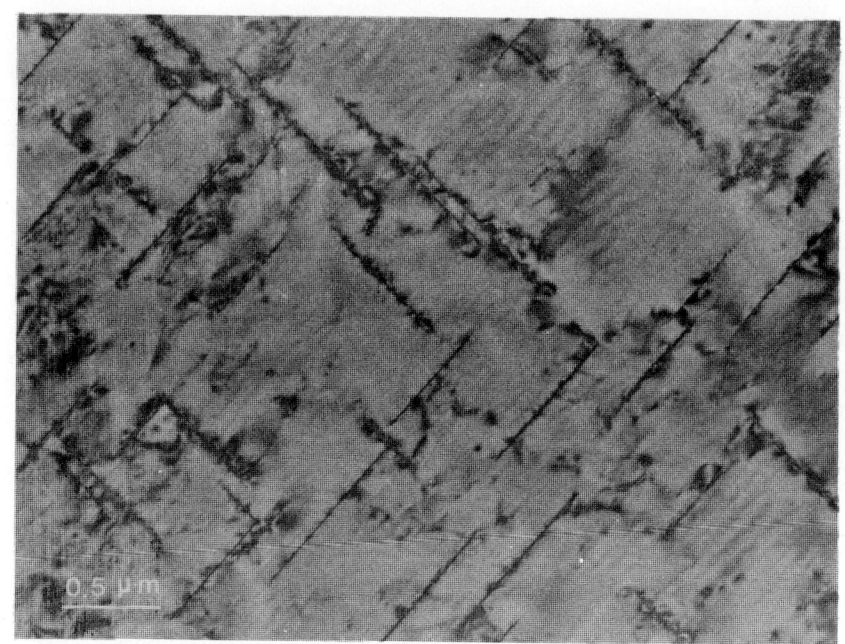

Fig.5: Al-1 at% Cu (θ⁻ phase), 26% deformation. Bright field/strong beam image, [100] orientation, $\vec{g}$ = [002].

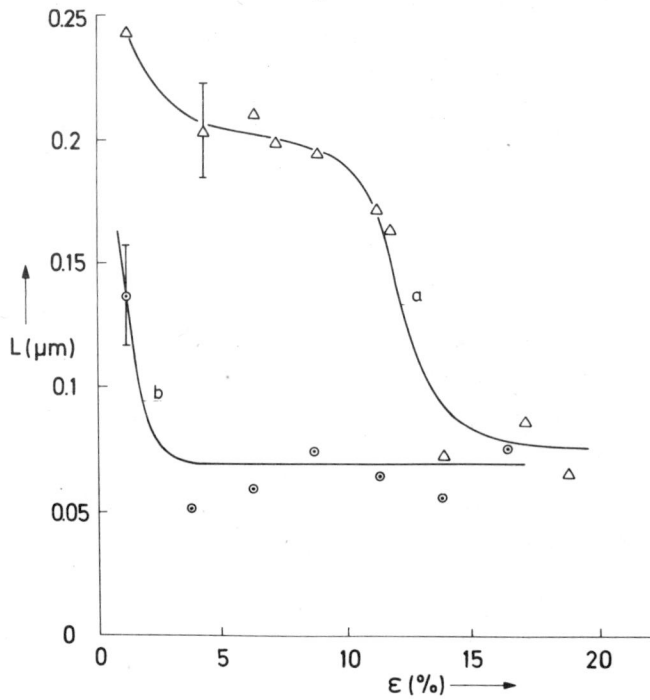

Fig.6: The mean jump distance measured by NMR as a function of strain ε in (a) Al-2.2 wt% Li aged at 245°C (115 hrs) and (b) Al-2.2 wt% Li aged at 215°C (1hr)

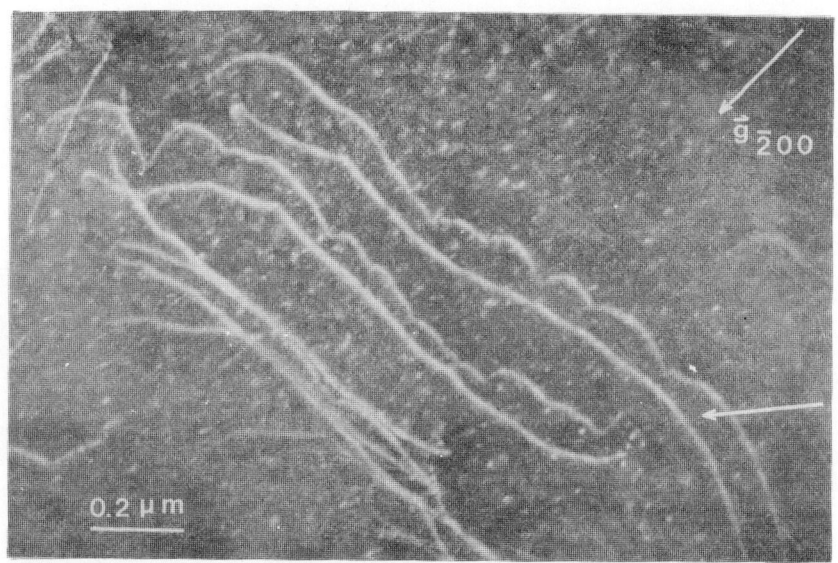

Fig.7: Al-2.2 wt% Li aged at 215°C (1hr) deformed 5% at 77 K. Dark field/ weak beam image, [011] orientation, $\vec{g} = [\bar{2}00]$.

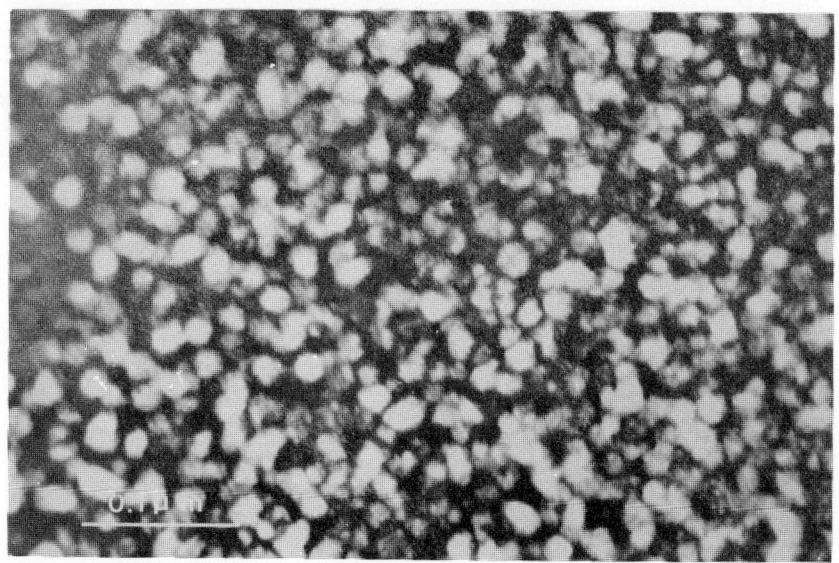

Fig.8: Al-2.2 wt%Li aged at 215°C (1hr) deformed till fracture. Dark field/ strong beam, [011] orientation, $\vec{g} = [001]$.

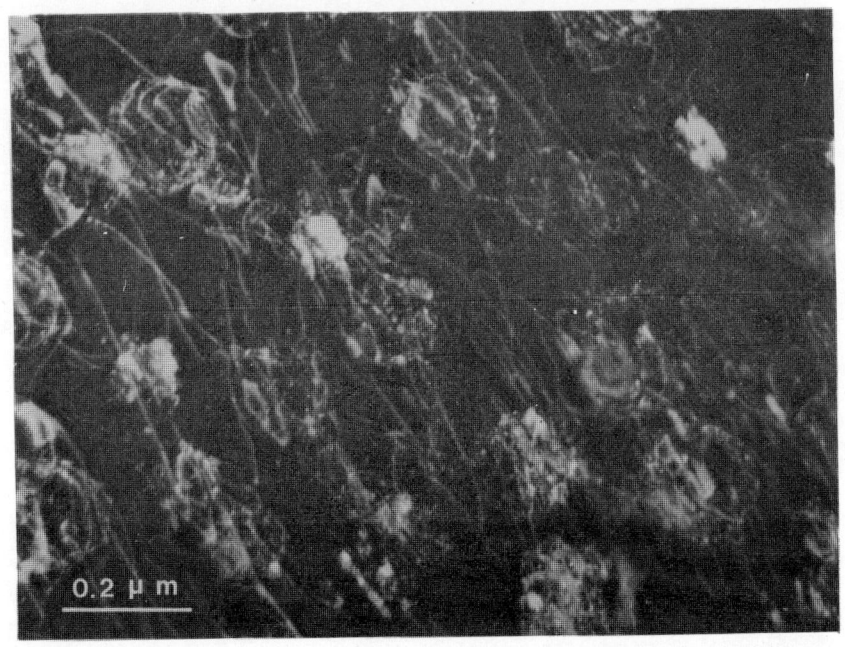

Fig.9: Al-2.2 wt% Li aged at 245°C (115hrs) deformed till fracture, dark field/weak beam, [211] orientation, $\vec{g} = [02\bar{2}]$.

TEMPERATURE DEPENDENCE OF STACKING FAULT ENERGY

T. Imura and H. Saka

Department of Metallurgy, Faculty of Engineering, Nagoya University, Furo-cho, Chikusa-ku, Nagoya 464 Japan

INTRODUCTION

Stacking fault energy (γ) of fcc metals and alloys is an important physical parameter which determines mechanical and physical properties. This γ depends not only on type and content of solute elements but also on temperature. It is known that γ decreases with increasing of electron atom ratio (e/a) in noble metal alloys but as for the temperature dependence unified view has not yet been established[1,2,3].

This paper presents the recent experimental results and a unified view obtained with the precise measurements of the intrinsic temperature dependence of γ in fcc alloys by means of in situ thermal cycling experiments carried out in an HVEM on pure Ag[4], Ag alloys[5] and Cu alloys[6].

EXPERIMENTALS

Foil specimens were examined in a Hitachi HU-1000D microscope at the accelerating voltage of 600kV or 400kV; the voltage was kept low to avoid electron-irradiation damage of the specimen. The weak beam electron microscopy was used for observation. Isolated, long, nearly straight dislocations lying in the plane parallel to the foil surfaces were investigated to reduce the influence of the surfaces or nearby dislocations during the in situ thermal cycling experiments.

The following precautions have been taken for γ determination:
(1) the determination of γ is made precisely by measuring the width Δ of extended dislocations lying separately in a plane parallel to free surfaces.
(2) to reduce scatter of data to a minimum, the observation of the same extended dislocations is made during thermal cycling experiment.
(3) the intrinsic temperature dependence is studied from the data of reversible component of the change of γ by repeating thermal cycling several times since it is probable that the change of γ in alloys results from not only an intrinsic parameter on the temperature dependence but also extrinsic parameters such as those on solute impedance

effect, Suzuki effect, electron-irradiation effect, short range order elastic constant and so on/6/ (details to exclude these; cf./6/).

Cu-Al ALLOYS

Fig.1 illustrates extended dislocations observed in Cu-13.43 at% Al alloy. The width Δ of extended dislocations is dependent on the orientation of the **total** dislocation and it becomes maximum in edge orientation and minimum in screw orientation. Fig.2 shows the plot of the width Δ against the orientation θ of the total dislocation. Comparing with theoretical curves/7/ the precise determination of γ has been made (in the case of Fig.2, $\gamma = 5.8 \pm 0.4$ mJm^{-2}). Fig.3 illustrates the results of observations of the change of Δ in the temperature range of 120K-773K for the same extended dislocation.

Fig.4 illustrates the change of Δ due to the thermal cycling of the specimen in an HVEM which was deformed at 77K. From this observation, the followings are found;
(1) no apparent change of Δ below 300K.
(2) the change of Δ has only been recognized after heating at about 430K. The Δ decreases rapidly in the range 430K-600K and above these temperatures Δ indicates a slight increase or no apparent change.
(3) during cooling, Δ expresses recovery but the value of Δ at room temperature after the application of thermal cycling is about 30% less than the value of after-deformation.
(4) temperature dependence of Δ after the thermal cycling is just the same as that of cooling cycle of the first thermal cycling experiment i.e., once the specimen was heated up above 600K, the change of Δ becomes reversible. This has been confirmed with the specimen annealed in bulky state.

The aforementioned experimental results are to be understood in the following way. The intrinsic temperature dependence of γ indicates the increase of γ up to 800K but below 400K, dislocations can not move easily due to solute impedance (although γ increases), no apparent change of Δ occurs. The reduction of Δ can be obtained only above 400K where dislocations overcome the solute impedance. The same happens during cooling cycle. Therefore, the values Δ for the specimens deformed below 400K represent those of γ at the deformation temperature rather than those of γ at the observation temperature. It is concluded that the reversible change Δ above 400K is attributable to the change of γ, so that the intrinsic temperature dependence can be obtained/6/.

Fig.5 indicates the presence of a peak of γ near 800K in the case of Cu-13.43 at% Al alloy. The similar experiments have been done on Cu-6.44 at% Al alloy and the results are also indicated in Fig.5. The value of γ decreases with the increase of Al content but $d\gamma/dT$ increases with Al content in the temperature range below 800K.

Ag AND Ag ALLOYS

Since the measurement of temperature dependence of γ has been already been obtained in pure Ag[4], it is more appropriate to examine the effects of solute addition to the temperature dependence of γ in Ag base alloys.

Fig.6 shows a typical sequence of the variation of dislocation dissociation during an in situ thermal cycling experiment carried out on Ag-15.0 at% Al. The actual separation of partial dislocations Δ was calculated from the experimental separation Δ_{obs} according to the equation proposed by Cockayne, Jenkins and Ray [8], and plotted against the orientation of a dislocation line θ, where θ is the angle between the dislocation line and the total Burgers vectors, for the temperature studied. Fig.7 illustrates an example. The width of a dissociated edge dislocation ($\theta=90°$) was determined by fitting the experimental points with theoretical curves predicted by anisotropy elasticity[7] and the corresponding value of the apparent stacking fault energy was determined; in this determination, the temperature dependence of the shear modulus was, of course, taken into account.
Here, the term 'apparent stacking fault energy' is used in case there is a possibility of the measured values of the stacking fault energy under consideration being affected by parameters other than the intrinsic temperature dependence of γ. The results on the variation of ($\theta=90°$) during thermal cycling experiments on Ag-15.0 at% Al are illustrated in Fig.8, where the variation is alike to the case on Cu-13.43 at% Al. Fig.9 indicates a typical example of the sequence of dissociation of dislocations during an in situ thermal cycling experiment carried out on Ag-9.6 at% Al.

Fig.10 illustrates a typical example of the sequence of dissociation of dislocations during a thermal cycling experiment on Ag-5.4 at% Al and Fig.11 indicates the results on the variation of the width during thermal cycling experiments on the same alloy. It can be seen from Fig.11 that the variation of the width in the dilute alloy like Ag-5.4 at% Al is different from that of the other more concentrated alloys; the width Δ in Ag-5.4 at% Al increased slightly on increasing temperature and the variation was reversible, while in the others, Δ decreased on increasing temperature and both reversible and irreversible variations of Δ took place. These features were very similar to those observed on Cu-Al alloys.

Fig.12 illustrates the change of Δ in an extended dislocation in pure Ag during thermal cycling experiments. In the case of pure metals, it is considered that the change of Δ may directly correspond to the change of γ, although the temperature dependence of the shear modulus has to be taken into consideration.

The γ-T curve obtained on Ag and Ag-Al alloys is illustrated in Fig.13. From this curve, it is seen that the values for pure Ag and dilute alloys decrease with temperature, whereas those for the high solute content alloys increase with temperature. The variation of Δ on Ag-Sn alloys is reversible when Sn content is less than 4 at% and it represents the variation of γ with temperature. Fig.14 illustrates the temperature dependence of γ on Ag and Ag-Sn alloys. The γ decreases slightly according to the increase of temperature in the case of Ag and Ag dilute Sn alloys, but in the case of higher solute content alloys (Ag-9 at% Sn[9]), γ increases with temperature. In other words, $d\gamma/dT$ indicates the tendency to increase systematically according to the content of Sn. This fact is the same as that on Ag-Al, Cu-Al and other alloys investigated in the present experiments.

To examine whether or not this tendency is generalized, $d\gamma/dT$ was plotted as a function of (e/a) and illustrated in Fig.15. The systematic increase of $d\gamma/dT$ is observed in the figure not only on Ag alloys but also Cu-Al alloys. This experimental finding is consistent with the Tisone's prediction in which $d\gamma/dT$ becomes positive above (e/a) = 1.14[10,11].

REFERENCES
/1/ Christian J.W.,Swann P.R.:Alloying Behaviour and Effects in Concentrated Solid Solutions, Ed. by Massalski,Gordon and Breach, N.Y.(1965)
/2/ Gallagher P.C.:Metall. Trans,1 (1970) 2429
/3/ Remy L.,Pineau A.,Thomas B.:Materials Sci. Eng. 36(1978) 47
/4/ Saka H.,Iwata T.,Imura T.:Phil.Mag. A 37,(1978) 291
/5/ Saka H.,Kondo T.,Imura T.:Phil. Mag. in printing
/6/ Saka H.,Sueki Y.,Imura T.:Phil. Mag. A,37(1978) 273
/7/ Teutonico L.J.:Acta Metall. 11(1963) 1283
/8/ Cockayne D.J.H.,Jenkins M.L.,Ray I.L.F.:Phil.Mag.24(1971) 1383
/9/ Ruff A.W.,Ives L.K.:Phys.Status Solidi (a)16 (1973)133
/10/Tisone T.C.:Met.Trans.,3 (1972) 427
/11/Tisone T.C.,Brittain J.O,Meshii M.,:Phys.Status Solidi 27(1968)185

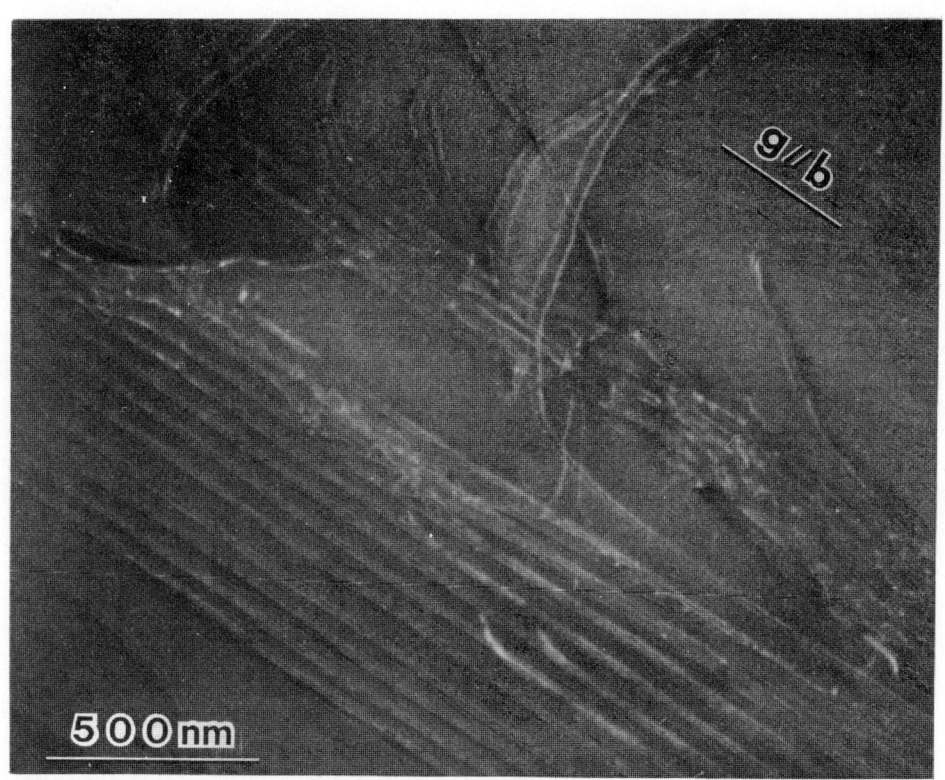

Fig.1 Extended dislocations in Cu-13.43 at% Al alloy observed by the weak beam method.

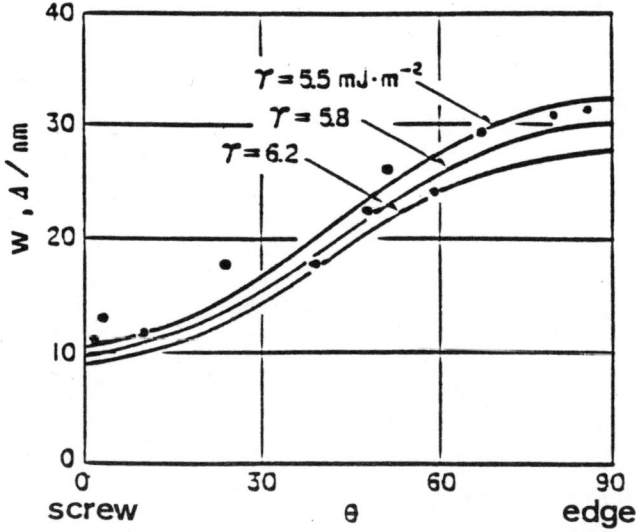

Fig.2 Width Δ of extended dislocations against orientation θ of the total dislocations.

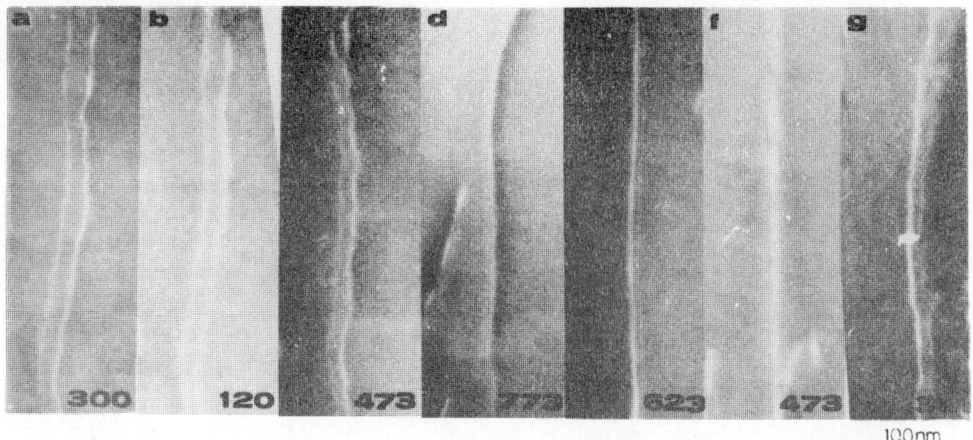

Fig.3 A typical example of the sequence of dissociation of dislocations during a thermal cycling experiment on Cu-13.43 at% Al deformed at 77K. The numbers refer to the temperature in K and letters in the upper left corners to the chronological order.

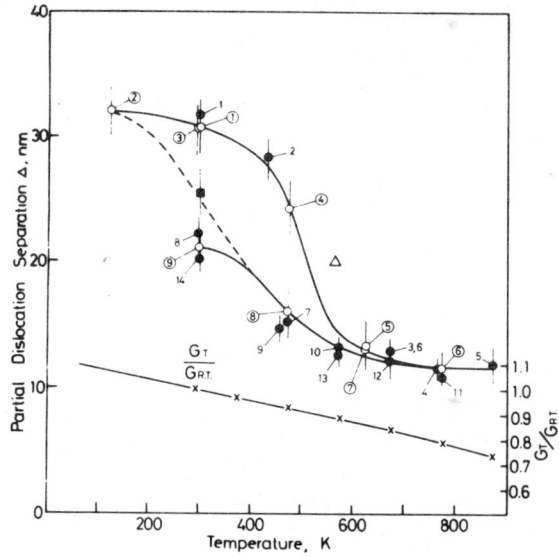

Fig.4 Variation of the width of extended dislocations with temperature during two series of in situ thermal cycling experiments carried out on Cu-13.43 at% Al deformed at 77K. Open circles indicate the data obtained in one experiment and closed ones in the other. The numbers refer to the chronological orders.

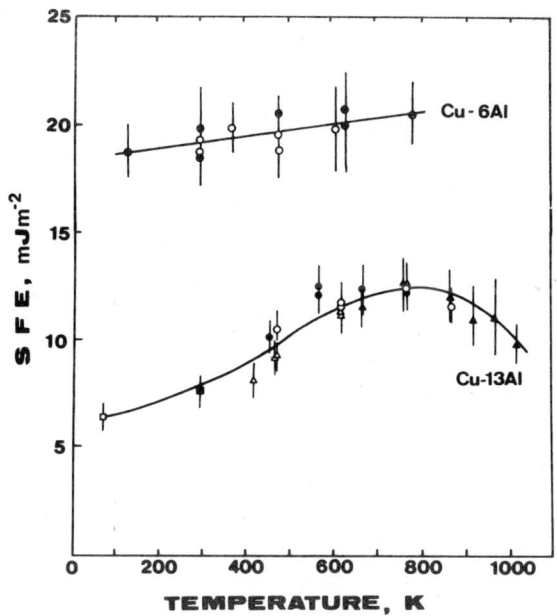

Fig.5 Intrinsic temperature dependence of stacking fault energy in Cu-13.43 at% Al and Cu-6.44 at% Al alloys.

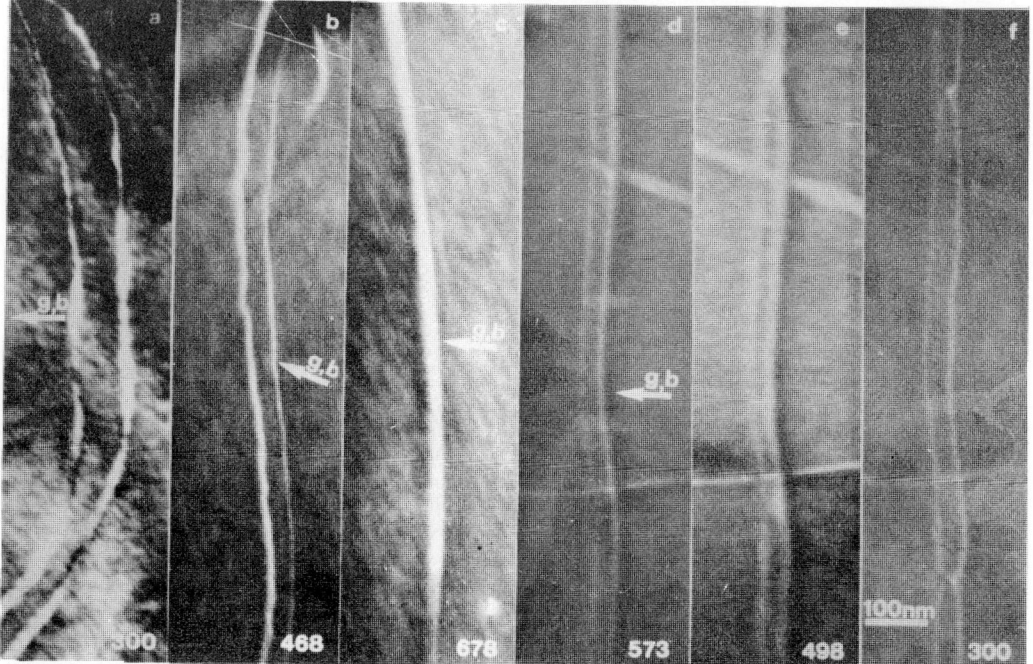

Fig.6 A typical example of the sequence of dissociation of dislocations during a thermal cycling experiment on Ag-15.0 at% Al.

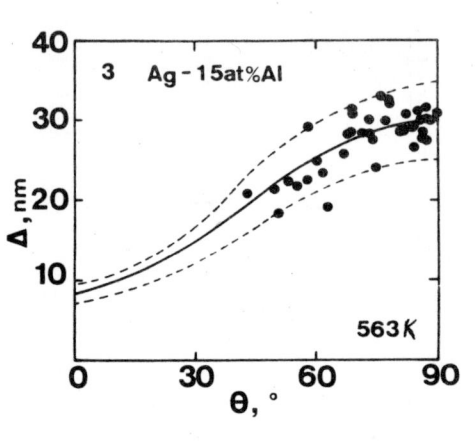

Fig.7 Width Δ of extended dislocations against the orientation of the perfect dislocation in Ag-15 at% Al alloy at 563K.

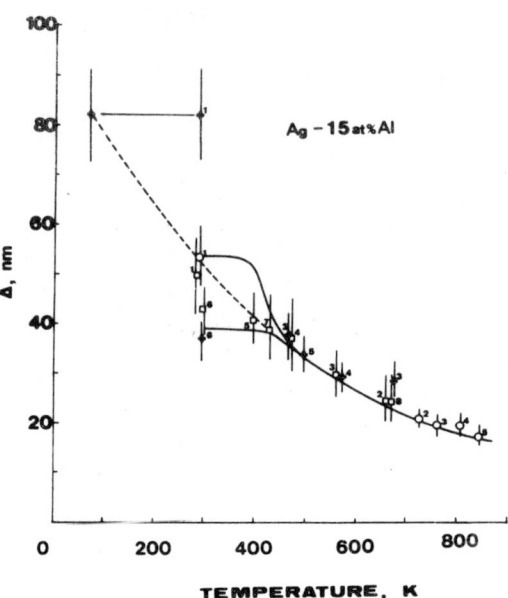

Fig.8 Variation of the width of extended dislocation with temperature carried out on Ag-15 at% Al deformed at 77K and 295K.

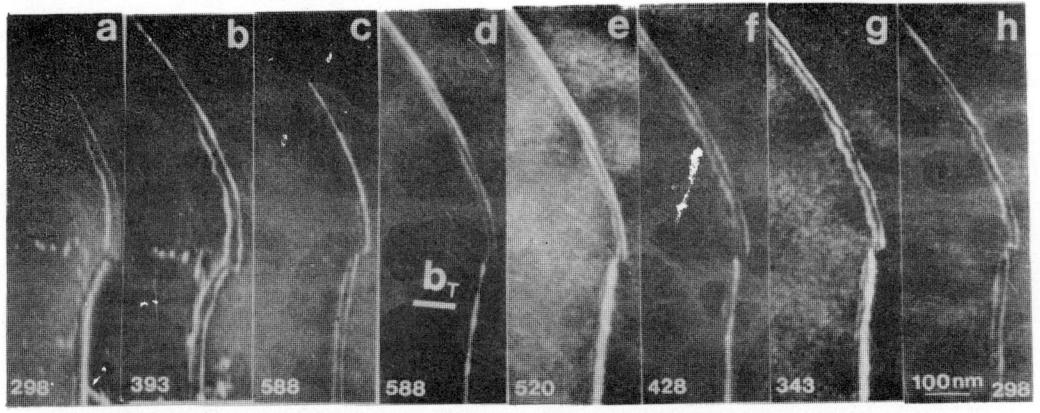

Fig.9 A typical example of the sequence of dissociation of dislocations during a thermal cycling experiment on Ag-9.6 at% Al. The numbers refer to the temperature in K and letters in the upper right corners to the chronological order.

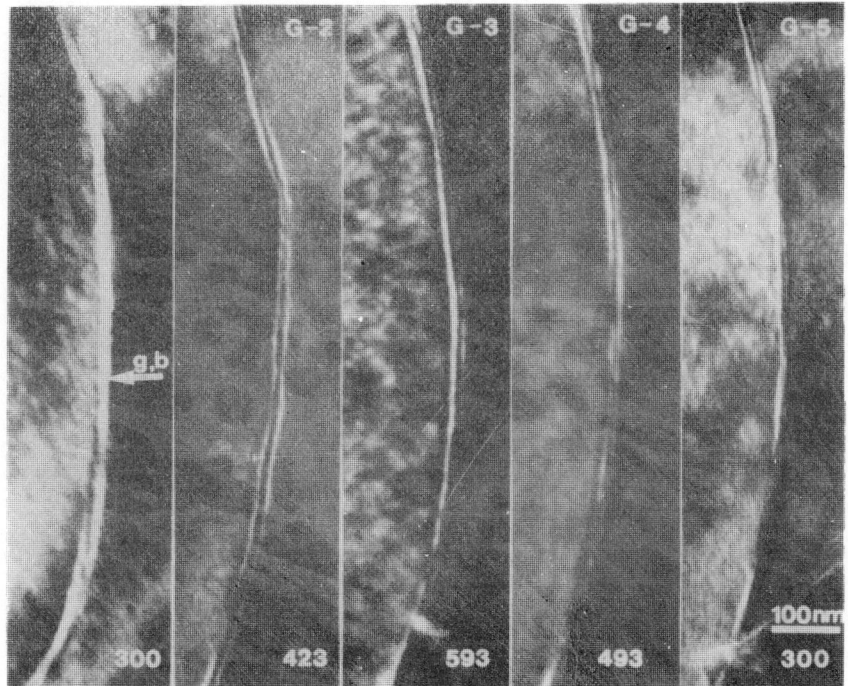

Fig.10 A typical example of the sequence of dissociation of dislocations during a thermal cycling experiment on Ag-5.4 at% Al. The numbers refer to the temperature in K.

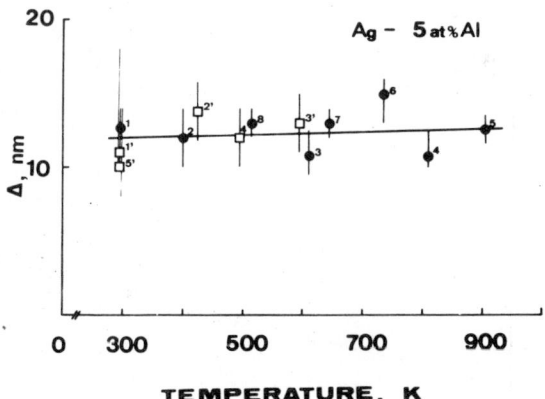

Fig.11 Variation of the width of extended dislocation with temperature during in situ thermal cycling experiments carried out on Ag-5.4 at% Al deformed at 295K.

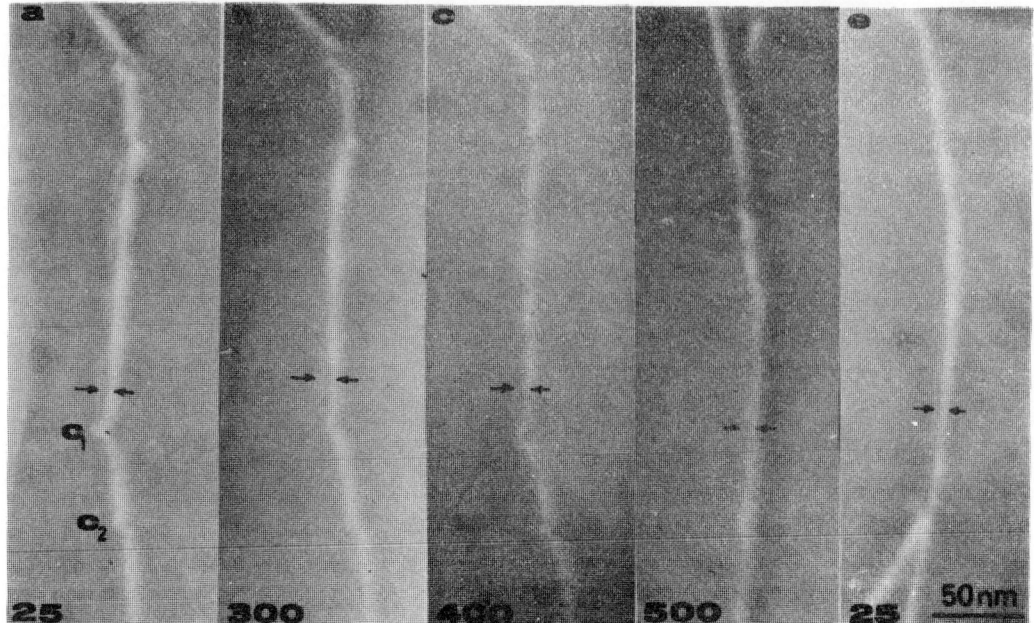

Fig.12 An example of the sequence of the variation of the width of a single dislocation in pure Ag during an in situ thermal cycling experiment.

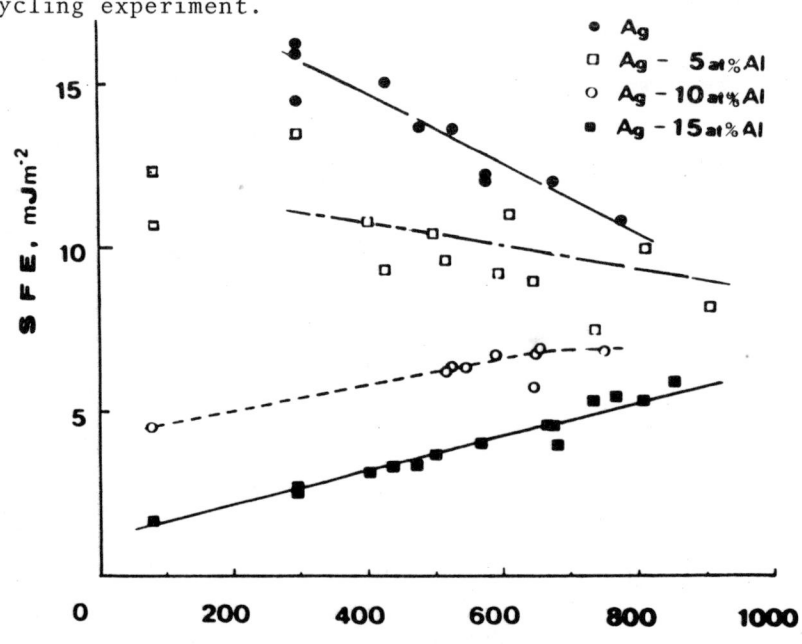

Fig.13 Intrinsic temperature dependence of γ in pure Ag, Ag-5.4 at% Al, Ag-9.6 at% Al and Ag-15.0 at% Al alloys.

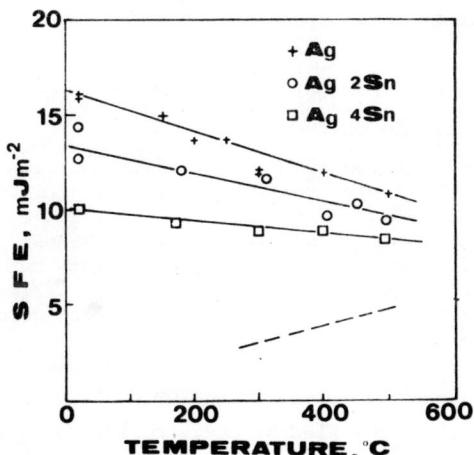

Fig.14 Intrinsic temperature dependence of γ in Ag, Ag-2 at% Sn and Ag-4 at% Sn. The broken line indicates the data by A.W. Ruff et al.[19] on Ag-9 at% Sn.

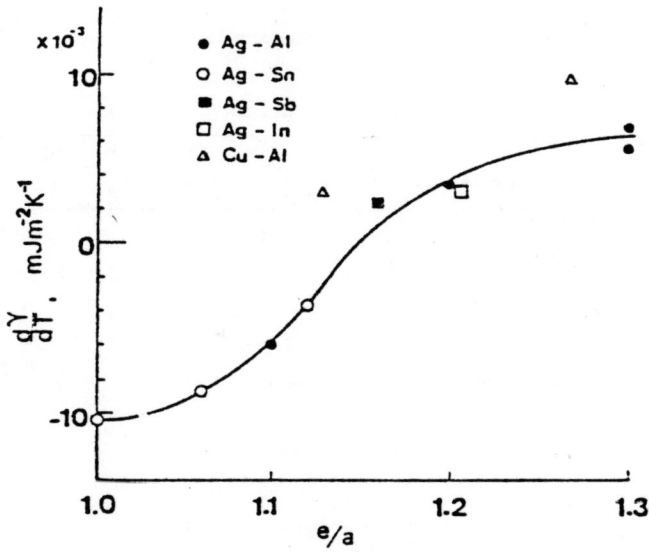

Fig.15 Effects of alloying element on the temperature dependence of γ, $d\gamma/dT$, in Ag, Ag-Al, Ag-Sn, Ag-Sb, Ag-In and Cu-Al. ($d\gamma/dT$ against e/a)

DISLOCATION CORE STRUCTURES IN CLOSE-PACKED-HEXAGONAL METALS

D.J. Bacon

Department of Metallurgy and Materials Science, The University of Liverpool,
P.O. Box 147, Liverpool L69 3BX.

Abstract. Computer simulation of model crystals has been used to investigate dislocation behaviour in h.c.p. metals, and research in this area is reviewed. Several interatomic potentials have now been used, and they suggest that stable stacking faults are possible on several distinct planes. $<11\bar{2}0>\{10\bar{1}0\}$ slip is preferred in the absence of a low-energy basal fault, but it is not clear that dislocations truly dissociate on the prism planes. Dislocations with $\underline{b} = \frac{1}{3}<11\bar{2}3>$ are believed to have a variety of complex core structures.

1. Introduction.

This paper is concerned with dislocation behaviour in the hexagonal-close-packed (h.c.p.) metals as revealed by their core structure. These metals are well-known for their technological importance and wide range of properties, and, despite the fact that they have been studied for many years, there is still much about them that is not understood. Although they share the same crystal structure, they do not have the ideal lattice-parameter ratio for close-packed spheres (c/a = $\sqrt{8/3}$), and their properties do not conform to a simple pattern. This is illustrated by the summary of preferred glide planes and loop-habit planes in Table 1, taken largely from the review of Jones and Hutchinson /1/,

Table 1. Data for c/a ratio, vacancy formation energy, basal stacking-fault energy, and principal glide and loop habit planes for h.c.p. metals. Basal $\equiv$ (0001), prism $\equiv \{10\bar{1}0\}$.

Metal	c/a (at 298K)	h_f^γ (eV)*	$\gamma(I_1)$ (mJm^{-2})	$\underline{a}$ glide plane	$\underline{c}+\underline{a}$ glide plane	loop habit plane
Be	1.568	-	≥395	basal	$\{11\bar{2}2\}$	prism
Y	1.571	-	-	prism	-	-
Hf	1.581	-	-	prism	-	-
Ru	1.582	-	-	prism	-	-
Ti	1.587	1.55	-	prism	$\{10\bar{1}1\}$	prism
Gd	1.590	-	-	prism	-	basal
Zr	1.593	≥1.23	-	prism	$\{10\bar{1}1\}$	prism
Re	1.615	-	-	basal	-	prism
Mg	1.624	0.58	125	basal	$\{11\bar{2}2\}$	basal
Co	1.628	-	16	basal	$\{11\bar{2}2\}$	prism
Zn	1.856	0.52	300	basal	$\{11\bar{2}2\}$	basal
Cd	1.886	0.41	175	basal	$\{11\bar{2}2\}$	basal

wherein references to the information are given. (Additional data on vacancy formation energy and stacking fault energy are also included.) The principal slip vector in all cases is the shortest lattice vector $\underline{a} = \frac{1}{3}<11\bar{2}0>$, and the preferred slip planes for dislocations with this Burgers vector are either the basal (0001) or first-order prism $\{10\bar{1}0\}$ planes. It should be noted that the 'basal-slip' metals can also exhibit prism slip, and vice-versa, but the critical resolved shear stress at room temperature is lowest for the plane indicated. Dislocations with Burgers vector $\underline{c}+\underline{a} = \frac{1}{3}<11\bar{2}3>$ compete with twinning in contributing to strain perpendicular to (0001), but the resolved shear stress required for slip is high. The preferred glide plane for these dislocations is of either the first-order pyramidal $\{10\bar{1}1\}$ or second-order pyramidal $\{11\bar{2}2\}$ type, as indicated. It is clear that analysis of dislocation behaviour in the h.c.p. metals is complicated by the fact that glide is not restricted to one system.

There is no clear explanation of why these metals behave as they do. Even a cursory glance at Table 1 indicates that lattice geometry is not the sole factor in determining dislocation structure, and that features of the interatomic forces, as yet unidentified, are of importance in many cases. The understanding of these effects requires a combination of experimental and theoretical study. The former involves, for example, detailed analysis of dislocation core structure and loop geometry using transmission electron microscopy. The latter requires development of interatomic potentials and their application in simulation by computer of dislocated model crystals. The technique of computer simulation has proved particularly fruitful in the study of cubic metals, and has probably been less widely applied to the h.c.p. case because of a lack of reliable potentials. There has been some progress in this area in recent years, and the purpose of the present paper is to summarize some of the results obtained. It revises an earlier discussion /2/ for which structures obtained with only one interatomic potential were known.

The potentials used to date for defect simulation in model h.c.p. crystals are reviewed in section 2. It is possible that the preference of dislocation glide and loop nucleation for certain planes is associated with the presence of stable stacking faults on those planes. Since direct experimental evidence for stacking faults is sparse, computer simulation can play an important role in establishing their structure and energy /3,4/, as discussed in section 3. Dislocations with $\underline{a}$ and $\underline{c}+\underline{a}$ Burgers vectors have now been simulated, and results for core structures in unstressed and stressed crystals are described in sections 4 and 5. Concluding remarks are made in section 6.

2. Interatomic Potentials.

Interatomic potentials $V(r)$ used for defect simulations should define a crystal that is stable under small to moderate homogeneous strain and has physical properties matching those of real crystals. The first condition is necessary, whereas the second is merely desirable and usually difficult to achieve. The potentials derived either from first-principles or by fitting to empirical data generally have limitations /5/, and in most cases it is not possible to completely match the properties of importance for defect modelling. Very few potentials have been reported for the hexagonal metals (see for example /6/), and many that have are limited in applicability. For example, the empirical potential for Mg of Doneghan and Heald /7/ produces lattice instability /8/; the empirical potentials for Mg, Ti and Co of Tomé et al. /9/, Johnson and Beeler /10/ and Beeler and Beeler /11/ respectively have short range and give zero energy for basal stacking faults; and the ion-ion pseudo potentials (e.g. /12/) are too long-ranged for dislocation simulation. It has therefore proved necessary to use potentials which simply describe stable h.c.p. structures rather than particular metals. This approach, which has proved so useful in the modelling of b.c.c. crystals /13/, provides a way of determining effects due solely to structure. It means, however, that we are still a long way from investigating in detail the differences between the individual h.c.p. metals referred to in section 1.

Most of the simulations reported to date have used the Lennard-Jones potential:

$$(1) \qquad V(r) = \varepsilon \left[\left(\frac{d}{r}\right)^{12} - 2 \left(\frac{d}{r}\right)^{6} \right].$$

It is shown graphically in Fig.1. It is possible to include in the total crystal energy a volume dependent contribution, representing to a first approximation the energy of the electron gas, and this enables the experimentally-observed Cauchy discrepancy in the elastic constants to be matched ($C_{13} \neq C_{44}$). However, it has been more common to use $V(r)$ alone. The two equilibrium conditions for the structure, namely that the normal stresses in and perpendicular to the basal plane of a perfect crystal be zero /14/, set the values of the lattice parameters a and c for a given potential range. The ratio c/a is not ideal unless the potential is truncated between the first- and second-neighbour shells. The calculated lattice parameters, vacancy formation energy, stacking-fault energy for the I_1 fault (section 3), and the five elastic constants, for the equilibrium crystal designated lj56 with $V(r)$ truncated between the 8th and 9th shells are listed in Table 2. The identification lj refers to Lennard-Jones and 56 is the number of atoms within the eight neighbour shells of another atom. (lj56 was denoted as lj6 in previous work /2,8/.)

Table 2. Some physical properties of crystals defined by the potential functions described in the text. <metals> refers to the mean value for six real metals. (Ω is the volume per atom, k is Boltzmann's constant, and T_m is the melting temperature.)

Crystal (units:)	c/a	h_f^V(relaxed) (ε)	$\gamma(I_1)$ (ε/a^2)	c_{11}	c_{12}	c_{13} (ε/Ω)	c_{33}	c_{44}
lj56	1.631	7.9	0.043	113	47	30	130	30
ti12	1.633	6.8	0	118	45	32	130	32
na56	1.620	7.0	0.110	104	56	30	136	30
bel34	1.616	0.5	0.346	112	41	37	137	37
(units:)		(kT_m)				(kT_m/Ω)		
<metals>	1.592	7.2	–	115	48	39	122	33

Three other potentials have been used by Liang and Bacon /3,4/. One is the short-range function chosen by Johnson and Beeler /10/ to represent titanium. Extending only to the nearest-neighbour shell of twelve atoms, it describes a crystal with ideal c/a. The second potential considered is the oscillatory potential for sodium derived from an orthogonalized plane-wave calculation by Basinski et al. /15/. The third potential is the non-local pseudopotential for beryllium derived by Duesbery and Taylor /16/. In their original forms, these potentials were developed for lattice parameters which were such that the crystals they describe are subjected to stresses. Although such effects can be taken to represent the electron gas if isotropic, they are of an uncertain origin and affect the simulation of defects. Thus, to be consistent with the lj potential, the potential functions have been used here in their equilibrium form, i.e. the model crystal has been taken to be in equilibrium under $\dot{V}(r)$ alone. Accordingly, the lattice parameters and potential range have been found which satisfy the criteria that (a) the perfect crystal is stress-free, (b) h_f^V and $\gamma(I_1)$ are ≥ 0, and (c) the perfect crystal is stable under homogenous strain. To meet these conditions, the sodium and beryllium potentials have to extend to eight and sixteen shells containing 56 and 134 neighbours respectively. In an obvious notation, the three functions are designated here as ti12, na56 and bel24. The potentials are shown in fig. 2 and properties they produce are listed in Table 2. The energies are measured in units of parameter ε, adjusted so that the elastic constants are close to those of lj56.

For comparison with real metals, the row labelled <metals> in Table 2 lists the mean values of the physical properties of six real metals, namely Y, Hf, Ti, Zr, Sc, Mg. It is seen that, as explained in /8/, a choice of $\varepsilon \approx 1kT_m$ produces model values not too dissimilar from real ones. A fifth equilibrium potential, referred to here as lj50, is the Lennard-Jones function truncated after 7 neighbour shells of 50 atoms. The elastic constants and vacancy formation energy are similar to those for lj56, but the basal fault energy is higher ($\gamma(I_1) = 0.165\varepsilon/a^2$) /8/. Finally, it should be emphasized that, despite the ti, na and be notation, the potentials are not considered to represent real metals. They simply describe model crystals which turn out to have rather similar c/a ratios and elastic constants, despite their markedly different forms.

3. Stacking Faults.

Basal-plane stacking faults are known to occur in some h.c.p. metals, but there is sparse evidence that faults occur on other planes. There has been, however, considerable speculation over the years about their possible existence, particularly in relation to dislocation motion on non-basal planes. The basal faults are easy to characterize in terms of hard-sphere packing. They are the intrinsic faults I_1 (with stacking sequence ...ABABCBCB...) and I_2 (...ABABCACA), and the extrinsic fault E(...ABABCABA...). On the basis of violation of the second-neighbour layer order, the ratio of energies $\gamma(E):\gamma(I_2):\gamma(I_1)$ should be 3:2:1. The I_2 fault is the most important as far as crystal plasticity is concerned, for the perfect dislocation can dissociate according to the reaction

$$(2) \qquad \tfrac{1}{3}<11\bar{2}0> \to \tfrac{1}{3}<10\bar{1}0> + \tfrac{1}{3}<01\bar{1}0>$$

into a ribbon of I_2 fault on the (0001) plane.

The preference for a-direction prism slip in some metals has led to suggestions that dissociation may occur on the $\{10\bar{1}0\}$ planes. One possibility inferred from the relative translation of hard spheres is /17,18/

$$(3) \qquad \tfrac{1}{3}<\bar{1}2\bar{1}0> \to \tfrac{1}{18}<\bar{2}6\bar{4}3> + \tfrac{1}{18}<\bar{4}6\bar{2}\bar{3}>.$$

Another reaction is

$$(4) \qquad \tfrac{1}{3}<\bar{1}2\bar{1}0> \to \tfrac{1}{9}<\bar{1}2\bar{1}0> + \tfrac{2}{9}<\bar{1}2\bar{1}0>,$$

and has been suggested /19/ on the grounds that the a/3 translation fault produces a thin layer of b.c.c. crystal, which is the high-temperature phase of some metals. On the basis of a hard-sphere model /1/, dislocations with $\underline{b} = \underline{c}+\underline{a}$ may dissociate on $\{10\bar{1}1\}$ planes by the reaction

$$(5) \qquad \tfrac{1}{3}<\bar{1}\bar{1}23> \to \tfrac{1}{9}<\bar{1}013> + \tfrac{1}{18}<\bar{2}6\bar{4}3> + \tfrac{1}{6}<\bar{2}023>$$

More general, non-planar dissociations on various pyramidal planes were discussed by Mendelson /20,21/.

The γ surfaces for translation faults on the (0001), $\{10\bar{1}0\}$, $\{10\bar{1}1\}$ and

$\{11\bar{2}2\}$ planes have been obtained /3,4/ for the four model potentials by computing γ for a grid of rigid translations lying in the fault plane. Fig. 3 shows these surfaces for planes in the crystals indicated. The γ surface for a particular plane has the same general form for all four crystals, but the height of the maxima and the existence of local minima corresponding to possible stable faults are potential-dependent. The position of the translations which define local minima are indicated by F in Fig.3. To identify these states as true stable faults, crystals containing up to 40 planes were faulted with translation vectors close to those shown, and the crystal energy was then minimised by relaxing the atom coordinates in one dimension. The energy of such faults is given in Table 3, together with the approximate translation, which is also potential-dependent, and the expansion at the fault plane. The basal faults I_1 and E were produced by multiple translations, and data for them is also included in the table.

It is possible for stable faults to exist on all the planes considered. The basal-fault energies scale approximately in the ratio 3:2:1, as expected, the ratio being exact for the potentials of short range. The small dilations for these faults also scale in roughly the same way, with the largest energies and expansions occurring in the bel34 crystal. Prism-plane faults were only detected for the simplest, hard-sphere type potentials. (A previous conclusion /2/ that a fault does not exist for lj56 is in error.) On the $\{10\bar{1}1\}$ planes, two stable faults occur in all crystals and three crystals have a fault on $\{11\bar{2}2\}$. The γ values for these faults in bel34 are comparable with those for the (0001) faults, but in the other crystals they are considerably higher and similar to each other. The volume expansions are uniformly high for the non-basal faults. The translation vectors lie in the fault plane, and for the non-basal faults with large dilations, they should be added to a small component normal to the plane in order to obtain the complete fault vector. If this is done, they approximate to the vectors anticipated from a hard-sphere model and the magnitudes of the expansions are roughly in the order expected from such a model.

Minonishi et al. /22-25/ reported the existence of stacking faults on $\{10\bar{1}1\}$ and $\{11\bar{2}2\}$ planes in model crystals with the lj56 potential. On translating by $\frac{1}{6}<11\bar{2}3>$ and relaxing, they found a stacking-fault energy of approximately $1.31\epsilon/a^2$ on both planes. Inspection of Fig.3(c) and Table 3 suggests that their crystal may have relaxed to the type II fault for the $\{10\bar{1}1\}$ case, but, as noted above, we were unable to detect a stable fault on $\{11\bar{2}2\}$ with lj56.

4. Dislocation Cores in Unstressed Crystals.

The dislocations simulated by Bacon et al. /2-4,8,26/ and Minonishi et al. /22-25/ are infinite straight lines with Burgers vector $\underline{b}$ equal to either $\underline{a}$ =

Table 3. Fault vector, stacking-fault energy and expansion at fault plane (as percentage of interplanar spacing) for translation faults in the four model crystals. *denotes no stable fault found.

Fault Plane	Translation Vector	Potential	Relaxed γ (ε/a^2)	Expansion %
$(0001)I_1$	multiple	ti12	0	0
		lj56	0.04	0.1
		na56	0.11	0.8
		bel34	0.35	1.4
$(0001)I_2$	$\frac{1}{3}<10\bar{1}0>$	ti12	0	0
		lj56	0.09	0.2
		na56	0.22	1.5
		bel34	0.66	2.0
$(0001)E$	multiple	ti12	0	0
		lj56	0.13	0.3
		na56	0.33	2.3
		bel34	0.99	2.7
$\{10\bar{1}0\}$	$\frac{1}{6}<\bar{1}2\bar{1}1>$	ti12	1.41	11.0
		lj56	1.18	10.6
		na56	*	*
		bel34	*	*
$\{10\bar{1}1\}I$	$\frac{1}{6}<\bar{1}012>$	ti12	1.19	10.8
		lj56	1.00	7.4
		na56	1.05	8.4
		bel34	0.68	10.8
$\{10\bar{1}1\}II$	$\frac{1}{12}<\bar{1}\bar{4}56>$	ti12	1.34	11.2
		lj56	1.31	13.4
		na56	1.75	14.4
		bel34	0.63	16.2
$\{11\bar{2}2\}$	$\frac{1}{9}<\bar{1}\bar{1}23>$	ti12	1.59	14.0
		lj56	*	*
		na56	1.30	8.5
		bel34	0.59	13.2

$\frac{1}{3}<11\bar{2}0>$ or $\underline{c}+\underline{a} = \frac{1}{3}<11\bar{2}3>$. For the former, dislocations along either $[0001]$ ('prism edge'), $<1\bar{1}00>$ ('basal edge') or $<11\bar{2}0>$ ('basal screw') have been modelled. For the latter, $<1\bar{1}00>$ ('edge') and $<11\bar{2}3>$ ('screw') orientations have been considered.

Prism edge. The computed core structure obtained in /8/ for the lj56 crystal is shown in fig.4. The Burgers vector is $\frac{1}{3}[2\bar{1}\bar{1}0]$, which is defined as the x direction, and figs.(a)-(c) show, respectively, (a) the (0001) projection of the atom positions in two adjacent basal planes, (b) the displacement difference ('disregistry') along the slip plane, i.e. Δu_x as a function of x, for the atom pairs linked by arrows in (a), and (c) the Burgers vector distribution $\rho_x = d(\Delta u_x)/dx$ in the slip plane. The unrelaxed starting configuration obtained using the displacements of linear elasticity theory is shown by the 'unrelaxed' curve in (b) and (c). The core obtained by atomic simulation is considerably wider than in the elastic solution, the width at half-peak height on the ρ curve more than doubling during relaxation. Despite this effect, which depends to a certain extent on the shape of the $\{10\bar{1}0\}$ γ surface /13/, the dislocation does not dissociate into two partials corresponding to reactions (3) and (4). The fault identified in section 3 could lead to reaction (3), but the partial spacing predicted from elasticity theory is only 1.9a, and simulations starting with the dissociated state relaxed to the form shown in fig.4.

The distribution of $\underline{b}$ along the slip plane for the prism edge in all four crystals is shown in fig.5. The cores in the na56 and til2 crystals are very similar in form to that in the lj56 model. Dissociation into a stable fault is again possible in the til2 case, but the partial spacing predicted is only 1.7a and the form shown has the lowest energy. The curve for bel34 has an unusual form because the disregistry is concentrated into a region approximately a wide. This is achieved by the dislocation forming a microcrack just below the extra half plane, as shown by the projection of atom positions in fig.6. Inspection of Table 2 shows that the vacancy formation energy is anomalously low for the bel34 potential - in fact, the energy is negative for truncation inside the 11th shell - and this possibly permits the crack to form and reduce strain energy.

Basal edge. This dislocation can dissociate into two Shockley partials as in reaction (2) because of the stable I_2 fault. The partial spacings predicted from elasticity theory are ∞, 27a, 9.5a and 3.2a for the potentials til2, lj56, na56 and bel34 respectively. Accordingly, only the latter two have been used and for both the core dissociates. The structure is similar to that found by Bacon and Martin /8/ using the lj50 potential. The relaxed core with minimum energy has a partial spacing of approximately 10a for na56 and 3a for bel34, so that, as in the case of lj50 where the predicted and observed spacings are 7a and 7.5a respectively, elasticity theory gives a good estimate of the spacing. The partial cores are wide, however, and a ribbon of true I_2 stacking fault exists only at the centre of the dissociated region in the na56 model.

Basal screw. Despite the nomenclature, this dislocation can glide on both the basal and prism planes. On the basis of elasticity, dissociation on (0001) should give Shockley partial spacings of ∞, 3.5a, 10a, 3a and 1.6 for til2, 1j50, 1j56, na56 and be134 respectively. The first case can be neglected, and the second and third produce a dissociation with a partial spacing close to the elastic estimate /8/. A similar agreement is found for the na56 crystal. The $(2\bar{1}\bar{1}0)$ projection of the relaxed structure in the 1j50 crystal is shown in fig.7(a). Here, the length of the arrows reveals the difference in $[2\bar{1}\bar{1}0]$ displacement between pairs of atoms. The Burgers vector distribution along the basal glide plane for both the screw (ρ_z) and edge (ρ_x) components are shown in fig.7(b). As in the basal-edge model, the partial cores are wide and a true I_2 stacking sequence is not obtained.

The screw dislocation can, in principle, dissociate on the prism plane, but γ is high (Table 3) and there is no tendency to do so with the 1j and na potentials. In fact, the relaxed core width along the prism plane is less than that given by the elastic displacement solution. In the be134 crystal, however, two stable core states have been found /3,4/. Their structure is demonstrated by the differential displacement maps projected on a plane perpendicular to the dislocation line in fig.8. In one (fig.8(a)) the disregistry is concentrated on the prism plane, whereas in the other (fig.8(b)) the core spreads on the basal plane. Both cores exhibit components of edge character in the basal plane. One or the other is obtained by varying the origin of the elastic displacement field used to generate the unrelaxed core.

c+a edge. Slip on the $<\bar{1}\bar{1}23>$ $\{11\bar{2}2\}$ system has been observed in a number of metals, and the core structure of the edge dislocation was first simulated by Minonishi et al. /22/. In a model crystal of the 1j56 potential, they found a distinctive configuration in which the basal planes are bent differently on each side of the core. The structure, reproduced by Liang /3/, is shown in fig.9(a). Minonishi et. al. interpreted this core as being equivalent to two microtwins. On the left of the core centre, the basal planes are reorientated and shifted parallel to the line to positions appropriate to a $\{11\bar{2}1\}$ twin. The twin is approximately 2b wide and seven planes thick, as shown by the outline in fig.9(a). On the right-hand side, the atoms in the area outlined represent a small $\{11\bar{2}2\}$ twin, for the two atoms in the middle of this region undergo a relative displacement parallel to the line which interchanges their symbols.

In a subsequent paper, Minonishi et al. /24/ established the existence of a second core configuration, consisting of two $\frac{1}{2}$(c+a) partials separated by a stacking fault. The occurrence of the two possible core structures was found to depend on the choice of initial, unrelaxed displacements. According to Table 3, the lj56 crystal does not have a stable fault on the $\{11\bar{2}2\}$ plane, so that the structure observed in /24/ may result from the creation of fractional dislocations. The $c+a$ dislocation should dissociate in the til2, na56 and bel34 crystal crystals, however. The Burgers vectors of the partials are predicted to be approximately $\frac{1}{3}(c+a)$ and $\frac{2}{3}(c+a)$, and the spacing should be 2.7b, 3.2b and 8.8b respectively. Relaxed structures approximating to those predicted are produced in simulations which start from a dissociated state /3,4/, as shown by the projection for na56 in fig.9(b). A stable, undissociated core is sometimes found in relaxations which start with the undissociated form, however. The result that the core has two possible states stabilized by either a $\{11\bar{2}2\}$ fault or $\{11\bar{2}1\}$ and $\{11\bar{2}2\}$ twins therefore appears to be general.

$c+a$ screw. This dislocation was also first modelled by Minonishi et al./23/ using the lj56 potential. Unlike the edge dislocation, twinned arrangements of atoms were not observed. Instead, a variety of stable, dissociated cores were found, the form of the relaxed core being dependent on the starting structure. In all cases, the displacement disregistry was concentrated over the $\{10\bar{1}1\}$ and/or $\{11\bar{2}2\}$ planes of the $<11\bar{2}3>$ zone. Minonishi et al. /23/ accounted for these effects by the existence of $\frac{1}{2}(c+a)$ translation faults with approximately the same energy on the $\{10\bar{1}1\}$ and $\{11\bar{2}2\}$ planes. As explained in section 3, the stable faults in an lj56 crystal may not have precisely this form, and the dissociation may therefore be to fractional dislocations. A similar variety of stable cores consisting of combinations of these elementary dissociations are found in other crystals, and in some cases fractional dislocations are also created on the $\{10\bar{1}0\}$ planes /3,4/. Three of the stable structures in the na56 crystal are shown in the projections of fig.10, where the arrows map the $c+a$ differential displacements. It is probable, therefore, that this complex geometry is a general phenomenon.

5. Dislocation Behaviour Under Stress.

The effect of applied shear stress on all the dislocations described in the preceding section has been simulated with the aim of investigating the crystallographic factors controlling plasticity. A comprehensive description of this work is to be presented elsewhere /4/, and only a summary of some aspects is given here.

Basal slip. As the applied shear strain is increased towards the critical value at which glide occurs, the distribution ρ of Burgers vector changes to reduce the partial spacing /26,3,4/. The edge dislocation glides at a lower stress than the screw in the same crystal, as might be expected for a wider core.

The critical shear strain for the basal screw is considerably lower (∼0.003) for na56 and be134 than in the 1j50 and 1j56 crystals (∼0.011-0.015), however, so the effect of an increase in $\gamma(I_2)$ is not as expected. There are other features of the interatomic potential that control the critical value.

Prism slip. In studies of glide of the prism edge in the 1j50 and 1j56 crystals and variants of them /2,26/, the critical shear strain was found to range from 0.007 to 0.029. The smaller values correspond to potentials for which the negative slope at the nearest-neighbour distance is largest. In recent work using the ti12 and na56 potentials /3,4/, the critical strain has been found to be approximately 0.02 and 0.003 respectively, suggesting again that the slope at $r \simeq a$ may be important. The cracked core in the be134 crystal (fig.6) does not glide; instead, the crack extends in a <11$\bar{2}$0> direction at 60° to the Burgers vector.

The <11$\bar{2}$0> screw dislocation can also glide on the prism plane, but, when dissociated on the basal plane, must first constrict. In the 1j50 and 1j56 crystals, this occurs with an asymmetry in which a contriction forms at the site of one partial: for example, the screw in fig.7 glides upwards on the plane shown by the dashed trace /26/. A similar effect is seen in the na56 crystal. For the two core states found with the be134 potential, the one shown in fig.8(b) adopts the form of fig.8(a) before gliding. The critical strain for 1j50, 1j56 and na56 is 0.05, 0.09 and 0.05, respectively, and is much higher than that for basal slip. In be134, on the other hand, it is only 0.002 and is lower. This probably reflects the low maximum on the γ surface for $\{10\bar{1}0\}$ in this crystal /3,4/.

c+a dislocations. The behaviour of these dislocations under a stress is more complicated. In the 1j56 crystal, changes in the two edge cores discussed above depend on the sense of the stress /24/. When it has a component producing tension along $[0001]$, i.e. the top surface is moved to the left in fig.9, the $\{11\bar{2}1\}$ twin on the left of the undissociated core in fig.9(a) extends along $(11\bar{2}1)$ and is fully developed at an applied shear strain of 0.075. The dissociated core, on the other hand, glides without significant change when the strain is increased to 0.025. Under a reverse stress, the undissociated core transforms to the dissociated state at a shear strain of 0.013, and this in turn glides freely when the strain reaches 0.025. The screw dislocation in the 1j56 crystal also behaves in a manner dependent on the sense of the stress, but without the complication of twinning /25/. Minonishi et al. find that, irrespective of which of the dissociated cores is used in the stress-free crystal, the application of a resolved shear stress producing compression along $[0001]$ results in glide on $\{11\bar{2}2\}$ (to the right in fig.10). Even when the stress-free core is spread mainly on a $\{10\bar{1}1\}$ plane and the maximum shear stress is on this plane, the core structure changes so that glide still occurs on the $\{11\bar{2}2\}$ system. The critical resolved shear strain is 0.025. Under the reverse shear stress, glide occurs on the $\{10\bar{1}1\}$ planes, again irrespective of the initial core state. On this system, the critical strain is 0.02. Under a compressive c-axis stress, therefore, both edge and screw dislocations glide on the $\{11\bar{2}2\}$ plane in a dissociated state, whereas under a tensile stress edge and screw dislocations behave differently.

Minonishi et al. /24,25/ compare their results with experimental observations and note that there are areas of agreement and some of uncertainty. The asymmetry of c+a slip is inherent in the lattice structure, whereas the factors controlling the choice of preferred slip planes in different metals is not understood. Also, the importance of normal stress in determining slip behaviour /1/, and the inter-relation between c+a slip and $\{11\bar{2}1\}$ twinning /24/ require further study. Recent simulations of these dislocations using the other potentials described here reveal similar effects to those found in the lj56 crystal, but there are also some important differences and they will be presented elsewhere /4/.

6. Concluding Remarks.

The results of computer simulations discussed here show that considerable advances have been made in recent years, but fundamental questions concerning the choice of slip plane remain unanswered. To this end, it will probably be necessary to develop many-body potentials which match particular metals. Nevertheless, the equilibrium potentials described here provide an important means of studying the variety of core structures that can now be anticipated to exist in the h.c.p. metals. They show that the cores of c+a dislocations are probably complex. The cores of b=a dislocations on $\{10\bar{1}0\}$ planes are not, however, and the preference for prism slip in some metals probably arises from an absence of a stable, low-energy stacking fault on the basal plane.

The conclusion that stable stacking faults on different crystallographic planes are likely to be commonplace is supported by a recent transmission-electron-microscope study of ruthenium irradiated with ions /27/. By carefully matching experimental images of the small (∼2nm) vacancy loops produced by displacement-cascade collapse to computer-generated ones, faulted loops on both prism and basal planes have been identified. Another experimental investigation has recently shed light on core structure of the prism edge dislocation with b=a in titanium /28/. de Crecy et al. used the technique of high-resolution electron microscopy to produce a lattice image for a foil containing the prism edge dislocation in the orientation of fig.4(a). The cores observed are planar with a width of about 4a. The experimental image was compared with images generated by computer for the three core structures given by (a) dissociation reaction (3), (b) dissociation reaction (4), and (c) the lj56 model potential (fig.4(a)). The partial spacings in (a) and (b) were chosen to match the observed width. The three images and the experimental one are shown in fig.11. The worst agreement is with (b), and de Crecy et al. conclude that (a) provides the best match. This corresponds to reaction (3) with $\gamma \simeq 155$ mJ m^{-2}, which is close to the value 145 mJ m^{-2} deduced from tensile tests /29/ and is approximately $0.47\ \varepsilon/a^2$ with $\varepsilon = kT_m$. This is considerably less than the value for 1j56 (Table 2), and it is probable that an atomistic model with $\gamma = 0.47\ \varepsilon/a^2$ would relax to a wider core than that observed. Also, the prism edge with potential na56, for which a stable fault could not be found, actually has a wider spread than that for 1j56 (fig.5). There are, therefore, many questions to be answered, and further results based on the method of de Crecy et al. are awaited with interest.

Acknowledgement.

The author gratefully acknowledges helpful discussions with, and assistance from, M.H. Liang. Dr. A. Bourret kindly provided the print of fig.11, and the be134 potential values were supplied by Dr. M.S. Duesbery.

References.
- /1/ Jones I.P. and Hutchinson W.B.: Acta Metall. 29 (1981) 951.
- /2/ Bacon D.J. and Liang M.H.: in Interatomic Potentials and Crystalline Defects (ed. J.K. Lee), AIME, New York 1981, 181.
- /3/ Liang M.H.: Ph.D. Thesis, University of Liverpool (to be submitted).
- /4/ Bacon D.J. and Liang M.H.: to be submitted for publication.
- /5/ deHosson J.Th.M.: in Interatomic Potentials and Crystalline Defects (ed. J.K. Lee), AIME, New York 1981, 3.
- /6/ Stoneham A.M. and Taylor R.: Handbook of Interatomic Potentials II Metals, AERE-R10205, Harwell 1981.
- /7/ Doneghan M. and Heald P.T.: Phys.Stat.Sol. (a) 30 (1975) 403.
- /8/ Bacon D.J. and Martin J.W.: Phil.Mag. A 43 (1981) 883.
- /9/ Tomé C.N., Monti A.M. and Savino E.J.: Phys.Stat.Sol. (b) 92 (1979) 323.
- /10/ Johnson R.A. and Beeler J.R.: in Interatomic Potentials and Crystalline Defects (ed. J.K. Lee), AIME, New York 1981, 165.
- /11/ Beeler J.R. and Beeler M.F.: in Interatomic Potentials and Crystalline Defects (ed. J.K. Lee), AIME, New York 1981, 141.
- /12/ Appapillai M. and Heine V.: Tech.Rep. No. 5 SST/7/1972, Cambridge Univ. 1972.
- /13/ Vitek V.: in Crystal Lattice Defects, 5 (1974) 1.
- /14/ Born M. and Huang K.: The Dynamical Theory of Crystal Lattices, Clarendon Press, Oxford 1954.
- /15/ Basinski Z.S., Duesbery M.S., Pogany A.P., Taylor R. and Varshni Y.P.: Canad.J.Phys. 48 (1970) 1480.
- /16/ Duesbery M.S. and Taylor R.: J.Phys.F: Met.Phys. 9 (1979) L19.

/17/ Churchman A.T.: Proc.Roy.Soc. Lond.A 226 (1954) 216.
/18/ Tyson W.R.: Acta Met. 15 (1967) 574.
/19/ Regnier P. and Dupouy J.M.: Phys.Stat.Sol. 28 (1968) K55.
/20/ Mendelson S.: in Strength of Metals and Alloys, Jap. Inst. Metals 9 (1968) 812.
/21/ Mendelson S.: J.Appl.Phys. 41 (1970) 1893.
/22/ Minonishi Y., Ishioka S., Koiwa M., Morozumi S. and Yamaguchi M.: Phil.Mag. A 43 (1981) 1017.
/23/ Minonishi Y., Ishioka S., Koiwa M., Morozumi S. and Yamaguchi M.: Phil.Mag. A 44 (1981) 1225.
/24/ Minonishi Y., Ishioka S., Koiwa M., Morozumi S, and Yamaguchi M.: Phil.Mag. A 45 (1982) 835.
/25/ Minonishi Y., Ishioka S., Koiwa M., Morozumi S.: Phil.Mag. A 46 (1982) 761.
/26/ Bacon D.J. and Martin J.W.: Phil.Mag. A 43 (1981) 901.
/27/ Phythian W.P.: University of Liverpool (unpublished work).
/28/ de Crecy A., Bourret A., Naka S. and Lasalmonie A.: Phil.Mag. A 47 (1983) 245.
/29/ Akhtar A. and Teghtsoonian A.: Met.Trans. A 6 (1975) 2201.

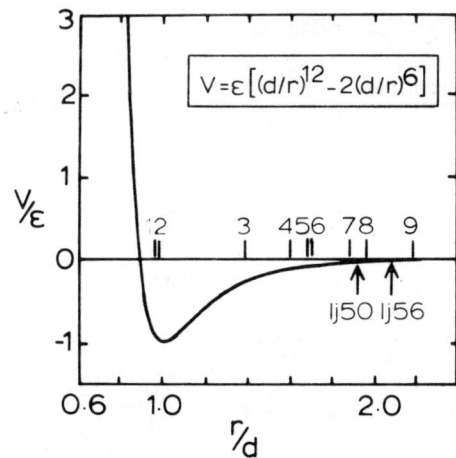

Fig. 1. The Lennard-Jones potential showing the approximate positions of the first nine neighbour shells in a perfect h.c.p. crystal in equilibrium. The ranges of the potentials lj50 and lj56 are indicated.

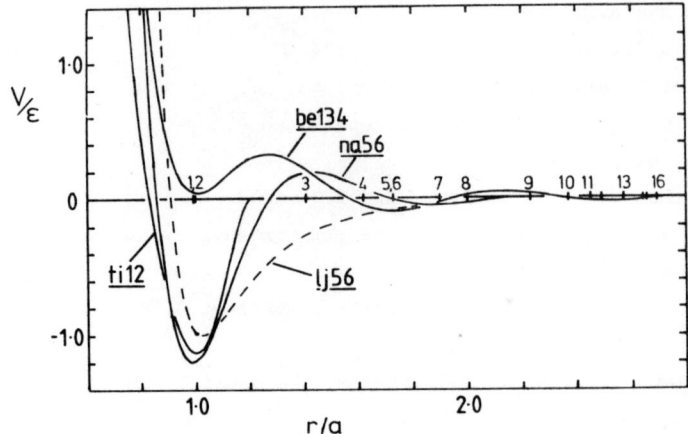

Fig. 2. The potentials described in the text showing the approximate positions of the first sixteen neighbour shells in an equilibrium h.c.p. crystal.

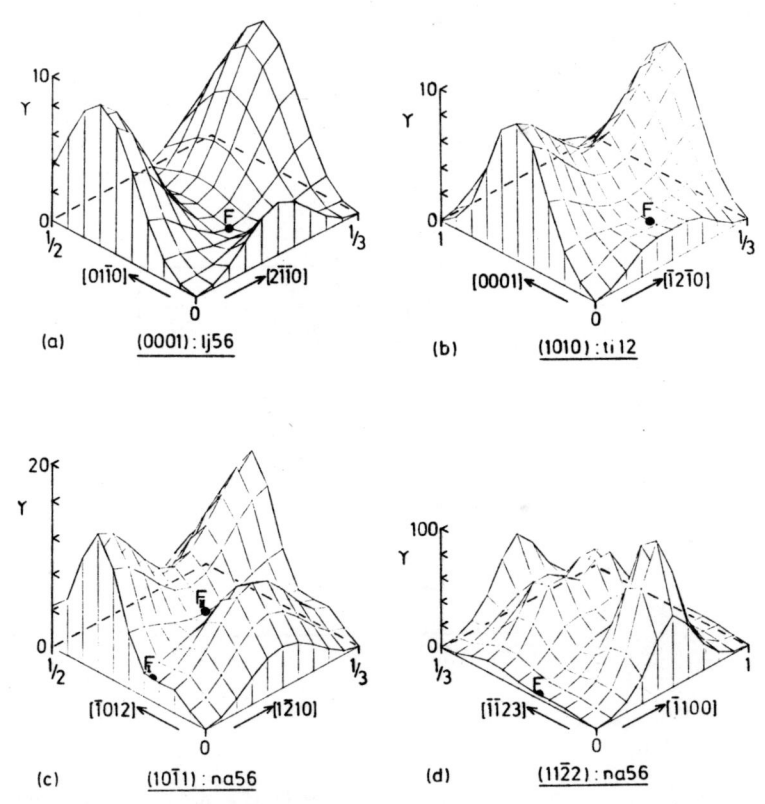

Fig. 3. Unrelaxed γ surfaces (units: ε/a^2) for the planes and potentials indicated.

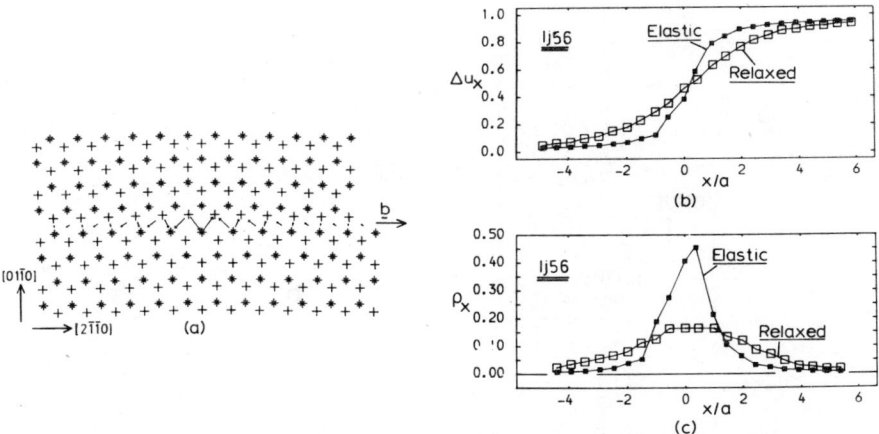

Fig. 4. The prism edge dislocation in the lj56 crystal /8/. (a) Atom projection on (0001), (b) and (c) relative $[2\bar{1}\bar{1}0]$ displacement and Burgers vector distribution along the slip plane (01$\bar{1}$0).

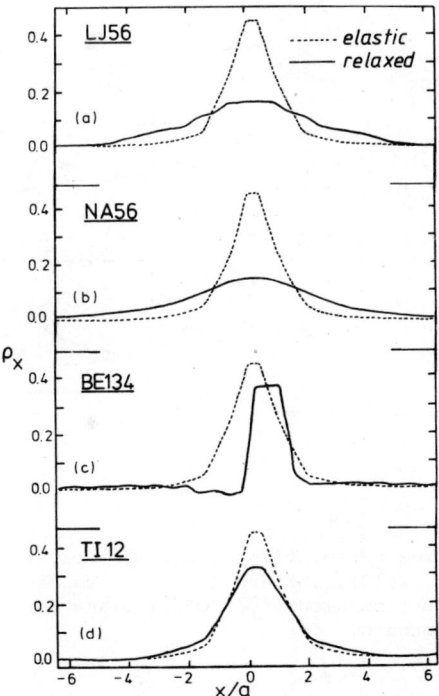

Fig. 5. Distribution of Burgers vector along the slip plane for the prism edge in the four crystals studied.

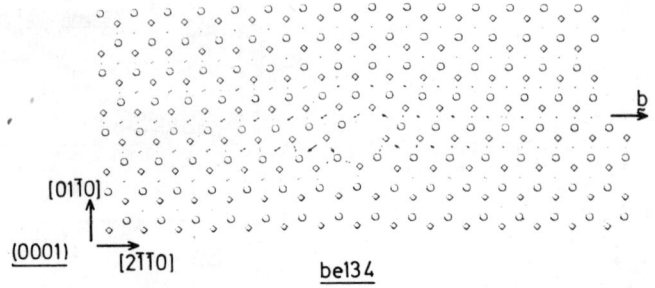

Fig. 6. (0001) projection of atom positions around the prism edge in the be134 crystal.

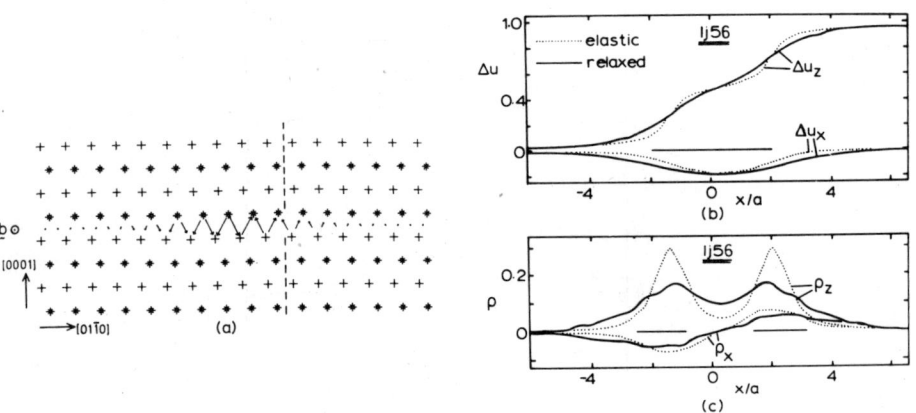

Fig. 7. The $[2\bar{1}\bar{1}0]$ screw dislocation in the 1j56 crystal /8/. (a) Atom projection on $(2\bar{1}\bar{1}0)$, (b) and (c) relative displacement and Burgers vector distribution along the (0001) plane for the screw (z) and edge (x) components.

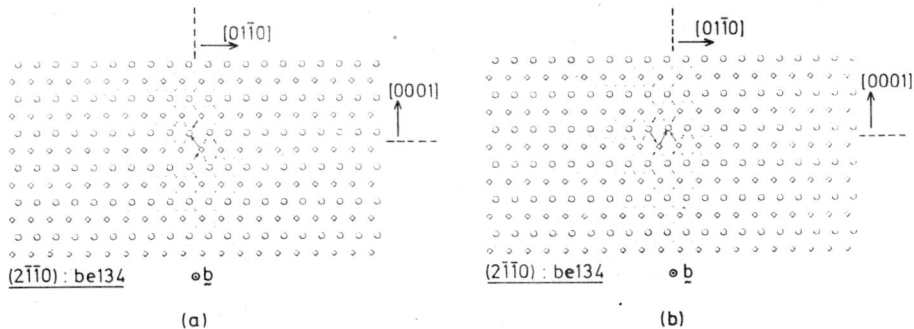

Fig. 8. ($2\bar{1}\bar{1}0$) projection of the two stable configurations for the $[2\bar{1}\bar{1}0]$ screw dislocation in the be134 crystal. The arrows denote the relative $[2\bar{1}\bar{1}0]$ displacement of pairs of atoms.

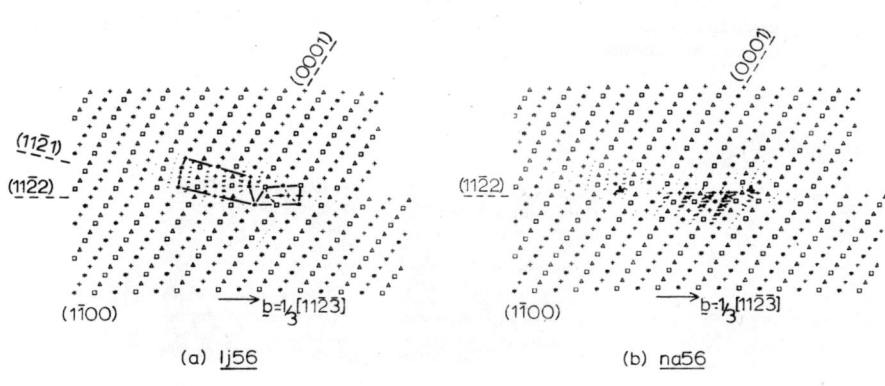

Fig. 9. ($1\bar{1}00$) projection of the two stable configurations for the c+a edge dislocation in (a) the lj56 crystal (after /22/) and (b) the na56 crystals. The arrows show the relative displacements of pairs of atoms in the direction perpendicular to the figure. The approximate positions of the partial cores are indicated in (b).

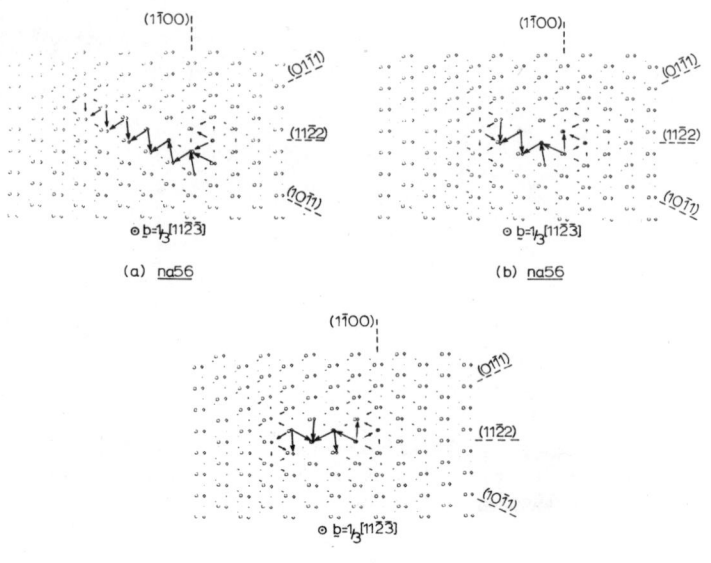

Fig. 10. Projection of atom positions on a plane perpendicular to the $[11\bar{2}\bar{3}]$ screw for three of the stable configurations possible in the na56 crystal. The arrows indicate the relative $[11\bar{2}\bar{3}]$ displacement of pairs of atoms.

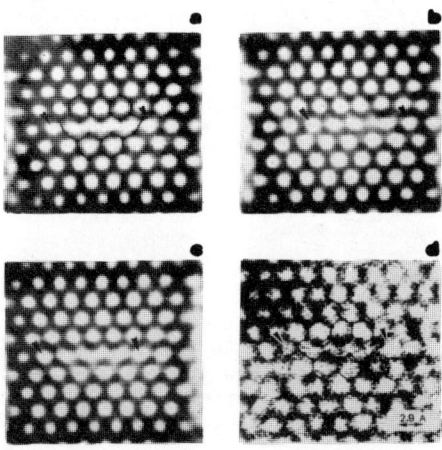

Fig. 11. Comparison of (a), (b), (c) real and (d) experimental images of the prism edge dislocation in titanium. (Courtesy: A. Bourret /28/).

MOTION OF DISLOCATIONS IN HCP METALS

P. Lukáč

Department of Metal Physics, Faculty of Mathematics and Physics, Charles University, Prague 2, Ke Karlovu 5, Czechoslovakia

1. Introduction

It is well known that the work hardening curves of hexagonal single crystals with low melting point (Cd, Zn, Mg) can be divided into three stages. The first stage A characterised by a low work hardening rate is followed by a relatively short stage B with a higher work hardening rate. In contrast to the f.c.c. metals the work hardening rates in both stages of the work hardening curve of hexagonal metals strong depend on temperature /1/. It is difficult to find a satisfying theoretical model explaining the observed strong temperature dependences of the work hardening rates. One can take into account the interaction between basal and forest dislocations /2/. Lavrentev and coworkers /3-5/ have shown that the density of forest dislocations affects significantly parameters of the work hardening curve of zinc and magnesium single crystals. Thus, for example, the length of stage A for zinc and magnesium single crystals deformed by basal slip decreases monotonically as the forest dislocation density in the pyramidal $\{2\bar{1}\bar{1}2\} \langle 2\bar{1}\bar{1}3\rangle$ slip system increases. The length of the stage A also depends on the initial orientation of the single crystal /6/. The work hardening curve parameters are also influenced by the concentration of solute atoms /7/. Fig. 1 shows the temperature dependence of the ratio of the shear stress at the end of stage A τ_A to the critical resolved shear stress τ_o for Cd-Zn alloy single crystals /8/.

Considering the above-mentioned experimental results one can conclude that the interaction between basal and forest dislocation should be considered /6,7/. The purpose of this paper is to point out some problems associated with motion of dislocations.

2. Principles of a work hardening model

In a previous paper /7/ we have suggested a model of work hardening in hexagonal metals with low melting points. According to this model the decrease of work hardening rate in stage A with temperature can be explained under assumption that the cross-slipping dislocation segments are more glissile at higher temperatures. The density of the forest dislocation produced after the cross-slip can increase. On the other hand the recombination segments are formed due to dislocation reactions.

The transition from stage A to stage B is assumed to be determined by the formation of sessile dislocations as obstacles for a gliding basal dislocation. These obstacles arise due to an interation between basal and pyramidal dislocations according to the following dislocation reaction

(a) $\qquad \frac{1}{3}\left[\bar{2}113\right] + \frac{1}{3}\left[2\bar{1}\bar{1}0\right] \longrightarrow \left[0001\right]$

The probability of this reaction is influenced by the micro-slip in the pyramidal slip system. The non basal dislocations will start to move when the stress in the pyramidal slip system reaches the value proportional to the critical resolved shear stress for this slip system. An appropriate stress concentration in the pyramidal slip systems can arise due to a pile-up of basal dislocations /9/. The dislocation velocity is a function of temperature, strain rate, and stress. The mobility of dislocations depends also on the kind of crystallographic plane in shich the dislocation moves /10,11/. It has been reported in a number of papers /11-18/ that the mechanism controlling the mobility of pyramidal dislocations in Zn is the surmounting the Peierls hills.

3. Calculation of the easy of gliding

Besides the dislocation reaction (a) the following dislocation reactions can occur

(b) $\qquad \frac{1}{3}\left[\bar{2}113\right] + \frac{1}{3}\left[11\bar{2}0\right] \longrightarrow \frac{1}{3}\left[\bar{1}2\bar{1}3\right]$

(c) $\quad \frac{1}{3}[\bar{2}113] + \frac{1}{3}[\bar{2}11\bar{3}] \rightarrow \frac{1}{3}[\bar{2}110] + \frac{1}{3}[\bar{2}110]$

These reactions are energetically advantageous. The elastic energy per unit length of a straight dislocation line has been calculated according to equation /19/

(1) $\quad E = \frac{Kb^2}{4\pi} \ln\left(\frac{r}{r_o}\right)$

where r is the radius of dislocation stress field, r_o is the radius of the dislocation core and K is a function of the elastic constants of the crystals and the orientation of both the Burgers vector and the dislocation line with respect to the crystal axes.

Eshelby /20/ defined a parameter

(2) $\quad \zeta/b = \frac{1}{2} KS_{66}' \, d/b$

as a measure of the easy of gliding of a dislocation, where d is the spacing of the crystallographic plane and S_{66}' is the transformed elastic compliance constant. Yoo and Wei /21, 22/ have applied the results obtained from the equations (1) and (2) to a discussion of slip modes of hexagonal metals.

The easy of gliding parameter can be influenced by temperature. The temperature dependence of the parameter $s = \zeta(T)b(T_o)/\zeta(o)b(T)$, where T_o is a reference temperature for edge dislocations in basal (2) and pyramidal (1) slip systems and screw dislocations in prismatic (3) slip system is shown in Fig. 2 and 3 for cadmium and zinc resp.

4. Comparison with experimental results

At the present time the dislocation structure in Mg and Zn single crystals in a wide temperature range during deformation is probably investigated the most fully /23-25/. It has been found that the transition from stage A to stage B of the work hardening curve is characterized by the presence of the forest dislocations in nonbasal slip systems. They are formed in prismatic planes in Mg and in the pyramical slip system in Zn. Motion of the basal dislocation is hindered by the forest dislocations. Therefore the length of stage A should decrease with increasing density of the forest dislocations as observed experimentally. A theoretical analysis of basal-pyramidal dislocation interactions and a calculation of their contribution to work hardening parameters for magnesium crystals has been made by Lavrentev and coworkers /4, 26/.

The motion of dislocations is also impeded by solute atoms. Dislocations in a pyramidal slip system can move if the resolved shear stress is higher than the critical resolved shear stress for this system. The applied stress may be lower than the corresponding critical resolved shear stress because the superdipole stress field has components into the secondary nonbasal slip (pyramidal and prismatic) /9/. The critical resolved shear stress in presence of solute atoms is higher than that for the pure metal. Thus the ratio of τ_A to τ_o should exhibit a similar temperature and concentration dependence as τ_{NB}/τ_o, where τ_{NB} is the critical resolved shear stress for nonbasal slip. Fig. 4 shows the temperature dependence of the ratio of the critical resolved shear stress for prismatic slip to that of basal slip in Mg-Zn single crystals. Data are plotted by the author from results of Akhtar and Teghtsoonian /28/.

The above-considered analysis indicates that the typ of dislocation interaction is a significant factor determining work hardening in hexagonal metals. It should be mentioned that the hardening mechanism at higher temperatures is influenced by recovery process (es). Then the motion of dislocations is a complex problem.

References

/1/ Wielke B.: Phys. Stat. Sol. (a) 33 (1976) 241.
/2/ Lukáč P., Trojanová Z., Svobodová A.: Czech. J. Phys. B 31 (1981) 133.
/3/ Lavrentev F.F., Vladimirova V.L., Gaiduk A.I.: Fiz. Met. Metalloved. 27 (1969) 732.

/4/ Lavrentev F.F., Pokhil Yu.A.: Mater. Sci. Engn. 18 (1975) 261.
/5/ Lavrentev F.F., Pokhil Yu.A.: Phys. Stat. Sol. (a) 32 (1975) 227.
/6/ Boček M., Lukáč P., Švábová M.: Phys. Stat. Sol. 4 (1964) 343.
/7/ Lukáč P.: Czech. J. Phys. B 31 (1981) 135.
/8/ Lukáč P., Rojko M.: Kovové materiály 13 (1975) 235.
/9/ Saxlová-Švábová M.: Metallkde 58 (1967) 266.
/10/ Adams K.M., Vreeland Jr.T., Wood D.S.: Mater. Sci. Engn. 2(1967) 37.
/11/ Adams K.H., Blish R.C., Vreeland Jr. T.: Mater. Sci. Engn. 2(1967) 201.
/12/ Blish R.C., Vreeland Jr.T.: J. Appl. Phys. 40 (1969) 884.
/13/ Lavrentev F.F., Salita O.P.: Fiz. Met. Metalloved. 23 (1967) 548.
/14/ Lavrentev F.F., Salita O.P., Vladimirova V.L.: Phys. Stat. Sol. 29 (1968) 569.
/15/ Soifer Ya.M., Shteinberg V.G.: Phys. Stat. Sol. (a) 6 (1971) 409.
/16/ Soifer Ya.M., Shteinberg V.G.: Phys. Stat. Sol. (a) 10 (1972) K 113.
/17/ Gektina I.V., Lavrentev F.F., Natsik V.D.: Zh. Eksp. Teor. Fiz. 79 (1980) 1927.
/18/ Gektina I.V.: Crystal Res. Technol. 18 (1983) 179.
/19/ Foreman A.J.E.: Acta Metall. 3 (1955) 322.
/20/ Eshelby J.D.: Phil. Mag. 40 (1949) 903.
/21/ Yoo M.H., Wei C.T.: J. Appl. Phys. 38 (1967) 4317.
/22/ Yoo M.H., Wei C.T.: Phil. Mag. 13 (1966) 759.
/23/ Pokhil Yu. A.: Kristall u. Technik 9 (1974) 1179.
/24/ Lavrentev F.F., Pokhil Yu.A., Sokolovsky S.V.: In: Strength of Metals and Alloys, Vol. 1., Pergamon Press, Toronto 1979, p. 163.
/25/ Lavrentev F.F.: In: Fizika deformatsionnogo uprochnenya monokristallov, Naukova Dumka, Kijev 1972, p. 128.
/26/ Lavrentev F.F., Pokhil Yu.A., Zolotukhina I.N.: Mater. Sci. Engn. 23 (1976) 69.
/27/ Lavrentev F.F.: Mater. Sci. Engn. 46 (1980) 191.
/28/ Akhtar A., Teghtsoonian E.: Acta Metall. 17 (1969) 1340 and 1351.

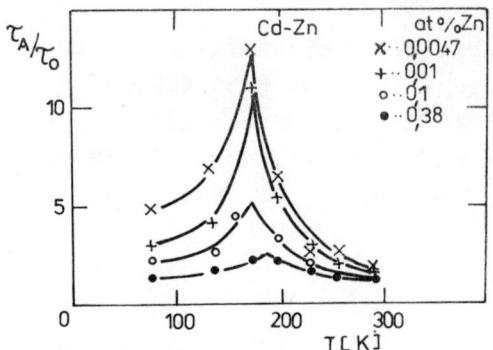

Fig. 1

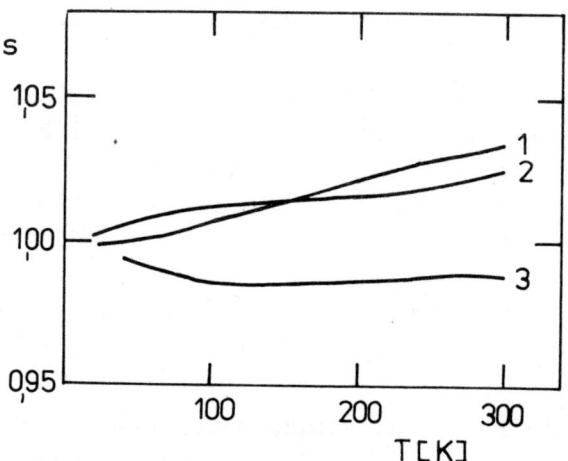

Fig. 2

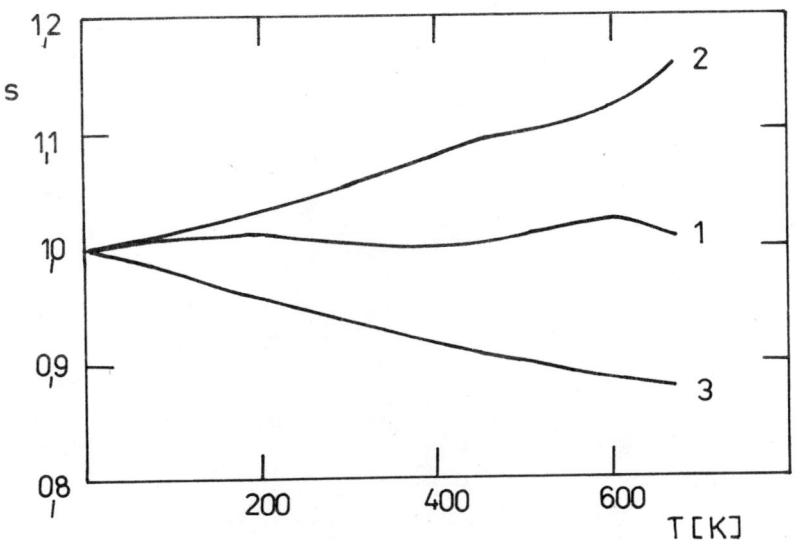

Fig. 3

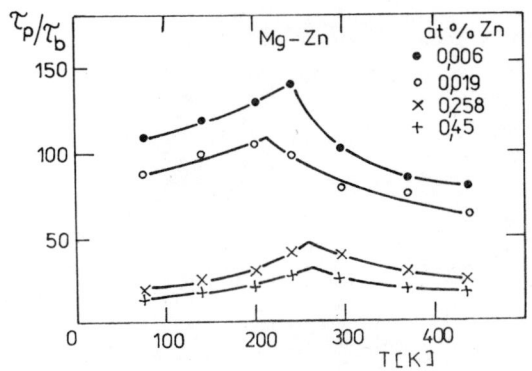

Fig. 4

- 127 -

SECTION 2

THE STRUCTURE AND PROPERTIES OF DISLOCATIONS IN METALS AND ALLOYS WITH A BCC LATTICE

DISLOCATIONS IN B.C.C. METALS AND ORDERED ALLOYS AND COMPOUNDS WITH
B.C.C.-BASED ORDERED STRUCTURES

M. Yamaguchi and Y. Umakoshi

Department of Materials Science and Engineering,
Faculty of Engineering, Osaka University,
Yamada-Oka 2-1, Suita, Osaka 565, Japan

Abstract

We first briefly review computer studies of dislocation core in the b.c.c. structure. Secondly, the atomistic calculations of the structure of antiphase boundaries and their stability in the B2, DO_3 and $L2_1$ structures are summarized and then a detailed description of the results of the calculations of both the core structure and motion behaviour of dislocations in B2 and DO_3 structures is given. Thirdly, we summarize the results of the recent deformation studies of ordered alloys and compounds with B2, DO_3 and $L2_1$ structures and discuss the deformation characteristics of these materials on the basis of the results of atomistic calculations.

1. Introduction

In materials in which no stable stacking faults exist or the stacking fault energy is too high, dislocation can not undergo well-defined dissociations into partial dislocations with smaller Burgers vectors, but usually possess cores with a somewhat extended configuration which is often non-planar and therefore gives rise to a limited mobility of dislocations. Thus, dislocations with such an extended core play an important role in the control of plastic properties of materials. The most well-known example of the dislocation core structure effects on mechanical properties is the low temperature deformation of b.c.c. metals, which has been known to be controlled by screw dislocations with an extended non-planar core structure (for reviews, see Christian [1], Sestak [2]).

Another well-known example is the deformation of ordered alloys and compounds with b.c.c.-based ordered structures such as B2, DO_3 and $L2_1$ types in which again no stable stacking faults other than antiphase boundaries (APB) exist [3, 4]. In these ordered alloys and compounds, slip occurs not only along <111> but also <100> and <110> directions. Of these three possible slip modes, the <111>-type slip in all three structures and the <001>-type slip in the DO_3 and $L2_1$ structures occur via the motion of superlattice dislocations dissociated into superpartials separated by APB's. The deformation behaviour is, however, very similar to that of b.c.c. metals, regardless of the type of slip; for example, the wavy nature of slip lines, failure of the Schmid law and orientation and temperature dependences of the flow stress and of the slip geometry are all commonly found in the B2, DO_3 and $L2_1$ ordered alloys and compounds (e.g.[5,6]). This analogy with b.c.c. metals leads to the conclusion that whichever of the three possible slip directions slip occurs along, it is screw dislocations which controls the deformation of these ordered alloys and compounds and screw dislocations possess cores such as those giving rise to a high Peierls type of stress.

In the present paper, we first summarize the results of recent atomistic studies of dislocations in b.c.c. and b.c.c.-based ordered structures and discuss the similarities and differences in the dislocation core structure and motion in these two classes of materials. Secondly, the recent deformation studies of ordered alloys and compounds with the b.c.c.-based ordered structures are presented. Then, the deformation characteristics of these materials, in particular, those typical of ordered alloys and compounds, are discussed in the light of the results of the atomistic studies of the dislocations in both b.c.c. and b.c.c.-based ordered structures.

2. Dislocations in b.c.c. metals

Since dislocations with Burgers vector of a/2<111>, in particular, those in screw orientation are of primary importance for the deformation of b.c.c. metals, their cores have been studied extensively (for reviews, see Vitek [7], Takeuchi [8], Puls [9], Vitek and Yamaguchi [10], Vitek and Duesbery [11], and Bullough and Tewary [12]). Besides a/2<111> dislocations, cores of a<100> dislocations and twinning dislocations on {112} twin boundaries have been also studied (e.g.[13-15]; for reviews, see [7,9,10,12]).

The core structures of a/2<111> dislocations have been calculated using various interatomic and interatomic row potentials. The most fundamental difference in the core structure between screw dislocations and non-screw dislocations with Burgers vector of a/2<111> is that the screw core is non-planar and the non-screw cores are always planar ([16,17]; for reviews, see [6,7]). This is obvious by comparison with the screw core in Fig.1(a) and a non-screw core in Fig.1(b), where structures are depicted using the method of the mapping of differential displacements originally introduced by Vitek, Perrin and Bowen [18] and the length of the arrows is proportional to the magnitude of the differential displacement, normalized to the range $\pm 1/2b$. This difference in the core structure reflects directly in the difference in the way of movement between screw and non-screw dislocation cores. The non-planar core of the screw dislocation must undergo a transformation from an originally sessile configuration to a glissile one before its movement can start. This gives rise to a high Peierls stress of screw dislocations.

Although various types of potentials have been used for atomistic studies of lattice defects, almost all of them, except for those for alkali metals calculated from first principles, were constructed empirically, for example, matching to the elastic constants. This means that the potentials used do not necessarily represent any real metal. Therefore, in the case of core structure calculations, it is important to sample a range of possible core structures and identify potential-independent effects [7,10,19]. The planarity is one of the important potential-independent properties of the core of 1/2<111> non-screw dislocations in b.c.c. metals and, of course, so is the non-planarity of 1/2<111> screw dislocation cores. The main features of the non-planar core of screw dislocations calculated using interatomic potentials have been summarized by Vitek as follows (see Fig.1(a))[7,10]:

(i) The core is spread mainly into three {110} planes intersecting along the dislocation line.

(ii) The displacements on {110} planes occur only on one side of the dislocation. This gives rise to the existence of two energetically degenerate core configurations related to each other by a {110} diad.

(iii) At the edge of the extended faults on the three {110} planes, displacements distribute asymmetrically onto the twinning {112} planes.

Such a non-planar core undergoes very significant changes, i.e. a sessile-glissile transformation before they start to move. Unlike the features of the stress-free core structure, the core transformation under an external shear stress have been found to be dependent on the interatomic potentials. This does not necessarily mean that the mode of the core transformation varies from potential to potential. Duesbery, Vitek and Bowen ([20]; for reviews, see [7,10]) have shown that only three distinct modes of core transformation exist:

(i) The transformation from one degenerate configuration to the other.

(ii) The formation of an extended multilayer fault on {112} planes.

(iii) The formation of an extended single layer fault on {110} planes.

The motion of the dislocation as a whole occurs along a {112} plane in the first and second cases.

When interatomic row potentials were used, somewhat different core structures of a/2<111> screw dislocations were obtained (for a review, see Takeuchi [8]). The stable core configuration was found to be either of degenerate type such as that shown in Fig.1(a) and of non-degenerate type which is similar to the linear elasticity solution. In the case of the non-degenerate core, the core being narrowly split on a {110} plane can be metastable and therefore the transformation of this type of core differs from that of the degenerate core. Masuda and Sato [21] also found the non-degenerate core stable using a tight binding type electronic theory.

3. Dislocations in B2, DO_3 and $L2_1$ structures

3.1 Antiphase boundaries and dislocation dissociation

Figure 2 shows a general description of the b.c.c.-based B2, DO_3 and $L2_1$ structures. As seen from the atomic arrangement in Fig.2, only one type of APB characterized by the displacement $\underset{\sim}{f}$=a/2<111> can exist in the B2 structure (a is the lattice parameter of the underlying b.c.c. structure), while in the DO_3 and $L2_1$ structures two types of APB's can be formed by displacements $\underset{\sim}{f}_1$=a/2<111> and $\underset{\sim}{f}_2$=a<100> which is equivalent to a<111>. This is obvious from crystallographic points of view. However, it is not clear a priori whether they are energetically always stable. Recently, a systematic investigation of the stability of planar faults in ordered alloys have been carried out using the technique which involves predicting the existence of stationary points in the γ-surface, i.e. a plot of the energy of a planar fault as a function of the displacement vector $\underset{\sim}{f}$ [7,22]. According to the results of this investigation, the stability of APB's in the three b.c.c.-based ordered structures is summarized as follows:

(i) The a/2<111> APB on {110} and {112} planes in the B2 structure is always stable.

(ii) The a/2<111> APB on {110} and {112} planes in the DO_3 and $L2_1$ structures are either unstable or stable with $\underline{f}$=a/2<111> + $\underline{f}$'. The magnitude of $\underline{f}$'may vary from material to material, but its direction must be along <001> for the APB on {110} and <111> for that on {112}.

(iii) The a<100> APB on {110} planes and the a<111> APB on {112} planes are always stable in both DO_3 and $L2_1$ structures.
The results of the γ-surface calculations for {110} and {112} planes in the B2 structure [4,6] and of those in the DO_3 structure by Paidar [3] are in full agreement with the above conclusion. At the same time, the γ-surface calculations confirmed that no stable stacking faults other than APB's exist in these structures.

Thus, a<111> superdislocations in the B2 structure are always dissociated into two a/2<111> superpartial dislocations joined by the stable a/2<111> APB. Similarly, 2a<100> superdislocations in the DO_3 and $L2_1$ structures are always dissociated into two a<111> superpartials. In the case of 2a<111> superdislocations in DO_3 and $L2_1$ structures, the dissociation scheme depends on the stability of the a/2<111>-type APB. When the a/2<111>-type APB is stable, the dissociation occurs as shown schematically by solid line in Fig.3 and when the a/2<111>-type APB is unstable, the dissociation would be like those shown by dotted lines in the figure. Kroupa and Paidar [23] calculated the energy of a superdislocation dissociated into four superpartials using elasticity theory and the results of γ-surface calculations [3] and found the solid-line scheme stable. 2a<111> superdislocations composed of four a/2<111> superpartials have been observed in Fe_3Al with the DO_3 structure [24].

3.2 Core structure and motion behaviour of dislocations

3.2.1 Superlattice screw dislocations with Burgers vector along <111> directions

The atomistic studies of core structure of a<111> superlattice screw dislocations in the B2 structure have been carried out by Takeuchi [25] using interatomic row potentials and by Umakoshi, Vitek and Yamaguchi [26] and Umakoshi, Yamaguchi and Vitek [27]. The calculations of Umakoshi et al. were performed using three different series of potentials constructed on the basis of J_o, J_1 and J_3 potentials employed in atomistic studies in the b.c.c. structure [20]. These potentials always represent a mechanically stable B2 lattice but lead to a large variation in the APB energy. In the calculations of both Takeuchi [25] and Umakoshi et al. [26,27], the core structure of a/2<111> superpartials was found to be, in general, very similar to that of a/2<111> screw dislocations in the b.c.c. lattice. The main features of the core structure of a/2<111> superpartial dislocations can be summarized as follows:

(i) Cores are again non-planar and spread into three intersecting {110} planes of the <111> zone.

(ii) Two core configurations, similar to the symmetry related ones found in the case of screw dislocations in the b.c.c. lattice, exist. However, these two core configurations are no longer energetically equivalent because of the presence of the APB.

(iii) Since the two core configurations are not equivalent, one of the two superpartials forming a pair possesses one core configuration and the other superpartial possesses always the other core configuration. Therefore, as seen from Fig.4(a) and (b), two combinations of configurations are possible, although the combination of Fig.4(a) is usually favoured [25].

When the combination of core configurations in Fig.4(b) occurs, the APB and the faults extended on {110} planes, formed inside the core and with the displacement vector of approximately a/6<111> overlap. Consequently, the faults with displacement vector, $f=a/3<111>$ and $f=2/3a<111>$ are formed. The energy of such faults is higher than the energy of the fault with $f=a/6<111>$, see Fig.5 which shows the section along <111> of the {110} γ-surface for a model B2 lattice. This is the reason why the combination of core configurations of Fig.4(a) is preferred to that of Fig.4(b).

The effect of an external shear stress upon the a<111> superlattice screw dislocations in the B2 structure have also been investigated in [25-27]. Three principle features of the superpartial dislocation motion are [26,27]:

(i) For almost all potentials used, the superpartials show a strong tendency to slip along the twinning {112} planes independently of the APB energy.

(ii) Except for the case where the APB energy is very low, the superpartial core transforms always in such a way that an extended multilayer fault is formed on the twinning {112} planes (see Fig.6).

(iii) Significant differences are usually found in the behaviour of the two superpartials. The trailing partial is, in general, more difficult to move than the leading one.

The most important factor controlling the motion of superpartials is their core structure and its transformations under the effect of the applied shear stress. In particular, it is the restoring force of the faults created under the effect of the applied shear stress which governs the core transformation [7,20]. Since the restoring force for a fault corresponding to a displacement $\underline{f}$ is given as $\underline{F}= - \text{grad } \gamma(\underline{f})$, the APB affects both the γ-surface and the restoring force. This is the reason why the APB has no direct influences on the motion of superpartials as mentioned in the first feature. The second feature may be understood when recognizing the following facts:

(i) The presence of APB leads to local minima in the restoring force surface for the faults on the {110} and {112} planes at $\underline{f}=a/6<111>$ and $\underline{f}=2/3a<111>$, and these local minima are usually more profound for the faults on {112} planes than for those on {110} planes. Fig.7 shows the section along <111> of the {112} restoring force surface calculated using one of potentials used.

(ii) The above described trend of the restoring force surface is found for almost all the potentials used; it seems to be characteristic of the B2 structure. The above mentioned two local minima in {112} restoring force surface are responsible for the movement of the superpartials along the twinning {112} planes and accompanied always by creation of multilayer faults on these planes.

Since APB exists, the restoring forces for the faults existing in the core region of the two superpartials are different. The third feature may be interpreted in terms of this difference in the restoring force as well as the elastic forces between the superpartials.

When the APB energy is very low, naturally the mode of the superpartial dislocation motion is the same as that of the screw dislocation in b.c.c. metals; both superpartials move along a {112} plane undergoing the core transformation characteristic of the potential on whose basis the potential for B2 lattice is constructed.

The local minimum of the restoring force for $\underline{f}=2/3a<111>$ on {112} planes is always much lower than the corresponding one on {110} planes. In the case of the fault with $\underline{f}=a/6<111>$, however, the restoring force on {110} planes can be little lower than that on {112} planes for some of the potentials constructed based on J_1. Such potentials usually give rise to lower values of APB energy and therefore a widely separated pair of $a/2<111>$ superpartial dislocations. When the stress is applied upon such a superpartial pair separated on a {110} plane, it is found that the leading partial moves along the {110} plane while the trailing one along a {112} plane in the twinning sense. Figure 8 shows an example of such a core behaviour. If such a cross-slip of the trailing superpartial occurs, the superlattice dislocation becomes immobilized. The role of such an immobilization of <111> superlattice dislocations will be discussed in § 4.1.

Some calculations of superlattice dislocations with Burgers vector 2a<111> in the DO_3 structure have been carried out [28]. When 2a<111> superlattice screw dislocations are dissociated into four a/2<111> superpartials the core structure of superpartials have been found to be again similar to that of a/2<111> screw dislocation in the b.c.c. structure. The effect of the applied stress on the superpartial cores have also studied. However, these results are still tentative.

3.2.2 Dislocations with Burges vector along <100> and <110> directions

Atomistic studies of the a<100> and the a<110> screw dislocations in the B2 and the DO_3 structure, respectively have been made by Yamaguchi and Umakoshi [13,28]. The core of these screw dislocations is spread on {110} planes. Thus, when they move on these planes, they experience the lowest Peierls stress. In the case of the a<100> screw dislocation, two energetically equivalent configurations exist since two orthogonal {110} planes intersect in the direction of dislocation line. When the stress is applied on the plane inclined more than 60° to the plane in which the core is spread, the transformation to the core spread onto another {110} plane which is perpendicular to the original {110} plane occurs. Therefore, the {hk0}<001> slip in some B2 compounds (e.g. [29-34]) may be explained in terms of the continual cross-slip of a<100> screw dislocations on two orthogonal {110} planes as suggested in [29]. In the case of a<110> screw dislocations in the DO_3 structure, no such equivalent core configurations exist. Therefore, the movement of the dislocation along planes other than {110} is then likely to be much more difficult. Although no ordered alloys and compounds with the DO_3 structure have been known to slip along <110>, Ni_2AlTi with the $L2_1$ structure deforms by the <110>-type slip at high temperatures [35,36]. According to the results of the deformation study on Ni_2AlTi [36], the critical resolved shear stress (c.r.s.s.) for the {110}<110> system is the lowest and the c.r.s.s. for the {100}<110> system is found to be about 40% higher than that for the {110}<110> system at about 1000K.

4. Deformation behaviour of b.c.c. metals and B2, DO_3 and $L2_1$ ordered alloys and compounds.

4.1 Deformation by slip along <111> directions.

We review briefly in this section the experimental results of recent investigations on the plastic behaviour of b.c.c. metals and B2, DO_3 and $L2_1$ ordered alloys and compounds deformed by slip along <111> directions.

As for transition metals, deformation studies on high purity Fe, Mo, Nb and Ta (e.g. [37-44]) are to be noticed. Kuramoto, Aono and Kitajima [37-39] have made a detailed measurement of Ψ-χ[+] and τ_y-χ relations for high purity Fe (RRR=5500-7200) and Mo (RRR= 3500-5000) at 4.2K and found that slip occurs on {110} planes independently of crystal orientations ($\Psi=0°$ for $-30°\leq\chi\leq30°$) and the τ_y-χ relation is of concave type.

Recently, the deformation behaviour of alkali metals and alloys such as Li [45], Li-Mg alloys [46], Na [47] and K [48] have been studied extensively. The mechanism of low temperature plasticity in these simple metals have been found to be the same as b.c.c. transition metals. However, Basinski, Duesbery and Murty [48] have reported that the orientation dependence of the low temperature flow stress in K is markedly different from that observed in b.c.c. transition metals; orientations near the three corners of the reference triangle exhibit essentially the same flow stress, while those in the centre of the triangle are much harder. This was explained by a computer model of a/2<111> screw dislocation core involving a potential calculated from first principles.

As for the plastic properties of B2 alloys and compounds, the Ψ-χ relation has been extensively investigated. Much of the work has been summarized in [6]. Although the Ψ-χ behaviour varies from one material to another, that $|\Psi|$ tends to degenerate to 30° at low

---

[+]The Ψ-χ dependence is commonly used to describe the slip geometry results. When the stress axis is referred to the standard [001]-[011]-[$\bar{1}$11] unit triangle, χ is the angle between the maximum resolved shear stress plane and ($\bar{1}$01), and Ψ is the angle between the macroscopic slip plane and ($\bar{1}$01).

temperatures is common to all the alloys and compounds with the B2 structure except for FeCo. This general trend of the low temperature Ψ-χ behaviour indicated that the most fundamental slip planes of a/2<111> superpartial pairs in B2 alloys and compounds are {112}. It is interesting to note that the {112} slip is favoured much more in B2 ordered alloys and compounds than in b.c.c. metals at low temperatures. Computer modelling of the a<111> superlattice screw dislocation core shows, in general, good agreement with slip plane observations in B2 ordered alloys and compounds at low temperatures.

The Ψ-χ relation for FeCo is shown in Fig.9 [49]. Slip is seen to occur exclusively on {110} planes ($\Psi=0°$) in the temperature range from 4.2-600K. Such a slip behaviour has been found so far only in FeCo. It may be explained on the basis of superpartial dislocation cores such as those shown in Fig.8. Although the overall movement of the trailing superpartial in the figure is on the twinning {112} plane, the elementary jumps occur always along a {110} plane. Therefore, it may be possible for the trailing partial to follow the leading one via a sequence of elementary jumps along the slip plane of the leading partial with the help of thermal activation.

When the trailing partial undergoes cross slip out of the slip plane of the leading partial, the motion of the superdislocation is strongly hindered, which then provides a hardening mechanism. In fact, an anomalous peak in flow stress has been known to occur in βCuZn at around 470K [50]. Figure 10 shows an example of the anomalous strengthening behaviour of βCuZn single crystals. In the range from room temperature to 470K, slip in βCuZn occurs exclusively on the {110}<111> system. The c.r.s.s. for slip on this system with increasing temperature and also with increasing the resolved shear stress on the {112} cross slip plane in the twinning sense. This orientation dependence of the anomalous strengthening behaviour could be explained in terms of the above mentioned mechanism involving cross-slip of the trailing superpartial dislocation. The anomalous strengthening has been also known to occur in FeCo, Fe_3Al (DO_3) (for a review, see Stoloff and Davies [51] and Ag_2MgZn ($L2_1$) [52]). However, the anomaly in these materials occurs just below the critical temperature of the corresponding ordered structure and does not show any crystal orientation dependences. The change in the degree of order rather than dislocation core effects is thought to be responsible for the strength anomaly of this type [50].

When compared with ordered alloys and compounds with the B2 structure, the systematic data on the slip behaviour in those with DO_3 and $L2_1$ structure are still lacking. The Ψ-χ relations have measured so far in Fe_3Al [53], Fe_3Si [53], $Fe_3(SiAl)$ [53], Ag_2MgZn [52] and Cu_2MnAl [54]. They are summarized in Fig.11. Although slip in these materials can occur on both {110} and {112} planes, the orientation region showing the former slip is wider than that showing the latter slip. Thus, in the case of ordered alloys with DO_3 and $L2_1$ structures, the {110} slip is seen to be given preference over the {112} slip. Such a preference for slip on {110} planes is likely to be rationalized in terms of the relative restoring forces for the faults on {110} and {112} planes, similarly in the case of the {112} slip in the B2 structure.

In DO_3 and $L2_1$ structures, the a/2<111>-type APB may be stable with displacement vector $\underline{f}$=a/2<111> + $\underline{f}'$. The additional displacement vector $\underline{f}'$ may affect the cross-slip of superlattice dislocations from a {110} plane to another {110} plane from the following reasons: (i) In order for the superpartial dislocation with Burgers vector $\underline{f}$ to cross-slip, it has to be dissociated into an a/2<111> screw dislocation and a non-screw dislocation with small Burgers vector $\underline{f}'$, but such a dissociation may be energetically unfavourable; (ii) The energy of the APB created behind the leading superpartial on the cross-slip {110} plane and with displacement vector a/2<111> is higher than the energy of the APB on the original {110} plane and with displacement vector a/2<111> + $\underline{f}'$.

4.2 Deformation by slip along <100> and <110> directions

Slip in <100> directions has been thought to be common in B2 compounds with high ordering energy such as NiAl (e.g.[29]) and AuZn [30]. Recently, however, the occurrence of the transition in the slip directions from <111> to <100> has been reported in AgMg [32,33], FeAl [34] and CuZn [55] at high temperatures. The transition can be interpreted in terms of the difference in temperature dependence of the c.r.s.s. between the two types of slip. Figure 12 shows the case for AgMg. The difference, in this case, has been suggested to be associated with the difference in the nature and the strength of two interactions-namely, the interaction between defects such as excess Ag atoms and the <001> dislocations and that between the defects and the <111> superdislocations [32]. The Ψ-χ relations for the {hk0}<001> slip in AgMg [32], FeAl [34] and AuZn [30] are summarized in Fig.13. The characteristics of the deformation by slip along <110> directions observed in Ni_2AlTi are given in the paper by the authors at this meeting.

Acknowledgements

The authors would like to thank Professor V. Vitek for invaluable discussions on this manuscript. The authers are also thank Professor T. Yamane for his encouragement.

References

[1] Christian J.W.: Proc. 2nd Int. Conf. on Strength of Metals and Alloys, ASM, 1970, p.31.
[2] Sestak B.: Proc. 5th Int. Conf. on Strength of Metals and Alloys, Pergamon Press, Oxford, 1979, p.1461.
[3] Paidar V.: Czech. J. Phys. B26(1976)865.
[4] Yamaguchi M., Pope D.P., Vitek V. and Umakoshi Y.: Phil. Mag. 43(1981)1265.
[5] Takeuchi S.: Proc. 5th Int. conf. on Strength of Metals and Alloys, Pergamon Press, Oxford, 1979, p.53.
[6] Yamaguchi M.: Mechanical Properties of BCC Metals, ed. Meshi M., TMS-AIME pub., 1982, p.31.
[7] Vitek V.: Crystal Lattice Defects 5(1974)1.
[8] Takeuchi S.: Interatomic Potentials and Crystalline Defects, ed. Lee J.K., TMS-AIME pub., 1981, p.201.
[9] Puls M.P.: Proc. Int. Conf. on Dislocation Modelling of Physical System, Special Acta Met./Scripa Met. Pub., 1981, p.249.
[10] Vitek V. and Yamaguchi M.: Interatomic Potentials and Crytalline Defects ed. Lee J.K., TMS-AIME Pub., 1981, p.223.
[11] Vitek V. and Duesbery M.S.: Mechanical Properties of BCC Metals, ed. Meshii M., TMS-AIME Pub., 1982, p.3.
[12] Bullough R. and Tewary V.K.: Dislocations in Solids Vol.2, ed. Nabarro F.R.N. North-Holland, Amsterdam, 1979,p.1.
[13] Yamaguchi M. and Umakoshi Y.: Phys. Stat. Sol.(a) 31(1975)101.
[14] Yamaguchi M. and Vitek V.: Phil. Mag. 34(1976)1.
[15] Bristowe P.D. and Crocker A.G.: Acta Met. 25(1977)1363.
[16] Yamaguchi M. and Vitek V.: J. Phys. F 3(1973)523; 5(1975)1, 11.
[17] Vitek V. and Yamaguchi M.: J. Phys F 3(1973)537.
[18] Vitek V., Perrin R.C. and Bowen D.K.: Phil. Mag. 21(1970)1049.
[19] Basinski Z.S., Duesbery M.S. and Murty G.S.: Acta Met. 29(1981) 801.
[20] Duesbery M.S., Vitek V. and Bowen D.K.: Proc. Roy. Soc. Lond. A 332(1973)85.
[21] Masuda k. and Sato A.: Phil. Mag. B37(1978)581.
[22] Vitek V.: Phil. Mag. 18(1974)773.
[23] Kroupa F. and Paidar V.: Phys. Stat. Sol. (a) 33(1976)555.
[24] Crawford R.C., Ray I.L.F. and Cockayne D.J.H.: Phil. Mag. 27 (1973)1.
[25] Takeuchi S.: Phil. Mag. 41(1980)541.
[26] Umakoshi Y., Vitek V. and Yamaguchi M.: to be published
[27] Umakoshi Y., Yamaguchi M. and Vitek V.: this symposium
[28] Yamaguchi M. and Umakoshi Y.: The 1982 Fall Meeting of Japan Institute of Metals, to be published
[29] Ball L. and Smallman R.E.: Acta Met. 14(1966)1517.
[30] Schulson E.M. and Teghtsoonian E.: Phil. Mag. 19(1969)155.
[31] Mitchell J.B., Aboelfotoh O. and Dorn J.E.: Met. Trans. 2(1971)3265.
[32] Murakami K., Umakoshi Y. and Yamaguchi M.: Phil. Mag. 37(1978) 719.

[33] Yamaguchi M. and Umakoshi Y.: Phil. Mag. 39(1979)33.
[34] Umakoshi Y. and Yamaguchi M.: Phil. Mag. 41(1980)573; 44(1981) 711.
[35] Strutt P.R., Polvani R.S., Ingram J.C.: Met. Trans. 7A(1976)23.
[36] Yamaguchi M., Umakoshi Y. and Yamane T.: this symposium
[37] Aono Y., Kitajima K. and Kuramoto E.: Scripta Met. 15(1981)275.
[38] Kitajima K., Aono Y. and Kuramoto E.: Scripta Met. 15(1981)919.
[39] Aono Y., Kuramoto E. and Kitajima K.: Proc. 6th Int. Conf. on Strength of Metals and Alloys, Melbourne, 1982.
[40] Matsui H., Moriya S., Takaki S. and Kimura H.: Trans. JIM 19(1978)163.
[41] Matsui H. and Kimura H.: Mater. Sci. Eng. 24(1976)247.
[42] Garratt-Reed A.J. and Taylor G.: Phil. Mag. 33(1976)577; 39A(1970)597.
[43] Nakagawa J. and Meshii M.: Phil. Mag. A 44(1981)1165;45(1982)983.
[44] Takeuchi S. and Maeda K.: Acta Met. 25(1977)1485.
[45] Sherry W.M. and Prinz F.: Acta Met. 28(1980)949.
[46] Saka H. and Taylor G.: Phil. Mag. A 43(1981)1377.
[47] Herke P., Kirchner H.O.K. and Schoeck G.: Proc. 4th Int. Conf. on Strength of Metals and Alloys, 1976, 1, p.151.
[48] Basinski Z.S., Duesbery M.S. and Murty G.S.: Acta Met. 29(1981)801.
[49] Yamaguchi M., Umakoshi Y., Yamane T., Minonishi Y. and Morozumi S.: Scripta Met. 16(1982)607.
[50] Umakoshi Y. and Yamaguchi M.: Acta Met. 24(1976)89; Scripta Met. 11(1977)211.
[51] Stoloff N.S. and Davies R.G.: Prog. Mater. Sci. 13(1966)29.
[52] Yamaguchi M. and Umakoshi Y.: J. Mater. Sci. 15(1980)2448; Scripta Met. 15(1981)605.
[53] Hanada S., Watanabe S., Sato T. and Izumi O: Trans. JIM 22(1981)873; Scripta Met.15(1981)1345.
[54] Yamaguchi M. and Umakoshi Y.: The 1983 Spring Meeting of Japan Institute of Metals, to be published
[55] Saka H., Kawase M. and Imura T.: The 1983 Spring Meeting of Japan Institute of Metals.

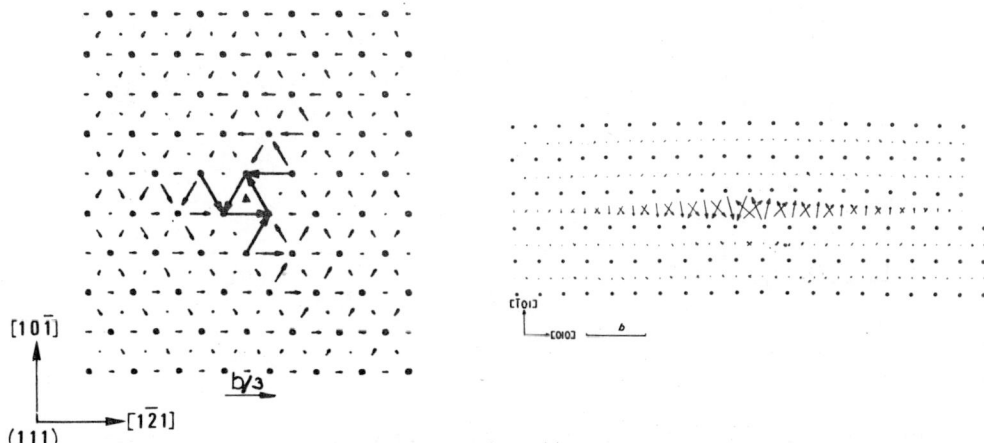

Fig.1 Core structures of 1/2<111> dislocations in the b.c.c. structure. (a) screw dislocation [7,20], (b) a non-screw dislocation lying along the [101] direction [7,16].

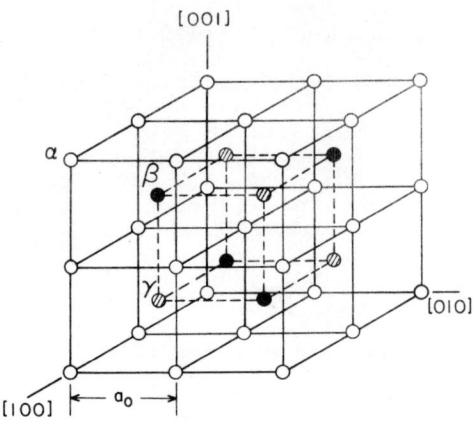
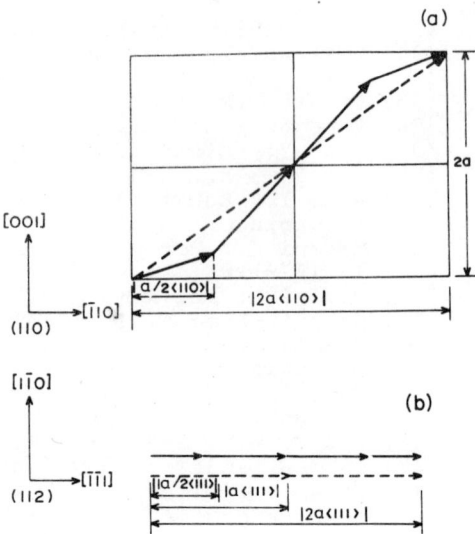

Fig.2 The b.c.c.-based B2, DO_3 and $L2_1$ structures. In AB(B2) alloys α sites are occupied by A atoms and (β, δ) sites by B atoms. In $A_3B(DO_3)$ alloys (α, β) sites are occupied by A atoms and δ sites by B atoms. In $A_2BC(L2_1)$ alloys α, β, δ sites are occupied by A, B and C atoms, respectively.

Fig.3 Possible dissociations of $2a\langle 111\rangle$ superlattice dislocations on (a) $\{110\}$ planes and (b) $\{112\}$ planes in DO_3 and $L2_1$ structures.

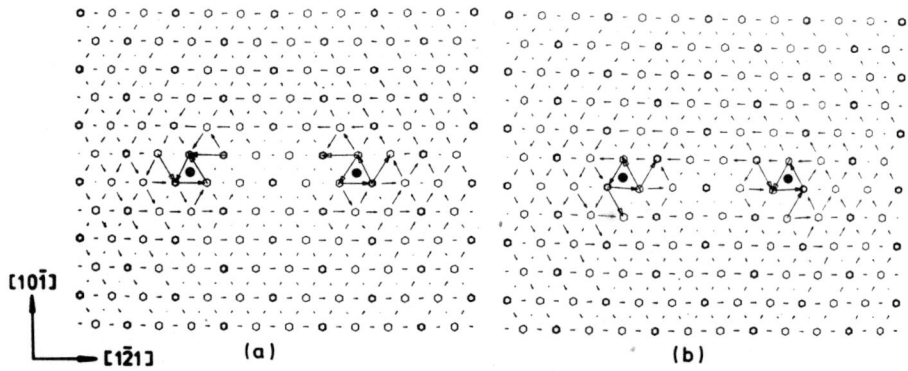

Fig.4 Two possible combinations of core configurations of $a/2 \langle 111\rangle$ superpartial screw dislocations in a B2 lattice.

- 144 -

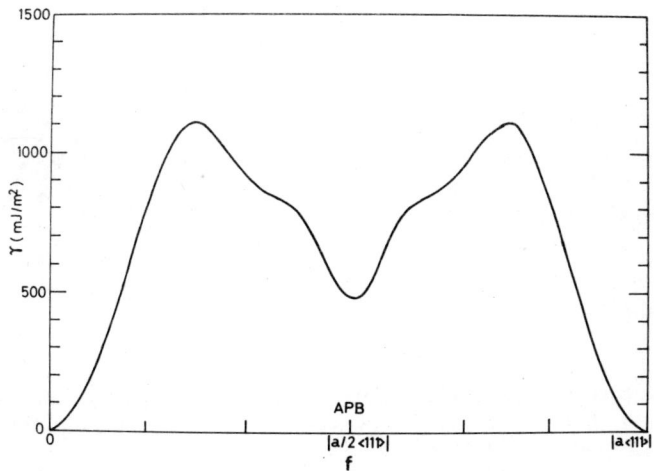

Fig.5 The section along $\langle 111 \rangle$ of the $\{110\}$ γ-surface for a B2 lattice.

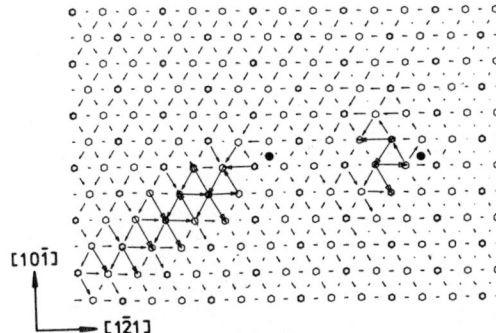

Fig.6 Core structures of $1/2 \langle 111 \rangle$ superpartials calculated for a J_1-based potential under a shear stress (0.07) applied on the $(10\bar{1})$ plane. The energy of APB on $\{110\}$ plane is 485 mJ/m^2.

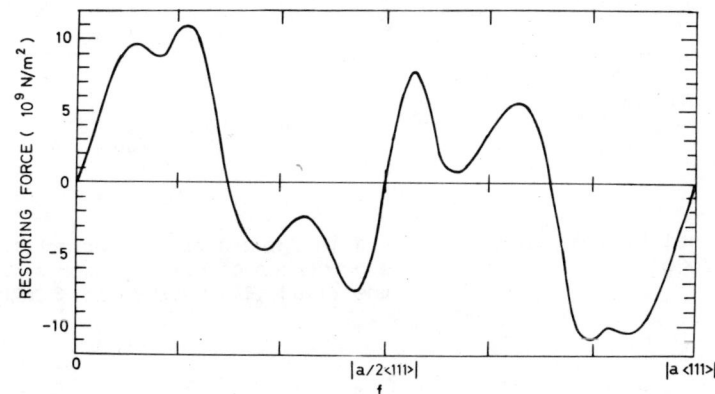

Fig.7 The section along $\langle 111 \rangle$ of the $\{112\}$ restoring force surface for a B2 lattice.

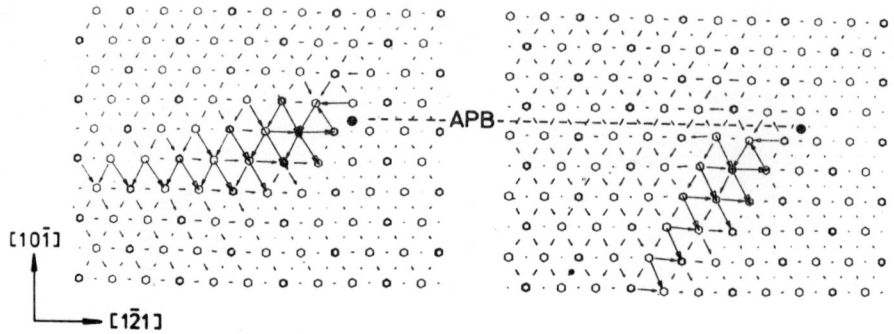

Fig.8 Core structure of 1/2 $\langle 111 \rangle$ superpartials calculated for a J_1-based potential under a shear stress (0.055μ) applied on the $(10\bar{1})$ plane. The energy of APB on $\{110\}$ planes is 95 mJ/m^2.

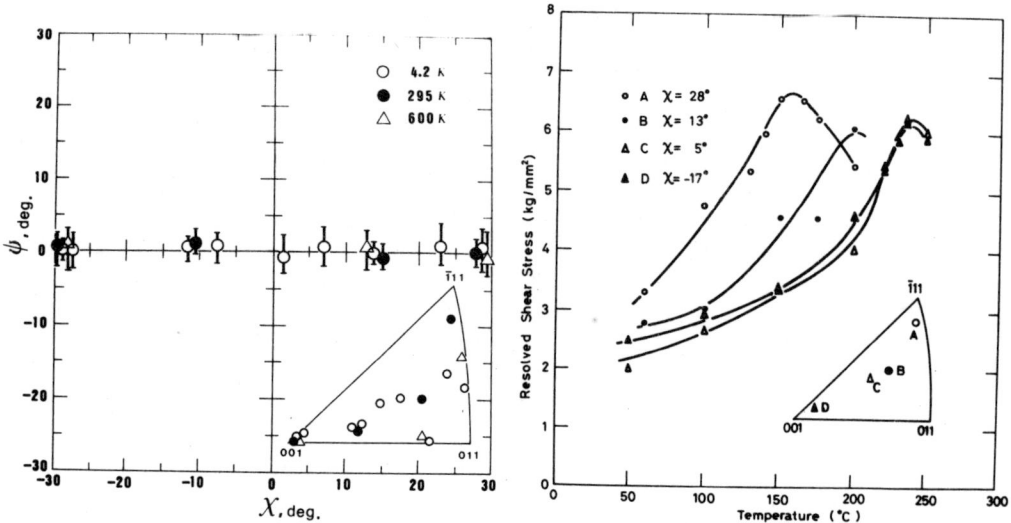

Fig.9 The $\psi - \chi$ relation for slip along $\langle 111 \rangle$ in FeCo.

Fig.10 Temperature and orientation dependences of c.r.s.s. for slip on the $\{110\} \langle 111 \rangle$ system in βCuZn.

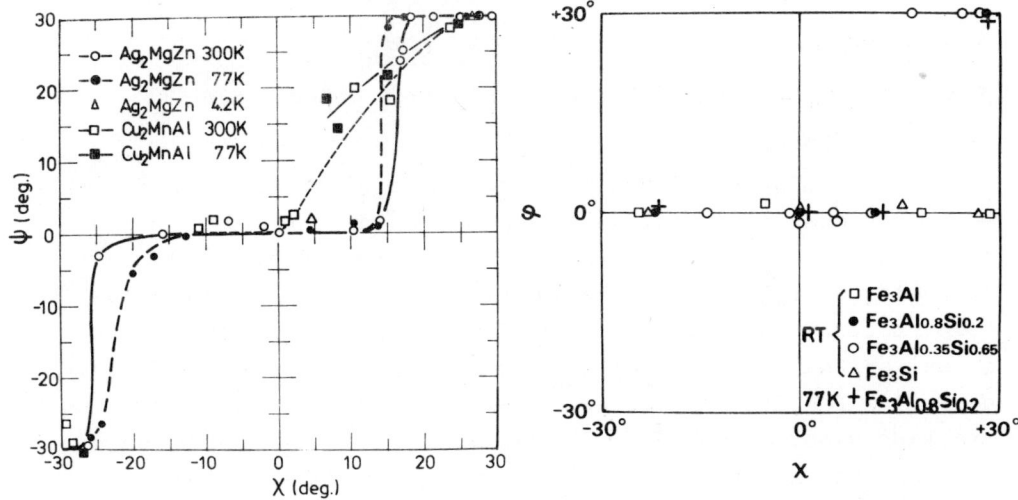

Fig.11 $\psi-\chi$ relations for slip along $\langle 111 \rangle$ in (a) Ag$_2$MgZn [52] and Cu$_2$MnAl [54], (b) Fe$_3$Al, Fe$_3$Si and Fe$_3$(AlSi) [53].

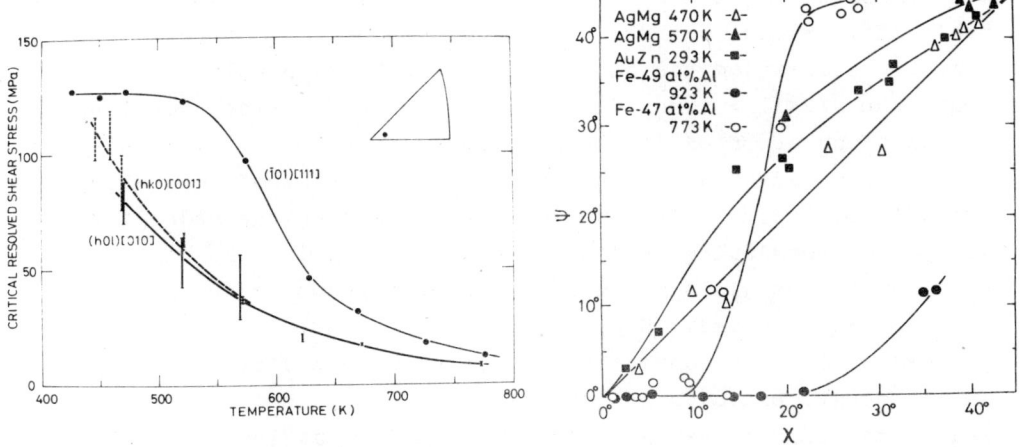

Fig.12 Temperature dependence of c.r.s.s. for slip along $\langle 111 \rangle$ and $\langle 100 \rangle$ directions in AgMg.

Fig.13 $\psi-\chi$ relations for slip along $\langle 001 \rangle$ in AgMg [32], FeAl [34] and AuZn [30]. Taking [001] as the slip direction, χ is the angle between the m.r.s.s. plane and (110) and ψ is the angle between the observed slip plane and ($\bar{1}$10).

KINKED SCREW DISLOCATIONS IN THE BODY-CENTRED CUBIC LATTICE

M.S. Duesbery

Division of Physics, NRC, Canada, Ottawa, Ontario K1A OR6

1. Introduction

In the history of research into crystal dislocations, the screw dislocation in solids crystallising in the body-centred cubic (bcc) structure occupies an unique position. While technologically important because of its part in the deformation processes of the refractory bcc metals, it has proved to be one of the most complex and physically interesting defects, depending for its properties on the details of the atomic stacking right at the dislocation core. Thus it is not surprising that a great deal of research effort has been expended over the past two decades in the experimental and theoretical study of the screw dislocation in bcc metals; the work reported below will be concerned principally with the theoretical aspects.

The early work is covered thoroughly by a number of excellent reviews /1-4/; more recent research has been reviewed by Kubin /5/. Because of the importance of the core effects, computer simulation has been the tool most frequently used to study the a/2<111> screw dislocation. With few exceptions, the calculations reported in the literature have been restricted to infinite, straight dislocations, simulated at zero temperature, a model obviously limited in scope but enjoying the redeeming virture of permitting periodic boundary conditions to be imposed parallel to the dislocation line, thereby reducing the amount of computation involved. Despite this constraint, it has been demonstrated quite convincingly that the screw dislocation core in bcc metals exhibits an intrinsically non-planar structure which can offer an explanation, in principle at least, of the large, strongly temperature and orientation-dependent flow stress and unusual slip geometry observed experimentally.

One of the most severe difficulties emerging from the computer simulation work on rigid dislocations, in the author's view, is the persistent discrepancy between the magnitudes of the calculated screw dislocation Peierls stress and the observed low-temperature limit of the metallic flow stress. Even in a direction comparison between theory and experiment for potassium /6/, a simple bcc metal for which a sound theoretical treatment is possible, the calculated Peierls stress is larger than the flow stress by a factor of three.

At finite temperatures the motion of screw dislocations is thought to proceed by way of formation and subsequent migration of kinks, rather than by translation of straight or nearly straight dislocations. Thus it seems natural to inquire into the properties of kinked dislocations, both to gain a deeper insight into thermally activated dislocation motion and to investigate whether the possibility of kink formation can modify the zero-temperature properties of the straight screw dislocations.

Gehlen /7/ has treated a kink in a screw dislocated model of α-iron. He reports a kink width of 4-5b, where b is the magnitude of the Burgers vector, a kink energy of order 0.8eV and an upper limit to the kink Peierls stress of G/500 (where G is the <111>{110} shear modulus); this latter value is of the same order as the flow stress observed at asymptolically low temperatures in iron and the refractory bcc metals. However, it is known /4/ that the screw dislocation can exist in degenerate but geometrically distinct forms, so that in principle there are several possible kinked states. Which of these is treated in /7/ is unclear, nor is it known whether the kink in /7/ is that of lowest energy. A more extensive study of a number of the possible types of kink, using a similar α-iron potential, has been made by Wüthrich and Seeger /8,9/, who find the kinks to have a width between 3b and 7b, with energies ranging from 0.6eV to 1.2eV. While these kink widths are compatible with that found by Gehlen /7/, the energies are an order of magnitude larger, a rather disturbing discrepancy. The work /8,9/ does not discuss the kink morphology or the kink Peierls stress.

The author /10/ has studied the morphology, energy and Peierls stress for the various possible kinks, using both a potassium model and an α-iron model as used in /8,9/. The work /10/ also considers kink interaction energies within a double-kink complex. In the text below, these results will be summarised and extended for the case of potassium.

2. Details of the Calculations

These will only be summarised; for fuller details reference should be made to /10/. In the calculations reported below, a model bcc lattice bound by a first-principles interatomic potential for potassium /11/ has been used. The model consists of a finite crystallite with boundaries fixed at the positions determined by linear anisotropic elasticity theory. Earlier studies /12/ using the same potential have shown that the structure and Peierls stress of the dislocation core are not affected by these rigid boundary conditions provided that the size of the model normal to the dislocation line is at least 30 x 30 atoms (28b x 28b). Accordingly this size was adopted as standard, while parallel to the dislocation line the crystallite was extended to a length of between 51b and 101b, depending on whether a single or double kink was being modeled. The model thus contains from 45,900 to 90,900 atoms and is substantially larger than either the largest (1900 atoms) used by Gehlen /7/ or that (600 atoms) used by Wüthrich /8/; this should permit a correspondingly more realistic simulation.

The numerical method employed involves a simple static relaxation technique /13/, during which the forces on individual atoms drop to the numerical limit imposed by the precision of the computer. In a typical relaxation, the forces, in units of eV per lattice parameter, drop from $O(10^{-2})$ to $O(10^{-7})$. The application of stress is simulated by deforming the crystallite through strains calculated from the applied stress using the full elastic compliance tensor.

The calculations were performed on a Floating Point Systems AP-120 array processor slaved to a Digital Equipment Corporation VAX 11/780 computer. Using an interatomic potential range of two lattice constants (64 neighbours) a processing rate of about 2000 atoms/sec. could be realised. Thus, one iterative pass over the entire crystallite took less than minute. Typically, full relaxation could be achieved in less than 50 passes.

3. Properties of Isolated Kinks

As first pointed out by Vitek /14/, the screw dislocation core in bcc metals does not have the full symmetry of the host lattice, existing rather in two degenerate but geometrically distinguishable forms, related by a diad operator normal to the dislocation line. The two types of a/2[111] screw dislocation core are shown in fig. 1(i) and (ii) using the different displacement /15/ display method; as indicated in fig. 1, a Cartesian reference frame is used with x_1 parallel to $[\bar{1}2\bar{1}]$, x_2 to $[\bar{1}01]$ and x_3 along [111]. The core shown in fig. 1(i) will be referred to as type A. The principle distinction between this core and the unrelaxed elastic core is that the central three atom rows

have been translated by approximately $b/6$ parallel to the
$-a/2[111]$ Burgers vector with respect to the long-range field.
This property, termed the "polarity" of the dislocation by
Seeger and Wüthrich /9/, reflects the decomposition of the total
dislocation into three fractional dislocations lying on {110}
planes, joined to the centre of the core by strips of generalised
stacking fault /16/. The core shown in fig. 1(ii), in which the
translation of the central atom rows is antiparallel to the
Burgers vector, will be called type B.

It can readily be seen that there are six possible elementary
kinks with line vector $\pm \frac{a}{3}[\bar{1}2\bar{1}]$ /8-10/. There are two kinks in
which the core configuration is the same on both sides of the
kink; termed homomorphous kinks /10/, these are denoted by the
sequences ApA and AnA, in which p, n indicate that the kink line
vector is a positive or negative $a/_3[\bar{1}2\bar{1}]$ step and the preceding
and trailing symbols indicate the type of the core on either side
of the kink. In addition, there are four possible heteromorphous
kinks ApB, BpA, AnB and BnA. Double kinks can be constructed by
combining any p-kink with any n-kink, provided that the juxtaposed
core configurations are the same. i.e. ApAAnA is a possible
double kink but ApABnA is not. This constraint can be removed by
introducing the defect which consists of a core configuration
change with no step in the dislocation line. There are two such
"flip" defects /17/, represented by the sequences AxB and BxA.
These defects are distinct states because of the above-mentioned
translation of the central three atom rows in the core. At the
site of the AxB flip both these translations are directed away
from the centre, suggesting a local density less than that of
the perfect lattice; conversely, a higher local density is
indicated for the BxA flip. It is worth noting that a similar
tendency is expected at the site of each heterokink, although the
effect should be less pronounced because in this case the
oppositely-translated rows do not meet head-on.

The detailed morphology of the various kinks is treated in
/10/, but will be ignored in this manuscript for reasons of space.
It is worth noting, however, that the kink widths are of order
16b. This value is more than twice that obtained by Wüthrich /8/
in his α-iron model; this is not surprising, since it is to be
expected that the potassium model should exhibit a smaller Peierls

potential. To confirm this point, some calculations were repeated using the same potential /18/ as Wüthrich: kink widths very similar to his quoted values were observed.

3.1 Kink Energies

The kink and flip defect energies are summarised in table I (for full details of the energy calculation, see /101/).

Table I

Defect	Energy(eV)	Defect	Energy(eV)
ApB	.038	ApA	.081
BnA	.038	AnA	.066
AnB	.111	AxB	.018
BpA	.059	BxA	.048

It is evident from table I that while the lowest-energy defect is the AxB flip, with an energy of 0.018eV, the double-kink complex of lowest-energy is the ApBBnA combination, with an energy of 0.076eV. The next-lowest energy double kink is the BnAAxBBpA complex, which has an energy of 0.115eV; this value is sufficiently far removed from the ApBBnA energy that at the temperatures involved (0-20 Kelvins), its relative contribution to a thermally activated process would be quite negligible.

The distribution of the kink energy is mainly confined to a cylinder concentric with the dislocation line of radius ~ 3b and length ~ 30b; further details are given in /10/.

3.2 The Kink Peierls Stress

As mentioned above, fixed boundary conditions for the size of crystallite used do not cause an appreciable error in the calculation of the Peierls stress of the rigid screw dislocation, which for pure shear stress on the $(\bar{1}01)$ plane is 0.94×10^{-2} G /13/. However, it is quite possible that the boundaries may exert a significant influence at the lower stress levels expected to be involved in kink motion. The boundary displacement field of the kinked dislocation is different on either side of the kink because of the change in site of the screw dislocation arms. The field can be considered as the sum of a large, constant field due to the presence of a single rigid screw dislocation at some average site and a small perturbative field due to deviations from the average site. The constant field cannot exert any force on the kink, for obvious reasons and can thus be neglected. However, if the perturbative field is held fixed while the kink moves, a retarding force in first order proportional to the kink displacement is to be expected. Thus when the kink is in equilibrium in the presence of external forces, its position is determined by a balance between the force due to the applied stress, the linear boundary restoring force and the force due to the kink Peierls barrier. The Peierls stress can be calculated by a simple variation of the method introduced by Woo & Puls /19/. If the applied stress is plotted as a function of kink displacement, the effect of the Peierls barrier, which must be periodic in b, should be visible as a modulation on the boundary force, which is not periodic: the deviations at the extremal points of the modulation then give the Peierls stress. In practice, it is found that the force-displacement curve of the kink, regardless of type, is closely linear to a stress of at least 0.35Mpa (2.6×10^{-4}G), corresponding to a displacement of 2.6b. The maximum deviation from linearity is 1 kPa (7×10^{-7}G), which figure can be taken as an upper limit on the magnitude of the Peierls stress.

This is in sharp contrast with the calculation /7/, which indicates a kink Peierls stress of 5×10^{-3}G for an α-iron model; to clarify this point, some of the calculations were repeated using a suitable α-iron potential /18/. The kink Peierls stress in this case was found to be 7×10^{-4}G, substantially larger than that found for potassium, but nevertheless an order of magnitude smaller than the value estimated in /7/ and than the observed low-temperature flow stress of α-iron. The high value obtained in /7/ can probably be attributed to the small size of block used. The difference in kink Peierls stress between the potassium and α-iron models confirms the expectation that narrow kinks, as in the α-iron model, should show a higher Peierls stress than wider kinks.

4. <u>Properties of Double Kinks</u>

The kink self-energies, treated above, are of paramount importance in the high-temperature limit of plastic deformation, when there is ample thermal energy for creation of pairs of widely separated kinks. At lower temperatures, while there may be insufficient energy for this process, double kinks with smaller separations may be generated, because the interaction between opposite kinks is attractive, so that the energy of the complex decreases with separation; however, for such an activation to be successful, there must exist an applied stress sufficiently large to overcome the kink interaction and force the activated complex to expand.

The elastic theory of kinks was developed by Eshelby /20/ and Seeger and Schiller /21/ and is reviewed in depth by Hirth and Lothe /17/. For separations large compared to the width of an isolated kink, the interaction energy should be inversely proportional to the separation, L, giving a force (from /17/)

$$(1) \qquad F = - \frac{a^2 b^2}{2L^2} \left[K(\beta) + \frac{\partial^2 K(\beta)}{\partial \beta^2} \right]$$

in which $K(\beta)$ is the energy factor of the kink and β is its "character angle" (i.e. the angle between the kink line and the Burgers vector): a is the length of the kinks. For kinks on a screw dislocation with sufficiently large separation, β can be taken to be $\pi/2$ regardless of the kink shape.

As was noted in the preceding section, the energy of the ApBBnA double kink is substantially lower than any other: therefore only this double kink need be considered in any detail.

4.1 The Shape of the Double Kink

The concept of a kink "shape", familiar from the elastic string picture of a dislocation, is not so clear when dealing with the kink on an atomic scale. The approach adopted in /10/ is to look at the change in relative displacements of neighbouring [111] rows as they pass through the kink. That these must undergo permanent change during this procedure can be seen easily by considering a pair of atom rows at a mean position vector $\underline{r}$ from the dislocation on the A side of an ApB kink: on the B side, the same pair of rows will lie at $\underline{r} + \underline{p}$ from the dislocation, where $\underline{p}$ is the displacement of the dislocation line across the kink. In general, the strains at these two positions will be different and hence there will be a change in the relative positions of the two atomic rows. Far from the dislocation line this difference will be small, but close to the core the effect is measurable and

is enhanced by the different core structures of the A and B
dislocation arms. The choice of which pair of atomic rows to
use is not critical, since very similar shapes are observed. The
pair actually chosen is that designated ℓ and n in fig. 1. In
fig. 1(i), the relative displacement of these two rows is about
$6/b$: in fig. 1(ii), if the core shown is imagined to be displaced
by $a/3\ [\bar{1}2\bar{1}]$, the relative displacement become $b/3$. Thus the
change, $b/6$, is quite large, enabling quite reasonable resolution.
In the case of a double kink, of course, the relative displacement
changes from one extreme to the other and then back, as long as
the kinks are widely separated.

Fig. 2 shows the calculated double kink shape in potassium
for a variety of kink separations. The separation was determined
as the distance between the two points at which the relative
displacement reaches the point midway between the two extremes,
i.e. in fig. 2, the points at which the curve intersects the
line $d = 0.25b$. This definition has some obvious drawbacks for
small separations; for example, in the smallest double kink
shown in fig. 2, the tip of the bulge does not even reach
$d = 0.25b$. An alternative procedure might be to define the kink
separation as the distance between the points at which the displacement is half the maximum. If this is done, a curious property
is apparent; for kink separations of less than about 20b, calculated by the first method, the separation determined by the
second method is constant, equal to $21.5b \pm 0.3b$. This suggests
that for separations less than 20b, or about 1.5 kink widths,
the double kink behaves more like a single defect with a shape
which depends only on the maximum extent of advance of the bulge
tip. This is in contrast with the case of large separations, for
which the shape of each individual kink remains constant. There
is a considerable transition region between the two regimes, as
can be seen from fig. 2. For the curve with the largest separation, 41b or about three kink widths, the peak displacement is
0.328b, measurably short of the asymptotic value of 0.333b.

The smallest double kink in fig. 2 corresponds to a stress
of 8Mpa, or $6 \times 10^{-3} G$, about two thirds of the Peierls stress of
the rigid screw dislocation.

4.2 The Energy of the Double Kink

The equilibrium pairs of applied stress and kink separation

(as measured by the first method above) are plotted in fig. 3(i) (curve I). The stress required to maintain equilibrium has a limiting value as the separation approaches zero of 7.8Mpa which, as mentioned above, is about two thirds of the Peierls stress of the rigid screw. As the separation increases, the stress drops only slightly out to a separation of ~ 8b, then rapidly to 1Mpa (7.6×10^{-4}G) for a separation of 22.5b and finally more slowly for larger separations. This curve can be integrated to give the energy of the complex as a function of separation (curve II in fig. 3(i)). Bearing in mind that there is still an appreciable interaction between the kinks at the largest separation shown, the estimated energy at this point of 0.059eV compares well with the calculated energy for inifinite separation of 0.076eV (table I).

The funtional dependence of the force on the kink separation can be seen more clearly by plotting the points on a logarithmic scale, the result of which is shown in fig. 3(ii). For kink separations > 8b, the force is given reasonably by an inverse square law (the straight line in fig. 3(ii)), as predicted by continuum elasticity (1). If the expansion (1) is fitted to the data of fig. 3(ii), a value for $\left|K + \frac{\partial^2 K}{\partial \beta^2}\right|$ of 1.33×10^3Mpa is obtained. The value of $K(\pi/2)$ for potassium, calculated using anisotropic elasticity theory, is 2.3×10^3Mpa; the second derivative of $K(\pi/2)$, estimated by numerical differentiation, is $-1.24 \pm 0.20 \times 10^3$Mpa. Thus the elastic value of $\left|K + \frac{\partial^2 K}{\partial \beta^2}\right|$ is $1.06 \pm 0.20 \times 10^3$Mpa, in fair agreement with the observed value. This agreement between modeling experiments and elasticity theory is not surprising, since the continuum expressions are vigourously correct for large kink separations. Of greater interest is the observation, from fig. 3(ii), that the inverse square law is valid for separations as small as 8b, or half the width of a single kink.

References

/1/ Sestak, B.: Proc. 3rd. Int. Symp. "Reinststoffe in Wissenschaft und Technik", Berlin, Akademie-Verlag 1970.

/2/ Christian, J.W.: Proc. 2nd. Int. Conf. "Strength of Metals and Alloys", Asilomar, ASM Press 1970.

/3/ Christian, J.W.: Proc. 3rd. Int. Symp. "Reinststoffe in Wissenschaft und Technik", Berlin, Akademie-Verlag 1970.

/4/ Vitek, V.: Crystal Lattice Defects $\underline{5}$ (1974) 1.

/5/ Kubin, L.P.: Rev. Def. Beh. Mat., (1983) in the press.

/6/ Basinski, Z.S., Duesbery, M.S. and Murty, G.S.: Acta Met. $\underline{29}$ (1981) 801.

/7/ Gehlen, P.C.: "Interatomic Potentials and Simulation of Lattice Defects", edited by P.C. Gehlen, J.R. Beeler and R.I. Jaffee, Plenum, New York (1972).

/8/ Wüthrich, C.: Phil. Mag. $\underline{35}$, 325:ibid. $\underline{35}$, 337 (1977).

/9/ Seeger, A. and Wüthrich, C.: Nuovo Cimento $\underline{33B}$ (1976) 38.

/10/ Duesbery, M.S.: Acta. Met. (1983) n the press.

/11/ Dagens, L., Rasolt, M. and Taylor, R.: Phys. Rev. $\underline{B11}$, (1975) 2726.

/12/ Basinski, Z.S. and Duesbery, M.S.: "Dislocation Modelling of Physical Systems", edited by M.F. Ashby, R. Bullough, C.S. Hartley and J.P. Hirth, Pergamon, New York 1981.

/13/ Duesbery, M.S.: Proc. R. Soc. Lond. (1983) in the press.

/14/ Vitke, V.: Proc. 2nd. Int. Conf. "Strength of Metals and Alloys", Asilomar, ASM press 1970.

/15/ Vitek, V., Perrin, R.C. and Bowen, D.K.: Phil. Mag. $\underline{21}$ (1970) 1049.

/16/ Duesbery, M.S., Vitek, V. and Bowen, D.K.: Proc. R. Soc. Lond. $\underline{A332}$ (1973) 85.

/17/ Hirth, J.P. and Lothe, J.: "Theory of Dislocations", 2nd. edition, Wiley, New York 1982.

/18/ Chang, R. and Graham, L.F.: Phys. Stat. Sol. $\underline{18}$ (1966) 99.

/19/ Woo, C.H. and Puls, M.P.: J. Phys. C. $\underline{9}$ (1976) L27.

/20/ Eshelby, J.D.: Proc. R. Soc. Lond. $\underline{266A}$ (1962) 222.

/21/ Seeger, A. and Schiller, P.: Acta Met. $\underline{10}$ (1962) 348.

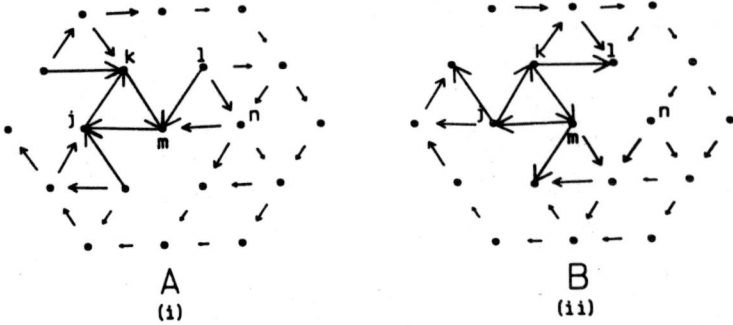

Fig.1 The stress-free dislocation core structures type A and B, shown in differential displacement form. The geometry of the projections is defined by the vectors drawn above the two cores.

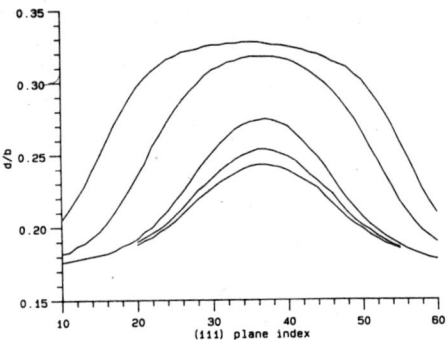

Fig.2 The shapes of double kink complexes with varying separations in equilibrium under an applied shear stress and the mutual attraction of the kinks.

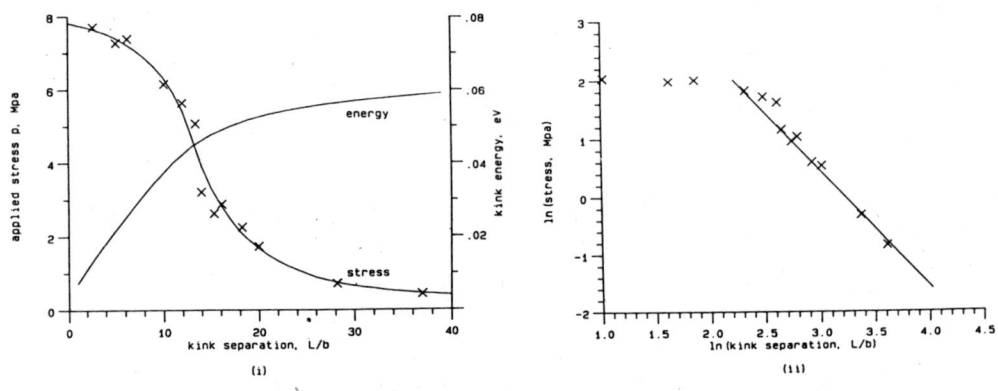

Fig.3 The kink-kink interaction force and energy. Fig.3(i) shows a linear plot of the force and energy on kink separation. Fig.3(ii) shows a logarithmic plot of the interaction force: the solid straight line indicates an inverse square law.

APPLICATION OF TIGHT BINDING TECHNIQUES TO CRYSTAL DEFECT CALCULATIONS

Donald M. Esterling
George Washington University
NASA-Langley Research Center
Hampton, VA 23665

The traditional approach to the computer simulation of defects in solids is to model the solid as a collection of "atoms" interacting via an assumed interatomic pair potential, subject to an appropriate boundary condition (e.g. displacements fixed by continuum theory beyond some distance from the defect center)/1/. A crucial issue has been, and remains, as to the viability of the assumed pair potentials in modeling real solids. Non-pair-potential contributions are well-known to be important in modeling point defects /2/. However the issue has been moot in the consideration of extended defects since the extension to more complex interactions has not, for the most part, been computationally tractable. In this paper, we will summarize an alternative - the tight binding method - that has some justification from first principle approaches and which has recently been recast in an efficient computational framework.

In an ideal computing environment, we could model a defect by considering many thousands of atoms whose equations of motion are governed by a relativistic, many body Schroedinger equation. Within the current paradigms of physics, such a solution would be an exact mirror of reality. In practice, as noted, empirical pair potentials are presumed to account for all relevant interatomic forces. Before presenting the tight-binding-method, per se, as a middle ground solution, a brief summary of our current understanding of bonding in metallic solids may be of value.

Pettifor /3/ has presented an excellent review of the current understanding of bonding in solids for simple metals (essentially the alkali series), bonding is described by a free-election-like contribution (density dependent, structure independent) and a pair potential contribution. The latter, however, only contributes about a third to the cohesive energy even for this special case. When the pair potential concept is extended to noble metals and transition metals, serious problems arise. For example, Gelatt, Ehrenreich, and Watson /4/ have produced a very good first principle description of copper and molybdenum reproducing the cohesive energy equilibrium volume, and bulk modulus. The method was then used to derive a unique pair potential by inverting the total energy as a function of atomic volume curve. The structural results (e.g. equilibrium lattice structure, phonon spectra) were unreliable. The problem is that the angular correlation of neighbors is ignored in a pair potential model. These correlations are primarily associated with the d-electron contributions. Others have also reached the conclusion that such angular correlations cannot be ignored in the context of twin and stacking fault instabilities /5/.

The tight-binding (TB) method is one of the oldest methods of calculating the electronic band structure /6/. Recently, there has been a resurgence of interest in the TB method. It has been shown that the model parameters may be obtained from other parameter free band structure calculations /7,8/. In addition, recursion techniques have been developed that enable the electron density of states to be calculated in an accurate yet efficient manner /9/. The method is particularly attractive for defect calculations in that, contrary to all other bandstructure techniques, the TB method is easily adapted to non-periodic structures. An abbreviated summary of the recursion/TB method is presented in the Appendix.

The TB method assumes the single electron wave function solution to the Schroedinger equation can be expressed as a linear combination of localized or atomic-like orbitals. This assumption works particularly well for d- and f-band electrons which reside in more localized states as opposed to the valence s or p electrons which are better described in the free electron picture. This is a point to which we will return. If, however, the electron states can be assumed to be a linear combination of states localized on various sites and if further the overlap of these states on different sites is small, then the eigenvalue or electronic bandstructure problem can be solved by diagonalizing a rather simple matrix of the Hamiltonian. For non-periodic solids, the problem becomes more complex due to the enhanced size of the matrix we must diagonalize. However the recursion methods rescue us here, producing accurate and efficient solutions for arbitrary atomic arrangements.

The recursion/TB method has been applied successfully to a variety of solid state problems. A recent review is provided by Heine, et al. /10/. This approach emphasizes the angular or structural component of the total energy, rather than the volume-dependent free electron-type terms. Hence it is most successful when treating atomic rearrangements under constant volume conditions. It follows that more or less volume conserving defects such as a screw dislocation are good candidates for this model whereas a crack would be problematic.

The most extensive application of the TB model to an extended defect is described in a series of papers by Sato and Masuda /11/. In addition, Masuda, et al. /12/ have investigated a grain boundary within this context. The (mostly attractive) d-electron contribution to the total energy is calculated within an abbreviated TB model. Specifically, the electron density of states is fixed as a Gaussian with parameters chosen to preserve up to the second moment of the true density of states curve. The repulsive s/p-electron and ion-ion contributions are modeled by a Born Mayer pair potential. Essentially the role of the Born Mayer potential is to fix the equilibrium lattice spacing and the bulk modulus. This latter approximation is not unreasonable. Pettifor /3/ has suggested that the s/p electron contributions are primarily responsible for these system characteristics, whereas the d-electron contributions control the more subtle rearrangements at constant volume.

The results of these applications of the TB model are interesting. The core structure for screw dislocations in various model bcc lattices differ from the canonical results obtained with a Johnson-like pair potential /13/. However many unnecessary assumptions were made in these treatises. Foremost is the crude approximation of the electronic density of states by a Gaussian. Many physical properties of a solid depend upon subtleties in the density of states. The tight-binding parameters are fixed by fitting the model elastic constants and equilibrium lattice parameter to certain chosen values - reminiscent of empirical pair potential techniques. Finally the relaxed core region is rather small - containing only about 100 atomic rows. For such a small region, boundary effects can dominate.

The TB parameters need not be chosen in such an arbitrary fashion. As mentioned above, they have been determined for periodic lattices from first principles bandstructure calculations. There is some question regarding the variation of these parameters as the interatomic spacing is varied - exponential versus power law.

However some recent studies re fixing this degree of freedom as well and indicate that the TB parameters decrease as a power law ($1/r^5$) for moderate separations (up to about 20% on expansion) and then decay exponentially /14/.

The other assumptions made by Sato and Masuda hinge upon the computational expense of the tight-binding model vis a' vis a pure pair potential model. An order of magnitude discussion may clarify. A more realistic electron density of states would be obtained by extending the scheme at least to about tenth or so order in the recursion technique - insteady of stopping at second order which produces a Gaussian density of states. The time to compute a complete electron density of states in the higher order scheme is relatively modest - about 8 seconds on a Cyber 175 using the code provided by the Cambridge Recursion Library. However, in order to compute the net force on one atom, such density of states calculation must be performed many times. The force in some direction may be obtained by computing the total energy of the lattice (with the defect) for the atom of interest at its desired location and again when moved a small amount in the given direction. The total energy calculation requires the density of states on all atoms in the "sphere of influence" of the atom of interest, both before and after the small displacement. Assume this sphere only includes nearest and next nearest neighbors (~ 14 atoms + the central atom). For d-electrons, the contributions from each atomic orbital on the central atom must be calculated, costing an additional factor of five. The vector force is obtained by small displacements in not one, but three, orthogonal directions producing another factor of four (three displaced calculations plus the original situation). In addition we are certainly interested in the force on more than one atom. Assume we relax a hundred atoms (another factor of 100). Lastly, the relaxation process requires these forces to be recalculated after each relaxation step. Assume this costs another factor of 20. When we finish, our modest execution time of 8 seconds has become

$$(8)*(15)*(5)*(4)*(100)*(20) \sim 5 \times 10^6 \text{ sec!}$$

Recently, Boswarva and Esterling /15/ have proposed a modification of the recursion/TB approach which reduces the computational cost by two orders of magnitude with only a mild loss of accuracy (about a 20% error). Further work /16/ has reduced the computational time by another two orders of magnitude, with no additional penalty in accuracy. Indeed, since a portion of the gain is associated with computing the forces analytically, rather than numerically, net improvement is obtained. In addition, the relaxed region is being modeled in a hybrid fashion. The region very close to the defect center is modeled with the modified tight binding method. This is the region which drives the relaxation effects elsewhere. A characteristic of essentially all computer simulation studies is that atoms more than a few lattice spacings from the defect center are relaxed only a small amount from the continuum situation. Their neighborhood resembles the perfect lattice. This is not to suggest that these small displacements can be ignored and set to zero. Their cumulative effects are substantial. Rather, in our model, we ask only that the lattice beyond some modest distance exhibit the correct atomistic "compliance" to small disturbances. Specifically, in this intermediate region the forces are obtained from an appropriate pair potential. In contrast to pure pair potential models, we do not require the resulting forces to be correct for arbitrary displacements - only small displacements from equilibrium. Such pair potentials already exist. An example of such a class are those obtained from fitting the phonon spectra /17/.

In conclusion, we suggest that our hybrid model, coupled with the modified recursion/tight binding method, will be a viable alternative to the traditional pair potential approach. This is a significant step towards realistic modeling of defects in solids.

REFERENCES

/1/ Lee, J.K. (Editor): Interatomic Potentials and Crystalline Defects, TMS-AIME, Warrendale, PA 1981.

/2/ Ho, P.S., Phys. Rev. $\underline{B3}$, 4035 1971

/3/ Pettifor, D.G. in: Atomistics of Fracture, Ed. by R.M. Latanision and J.R. Pickens, pp. 281-307, Plenum, New York 1983.

/4/ Carlsson, A.E., Gelatt, C.D., and Ehrenreich, H., Phil. Mag. $\underline{41A}$, 241, 1980.

/5/ Papon, A.M., Simon, J.P., Guyot, P., and Desjonqueres, M.C., Phil. Mag. $\underline{B40}$, 159, 1979.

/6/ Bloch, F., Z. Phys. $\underline{52}$, 555, 1928.

/7/ Pettifor, D.G., J. Phys. C.: Solid St. Phys. $\underline{2}$, 1051 1969; $\underline{5}$, 97, 1972.

/8/ Moriarty, J.A., J. Phys. F: Metal Phys. 5, 873, 1975.

/9/ Haydock, R., Heine, V., and Kelly, M.J., J. Phys. C: Sol. St. Phys. 5, 2845, 1972; 8, 2591, 1975.

/10/ Heine, V., Bullett, D.W., Haydock, R., and Kelly, M.J., in: Solid State Physics Vol. 35, Ed. by H. Ehrenreich, F. Seitz, and D. Turnbull, Academic Press, New York, 1980.

/11/ Sato, A. and Masuda, K., Phil Mag. 43, 1981.
Masuda, K. and Sato, A., J. Phys. Soc. Japan 50, 569, 1981.
Masuda, K., and Sato A., Phil Mag. 44, 799, 1981.

/12/ Masuda, K., Hashimoto, M., Ishida, Y., Yamamoto, R., and Doyama, M., J. Phys. Soc. of Japan, 51, 3990, 1982.

/13/ Vitek, V., Crystal Lattice Defects 5, 1 1974.

/14/ Esterling, D. and Bagayoko, D., personal communication.

/15/ Boswarva, I.M. and Esterling, D.M., J. Phys. C: Sol. St. Phys. 15, L729, 1982.

/16/ Boswarva, I.M. and Esterling, D.M., personal communication.

/17/ Stonham, A.M. and Taylor, R. (Editors): Handbook of Interatomic Potentials II Metals Available from AERE Harwell, Oxfordshire, England as Report AERE-R 10205, 1981.

APPENDIX

The electron density of states, n(E), describes the available energy levels in a one-electron band picture. The total electronic energy is then given by the expression

$$U = 2 \int_{-\infty}^{E_F} E \, n(E) \, dE \qquad (A1)$$

Here E_F is the Fermi energy and the factor of two accounts for the two electron spin states. As mentioned in the text, the force on an atom can be calculated by evaluating $U=U^{(0)}$ for the given atomic geometry and again when the atom of interest is displaced by a small amount (e.g. Δx in the x direction) giving $U=U^{(1)}$. The force on the atom of interest is then

$$F_x = [U^{(0)} - U^{(1)}] / \Delta x \qquad (A2)$$

These forces can then be used in a standard relaxation code. Note that, in general, the resulting forces are inherently non-central. It is possible to break the total energy U into contributions from individual atoms. However the contribution from one atom to the force on a second atom depends, in general, on the atomic coordinate not just in a pairwise fashion.

The density of states can be obtained via a sequence of steps. Start with the model Schroedinger equation for the solid

$$H \psi_i = E_i \psi_i \qquad (A3)$$

where H is the energy operator or Hamiltonian, ψ_i is an eigenfunction and E_i is the associated eigenvalue. Define the matrix elements H_{ij} as

$$H_{ij} = \int d^3r \, \psi_i H \psi_j \qquad (A4)$$

Further define the "Green's function" as

$$G(E) = [E - H]^{-1} \qquad (A5)$$

i.e. the inverse of the matrix $E\delta_{ij} + H_{ij}$, where δ_{ij} is the usual Kroneker delta function.

At last the density of states is obtained as

$$n(E) = -\frac{1}{\pi} \operatorname{Im} \sum_i' G_{ii}(E + i\delta) \qquad (A6)$$

where "Im" refers to the imaginary part, δ is a infinitesimally small, positive number, and the sum i is over individual atomic sites.

All of this formalism simply defers the force calculation to evaluating the Green's function. A series expansion for G_{ij} can be obtained from (A5) as

$$G_{ij}(E) = \frac{\delta_{ij}}{E} + \frac{H_{ij}}{E^2} + \frac{H_{i\ell} H_{\ell j}}{E^3} + \frac{H_{i\ell} H_{\ell m} H_{mj}}{E^4} + \ldots \qquad (A7)$$

There is an implied sum over repeated indices. Hence as we know the matrix elements, H_{ij}, we may evaluate G_{ij} and hence n(E). Unfortunately, the series expansion must be summed, at least approximately, to infinite order to get sensible results. In passing, we should note that the approximation of Sato and Masuda, et al. correspond to including only the first three terms exactly and making rather crude approximations for the remaining terms in the infinite series.

The recursion method/9,10/ is a nifty way to approximate the sum in equation (A7) which is both computationally efficient and which preserves certain exact properties of the density of states to very high order. In essence the Green's function is approximated by a continued fraction

$$G_{ii}(E) = \cfrac{1}{E - a_0 - \cfrac{b_1}{E - a_1 - \cfrac{b_2}{E - \ldots}}} \qquad (A8)$$

where a_0, b_0, a_1, b_1, etc. can be obtained from the matrix elements H_{ij} by well-defined recursion relations. With this new form for the

Green's function, it is possible to truncate the series at some finite order and now obtain a sensible density of states. As usual, each truncation at a higher order carries a certain extra computational price. In the text, the computational times refer to truncating the series at the eleventh order. This order reproduces many of the important features in the exact density states.

Boswarva and Esterling /15,16/ introduced a number of simplifications into this TB/recursion method. One important simplification was to avoid many of the computational steps in proceeding from (A8) through (A6) and (A1) to finally evaluating the forces with (A2). They recast the expression for the forces as an analytical function of the recursion parameters which allows a direct evaluation of the forces once the parameters are known.

The second simplification was predicated upon the following observations. First, it can be shown that the higher order recursion parameters depend essentially upon the crystal geometry in regions which are successively further and further removed from the site of interest. The near site contributions decrease in importance as the order increases. Second, as noted in the text most defects "heal" rather rapidly in that the crystal geometry away from the defect center mimics a perfect crystal. Using these ideas, Boswarva and Esterling proposed only to calculate the lowest order recursion parameters (a_0, b_0, a_1, b_1) exactly. The higher order parameters were fixed at their perfect crystal values. These latter can be computed once and for all and then stored for retrieval. The low order parameters can be evaluated rather quickly for arbitrary atomic arrangements. This second simplification was checked in a variety of test cases for various numbers of d electrons per atom. The worst case deviation was about 20%. A more systematic check is underway with an attempt to obtain insight into the circumstances under which this latter approximation breaks down. However, as noted in the text, the several orders of magnitude improvement in computation time now renders the TB method as a feasible alternative to the empirical pair potential approach.

*Research supported by the National Science Foundation

MOTION OF DISLOCATIONS IN BCC METALS AT LOW TEMPERATURES

S. Takeuchi, T. Hashimoto and K. Maeda

Institute for Solid State Physics, University of Tokyo
Roppongi, Minato-ku, Tokyo 106, Japan

§1. Introduction

In comparison with fcc metals and alloys, the plastic behaviour of bcc metals in general exhibits characteristic features at low temperatures; a strong temperature dependence of the yield stress and a characteristic orientation dependence of slip [1]. In the last two decades, many efforts have been devoted to the understanding of the above features both from the experimental and theoretical investigations. As a result, it seems now widely accepted that the plasticity of bcc metals at low temperatures is governed by an intrinsic resistance to the motion of screw dislocations. However, there exist two conceptually different views as to the origin of the lattice resistance in spite of a number of computer-simulation studies on the screw dislocation in bcc lattices [2]; one attaches importance to the sessile dissociation of the dislocation core and the other to the genuine Peierls potential. In the next section, based on our computer modelling of the screw dislocation motion [3], discussion will be made as to the distinction of the above two views.

Irrespective of the detailed mechanism of the activation process of dislocation motion, the thermal-activation analyses of plastic deformation have shown that the Arrhenius type strain-rate equation is obeyed for a wide temperature range for a variety of materials [4]. At very low temperatures typically below 50 K, however, deviation from an extrapolation from higher temperatures has been observed rather commonly in fcc metals and alloys as reviewed recently by Parkhomenko and Pustovalov [5]. For various bcc metals, the present authors have performed detailed experiments around helium temperatures and also found out a marked deviation from the Arrhenius rate equation below a few tens of kelvin [6]. In §3, experimental results will be presented on the precision measurements of the temperature and strain-rate dependences of the flow stress of β-CuZn single crystals down to below 1 K and the results are interpreted based on a simple treatment of the quantum mechanical oscillation of the dislocation.

§2. Peierls or Pseudo-Peierls Mechanism?

Earlier sessile dissociation models of the screw dislocation in the bcc lattice, typically the three-fold symmetric dissociation into three partials with b = 1/6[111], assumed the existence of stable stacking faults e.g. on {112} plane. Later computer-simulation studies generally disproved the earlier distinct-dissociation models, but very often they still yielded a three-fold symmetric core-extension, i.e. the Burgers vector is distributed into fractional ones around the centre [2]. Thus, the sessile dissociation concept survives in a modified sense. On the other hand, Suzuki was the first who pointed out that the geometrical characteristics of the bcc lattice necessarily produce the low-energy and high-energy positions of a screw dislocation alternately in the lattice, which give rise to a high Peierls potential [7]. Thus, there exist two concepts as to the origin of the lattice resistance to the screw dislocation; the dislocation motion governed by the former origin is often referred to as the pseudo-Peierls mechanism. It may be difficult to distinguish the two types of the mechanism for real crystals, but as far as our models are concerned, the ordinary Peierls mechanism is more appropriate to describe the dislocation motion for the following reasons:

(1) Depending on the interatomic potential, the stable core structure can be isotropic without exhibiting three-fold symmetric spreading [8]. Examples of the two types of the core are shown in Fig. 1 by the displacement map representation. In the left type of the core which may be called the polarized type, the central three atomic rows (denoted by P in the figure) displace either upward or downward with respect to the unpolarized state of the right type and as a result the strain extends in three directions. Using simple models based on inter-atomic-row potentials, one of the present authors (ST) obtained a criterion for the unpolarized core to be stable [8]. He calculated the Peierls stress for a number of models in which the stable core type is either the polarized or unpolarized type [3]. The calculated values distributed in a wide range from 0.0015μ to 0.045μ (μ: the shear modulus) but an important fact is that the distributed Peierls stresses are

even higher for the unpolarized cores than for the polarized cores†; namely, the high Peierls stress is not associated with the initial core extension.

(2) In the original meaning of the pseudo-Peierls mechanism, the spreading part of the strain field (generalized stacking fault) must be constricted before the core translates to the next stable position. In our polarized cores, even under a high stress just below the Peierls stress the spreading nature of the strain-field is essentially unchanged in most cases. An example is shown in Fig. 2. This fact implies that the Peierls stress is not determined by the stress required for the constriction of the extended strain field.

Thus, from these results of the computer-simulation studies it seems most natural to consider that the high resistance to the motion of screw dislocation in bcc metals is due to the high Peierls potential in the usual sense, and not necessarily related to the extension of the strain field as realized in polarized cores. Furthermore, as pointed out previously [8], the glide behaviour of high purity iron and molybdenum [10] is reasonably explained if the core structure is of the unpolarized type.

§3. Peierls Mechanism at Very Low Temperatures

3.1. Experiment

Since the screw dislocation motion is considered to be governed by the ordinary Peierls mechanism, it is interesting to investigate the quantum effect on the Peierls mechanism by detailed experiments at very low temperatures down to below 1 K. For this purpose, β-CuZn (ordered bcc crystal) has been selected for the following reasons: Because the stress level for slip at helium temperatures is rather low compared with elemental bcc transition metals, β-CuZn single crystals undergo stable deformation, without exhibiting geometrical necking, up to a high strain; this enables us to obtain reliable data in the stress and temperature change tests at helium temperatures. Also due to the low stress level, the thermal instability deformation which results in the serrated

---

† The same result has been obtained for models based on Johnson-Wilson potentials for five bcc metals [9].

flow is not liable to take place compared with transition bcc metals. Furthermore, twinning deformation is suppressed due to the ordered structure.

Even if the macroscopic thermal instability deformation does not take place, the localized slip deformation may induce a temperature rise at the slip band. To minimize the possible temperature rise, deformation experiments have been performed at very low strain rates under creep condition. The accurate strain measurement has been done by use of a special capacitance type extensometer which was employed previously for the precise stress-strain measurements of metallic glasses [11].

Specimens used were the same as those used previously [12]. The orientation selected is shown in the standard stereographic triangle given in Fig. 3. The primary slip system of this orientation has been found to be the twinning {112} plane at low temperatures, and the yield stress of it shows the minimum value. After a small amount of pre-strain of $\sim 0.5\%$, the same specimen was crept at different temperatures between 1.8 K and 77 K and under different stress levels; at a fixed temperature the stress level was increased stepwise by a small amount of 0.3 MN/m^2 and the creep rate was measured in the strain-rate range of $5 \times 10^{-7} \sim 5 \times 10^{-5} \mathrm{s}^{-1}$ and thus the stress dependence of the strain-rate was measured. In this procedure, the effect of the strain-hardening on the creep rate was corrected by a stress-reversal experiment. The experiment below 1.8 K in a ^{3}He cryostat was done under a constant strain-rate and with a stress-relaxation test.

3.2. Analysis

The temperature dependence of the flow stress normalized to a shear strain-rate of $10^{-5} \mathrm{s}^{-1}$ and of the value of $\partial \tau / \partial \ln \dot{\gamma}$ are shown in Fig. 3. From these data, one can obtain the activation volume v^* and the activation enthalpy ΔH in the Arrhenius type strain-rate equation according to the conventional procedure. The value of exponent $\Delta H/kT$ thus obtained for the strain-rate of $10^{-5} \mathrm{s}^{-1}$ is plotted against temperature in Fig. 4. If the Arrhenius rate equation holds, $\Delta H/kT$ should be a constant value. The result shows that the Arrhenius rate equation is obeyed above 15 K but breaks drastically below that. Such an anomaly comes from the fact that the slope of the τ-T curve decreases on lowering the temperature while the $\partial \tau / \partial \ln \dot{\gamma}$ value does not tend to zero, as seen in Fig. 3.

3.3. Origin of the anomaly

The anomalous temperature dependence of the yield stress at low temperatures ($\lesssim 50$ K) observed in fcc and hcp metals and alloys has most successfully been interpreted in terms of the dynamical effect on the dislocation motion (see [5]). This effect, however, is not applicable to bcc metals whose deformation is controlled by the Peierls mechanism at low temperatures. The most plausible origin is the quantum mechanical effect on the dislocation motion, which was first suggested by Mott as a tunneling of a dislocation through point obstacles [13]. In this paper, the quantum penetration of a dislocation through a Peierls potential will be treated by a simple treatment of the quantum mechanical oscillation of the dislocation lying in the Peierls valley.

The probability distribution of the position q of an oscillating dislocation with a frequency ω at a temperature T in the harmonic approximation is given by the Bloch formula expressed by

$$P(q) \propto \exp\left[-q^2 \bigg/ \left\{\frac{\hbar}{m\omega} \coth\left(\frac{\hbar\omega}{2kT}\right)\right\}\right], \qquad (1)$$

where m is the effective mass of the oscillating dislocation segment. The probability that the dislocation position exceeds a critical value q* corresponding to the potential maximum E* which is a function of the stress is approximated for large value of the exponent ($\gg 1$) by

$$\int_{q^*}^{\infty} P(q)\,dq \propto \frac{1}{2q^*} \exp\left[-q^{*2} \bigg/ \left\{\frac{\hbar}{m\omega} \coth\left(\frac{\hbar\omega}{2kT}\right)\right\}\right].$$

Using the relation $q^* \simeq \sqrt{2E^*/m}/\omega$ and putting $\theta \equiv \hbar\omega/k$, the probability is proportional to

$$\frac{1}{\sqrt{E^*}} \exp\left[-E^* \bigg/ \left\{\frac{k\theta}{2} \coth\left(\frac{\theta}{2T}\right)\right\}\right]. \qquad (2)$$

The exponent tends to the classical value of $-E^*/kT$ for $T \gg \theta$ and to a constant of $\exp(-2E^*/k\theta)$ for $T \to 0$. The latter fact, which is a natural consequence of the uncertainty principle, leads to the fact that the strain-rate dependence does not disappear as the temperature tends to zero, as observed experimentally. From eq. (2), the experimental value of the exponent analysed according to the conventional procedure is temperature dependent following the relation

$$(\theta/T)\operatorname{cosech}(\theta/T). \qquad (3)$$

The curve drawn in Fig. 3 corresponds to the above relation for $\theta = 7$ K; this value results from $\omega \sim 10^{12} s^{-1}$, which seems to be a reasonable value for the kink pair formation at high stress near the Peierls stress. Thus, the anomaly, in the sense of the classical rate process, observed at very low temperatures seems to be a natural consequence of the quantum mechanical effect of the dislocation oscillation.

References

/1/ See, e.g., Christian J.W.: Strength of Metals and Alloys (ICSMA 2), Amer. Soc. Metals, Metals Park, Ohio 1970, p.31; Kubin L.P.: Review of the Deformation Behaviour of Materials, Freund Publishing House Ltd., Tel-Aviv 1975, Vol. 1, p. 244.
/2/ E.g., Vitek V.: Crystal Lattice Defects 5 (1974) 1.
/3/ Takeuchi S.: Interatomic Potentials and Crystalline Defects, edited by J. K. Lee, The Met. Soc. AIME, Warrendale, Pa. 1981, p. 201.
/4/ See references in /6/.
/5/ Parkhomenko T.A., Pustovalov V.V.: Phys. Stat. Sol. (a) 74 (1982) 11.
/6/ Takeuchi S., Hashimoto T., Maeda K.: Trans. Jpn. Inst. Metals 23 (1982) 60.
/7/ Suzuki H.: Dislocation Dynamics, edited by A. R. Rosenfield, G. T. Hahn, A. L. Bement, Jr. and R. I. Jaffee, McGraw-Hill, New York 1968, p. 679.
/8/ Takeuchi S.: Phil. Mag. A 39 (1979) 661.
/9/ Kuramoto E., Aono Y., Tsutsumi T.: Strength of Metals and Alloys (ICSMA 6), edited by R. C. Gifkins, Pergamon Press, Oxford 1982, Vol. 1, p.69.
/10/ Aono Y., Kuramoto E., Kitajima K.: Ibid. p. 9.
/11/ Hashimoto T., Maeda K., Takeuchi S.: Ibid. p. 173.
/12/ Hashimoto T., Takeuchi S.: Acta Met. 30 (1982) 513.
/13/ Mott N. F.: Phil. Mag. 1 (1956) 568.

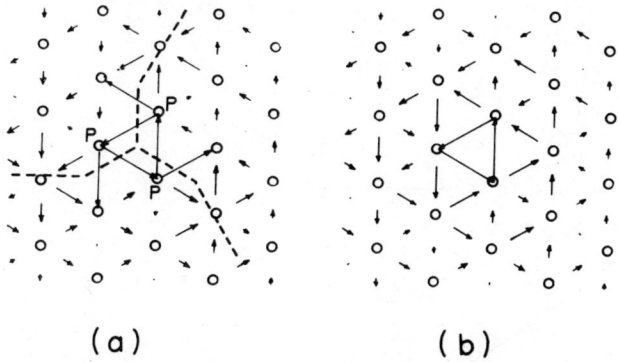

Fig. 1. Two types of the core structure of a screw dislocation in the bcc lattice as represented by the displacement map: (a) polarized core, (b) unpolarized core.

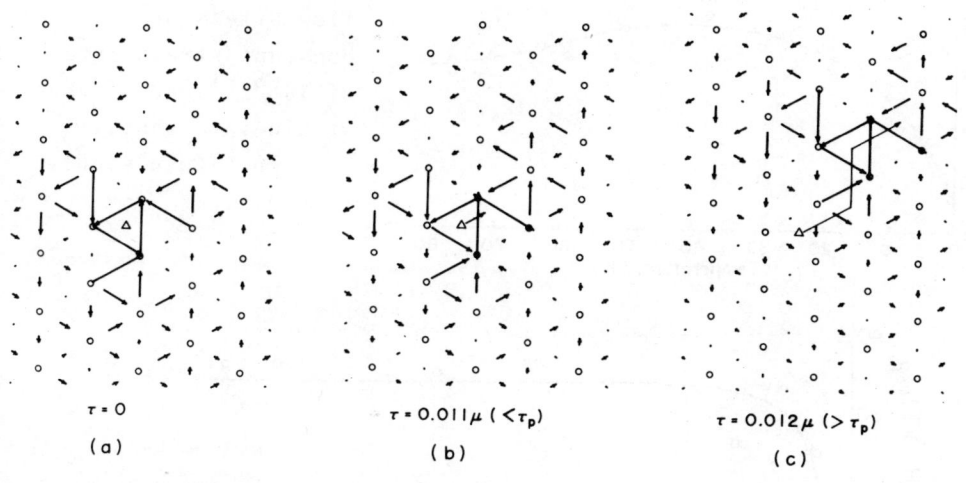

Fig. 2. Example of core translation behaviour under stress (model due to $\phi[2.5-2]$ potential in a previous paper [3]): (a) under no stress; (b) under a stress just below the Peierls stress; (c) under a stress higher than the Peierls stress, so that the core is translating.

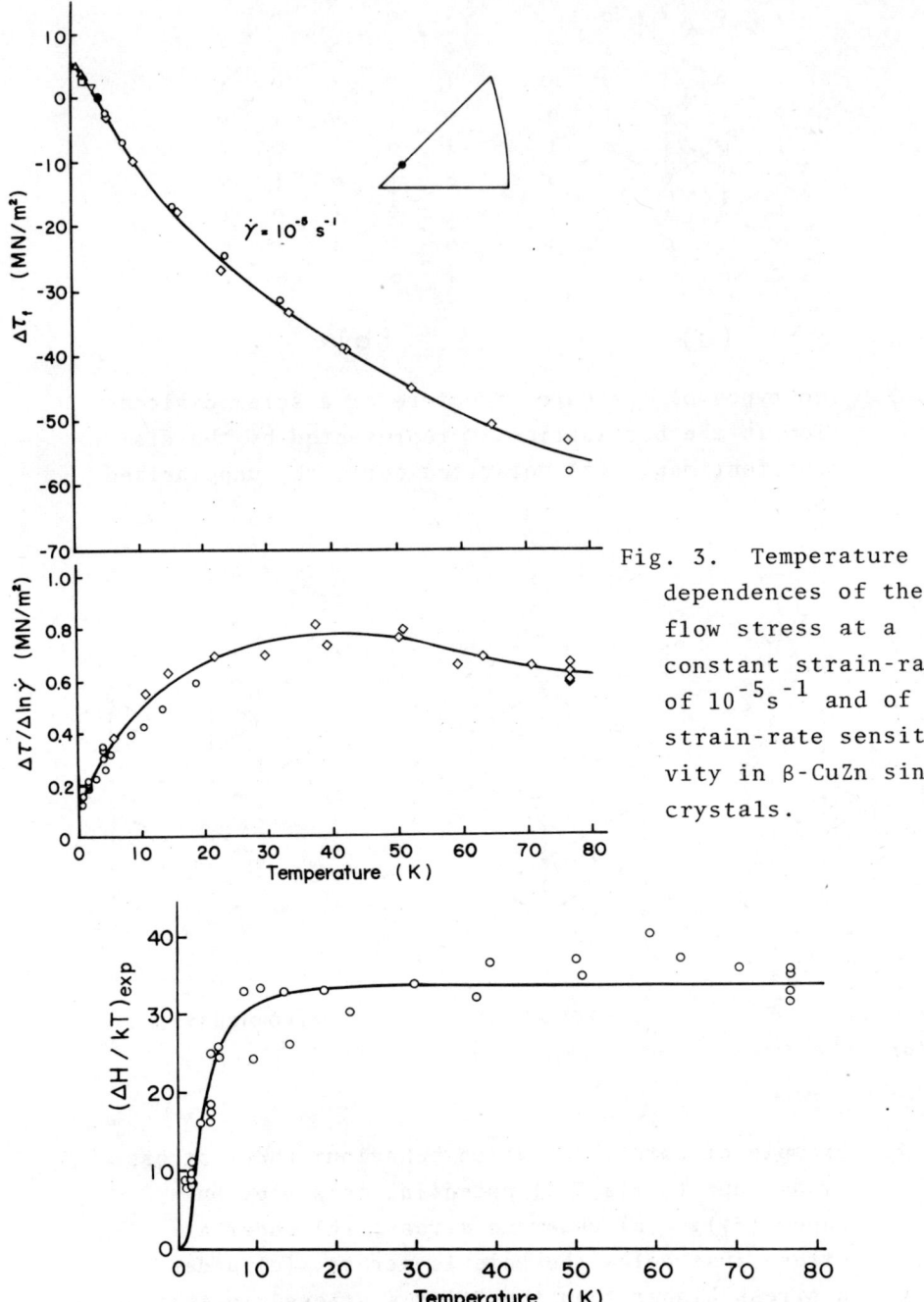

Fig. 3. Temperature dependences of the flow stress at a constant strain-rate of $10^{-5} s^{-1}$ and of the strain-rate sensitivity in β-CuZn single crystals.

Fig. 4. ΔH/kT value in the Arrhenius rate equation analysed according to the conventional procedure. The curve shows the dependence of eq. (3) with θ = 7K.

THE LOW-TEMPERATURE FLOW STRESS OF HIGH-PURITY α-IRON SINGLE CRYSTALS

D. Brunner, J. Diehl, and A. Seeger

Max-Planck-Institut für Metallforschung, Stuttgart, Germany (F.R.)

Introduction

It is now generally accepted that the pronounced increase of the flow stress of pure bcc metals towards low temperatures (below the "knee" temperature T_k) and the strong strain-rate sensitivity associated with it are caused by the low low-temperature mobility of screw dislocations in this crystal structure. It should therefore be possible to obtain information on the properties and the behaviour of the screw dislocations from the analysis of the low-temperature flow-stress of high-purity bcc metals. Such an analysis has to take into account that the low-temperature increase of the flow stress does not obey a uniform law /1,2/. This complication offers the possibility to gain more information than one might hope to derive from simpler situations. The appropriate theoretical framework appears to be the formation of pairs of kinks of opposite sign and the diffusion of kinks on the screw dislocations /2-5/.

Experimentally, the non-uniformity just mentioned is documented on the one hand by "the hump" (an inflection point in the temperature dependence of the flow stress observed on several bcc metals in different laboratories), on the other hand by a second transition between different laws occuring at lower temperatures /1/. The temperature region near and above "the hump" has been investigated by Zwiesele and Diehl /6/ by means of yield-stress measurements on high-purity α-Fe single crystals and in particular detail by Ackermann et al. /7,8/ by flow-stress measurements on various cyclically deformed bcc metals (Nb, Ta, Mo and α-Fe). The present communication is primarily intended as a progress report on the extension of the work of Zwiesele and Diehl /6/ to lower temperatures and as a first attempt to analyse the low-temperature non-uniformity in terms of the kink picture.

Experimental Procedures and Results

Rod-shaped α-iron single crystals with 2.2 mm in diameter and 40 mm measuring length were prepared as described by Zwiesele and Diehl /6/ (strain-anneal method; Johnson-Matthey iron purified in dry H_2, vacuum degassed) and with a similar orientation (angle χ between (110) plane and plane of maximum shear stress + 18°). The tensile tests were carried out with the tensile machine /9/ in the low-temperature irradiation facility at the Karlsruhe research reactor FR2 (without irradiation) at a shear strain rate $\dot{\varepsilon} = 8.5 \cdot 10^{-4} s^{-1}$.

The temperature dependence of the <u>macro</u>-yield stress was determined in successive tests at different temperatures according to the criteria and correction methods described earlier /6/; the results obtained in this way were in agreement with those on virgin crystals. The strain-rate sensitivity of the flow stress was obtained from stress-relaxation tests. The Schmid factor for $\{110\}$, $[1\bar{1}1]$ slip was used to deduce resolved shear stresses τ from the tensile-stress data. Fig. 1 shows the temperature dependence of the effective critical resolved shear stress $\tau^* = \tau - \tau_G$, where the athermal stress component τ_G has been adjusted to the τ value at the highest measuring temperature of Zwiesele and Diehl (410K) /6/. Fig. 2 gives the temperature dependence of the temperature sensitivity $(\partial\tau/\partial T)_{\dot{\varepsilon}} \simeq (\partial\tau^*/\partial T)_{\dot{\varepsilon}}$ and of the strain-rate sensitivity $(1/T)(\partial\tau/\partial \ln \dot{\varepsilon})_T = (1/T)(\partial \ln\tau^*/\partial \ln \dot{\varepsilon})_T$ of the resolved macro-yield stress.

Discussion

Qualitatively speaking, the temperature variation of the temperature sensitivity and of the strain-rate sensitivity of the macro-yield stress shown in Fig. 2 confirm the conclusions presented earlier /1,6/. It is evident that non-uniformities occur not only between 220 and 250 K but also at about 130 K. For the time being we distinguish the three regimes above, in between, and below these temperatures by roman numerals I, II and III.

The theoretical background required for the quantitative analysis of the data in terms of the formation of kink-pairs on screw dislocations may be found in the literature /2-5,7/. The key quantity in the analysis is the enthalpy of kink-pair formation, $H_{kp}(\tau^*)$, as a function of the effective stress τ^*. A preliminary inspection of the data shows that the parameter x introduced by Ackermann et al. /7/ is large compared to unity so that in the treatment of the kink-pair formation rate the so-called transition state theory may be used. This means that we may write the plastic strain rate as (k_B = Boltzmann's constant)

$$\dot{\varepsilon} = \dot{\varepsilon}_o \exp(S_{kp}/k_B) \exp[-H_{kp}(\tau^*)/k_B T], \qquad (1)$$

where $\dot{\varepsilon}_o \propto T^{-1/2}$. The temperature and strain-rate dependence of the kink-pair formation entropy S_{kp} becomes negligible at higher temperatures. In the following analysis, which in this respect must be considered preliminary, we disregard these dependences and absorb $\exp(S_{kp}/k_B)$ as a constant factor in $\dot{\varepsilon}_o$.

I) It has been demonstrated in detail /2,7,8/ that at effective shear stresses $\tau^* < \bar{\tau}$ ($\bar{\tau}$ to be discussed below) the long-range elastic interaction of the kinks accounts well for the stress-dependence of the kink-pair formation enthalpy. This interaction leads to

$$H_{kp}(\tau^*) = 2H_k - 2\alpha \tau^{*1/2}, \qquad (2)$$

where H_k is the energy of formation of an isolated kink and

$$\alpha^2 = a^3 b \gamma_o/2. \qquad (3)$$

In (3) a denotes the "height" of the kinks (i.e., the distance of the Peierls valleys connected by a kink), b the dislocation strength and γ_o the prelogarithmic factor of the line-tension γ_d of the dislocation. γ_o/b^2 is determined entirely by the elastic moduli of the material.

Under the assumptions stated above the parameters of (2) may be derived from the experimental data of Figs. 1 and 2 as follows /7/:

$$2H_k = -\frac{k_B T}{(\partial \tau^*/\partial \ln \dot{\varepsilon})_T} \left\{ 2\tau^* - T(\partial \tau^*/\partial T)_{\dot{\varepsilon}} \right\} + k_B T/2 \qquad (4)$$

$$\alpha^2 = \tau^* \left\{ k_B T/(\partial \tau^*/\partial \ln \dot{\varepsilon})_T \right\}^2. \qquad (5)$$

For the purpose of deducing $2H_k$ and α^2 from the present experiments by means of (4) and (5) we may treat $\dot{\varepsilon}_o$ as a constant. Theory then predicts

$$\tau^* = A^2 (T_k - T)^2; \quad (\partial \tau^*/\partial T)_{\dot{\varepsilon}} = 2A^2 (T_k - T) \qquad (6,7)$$

$$\frac{1}{k_B T} \left(\frac{\partial \tau^*}{\partial \ln \dot{\varepsilon}} \right)_T = B(T_k - T), \qquad (8)$$

and, with (4) and (5),

$$2 H_k = (2A^2 T_k/B) + k_B T/2; \qquad \alpha = A/B . \qquad (9,10)$$

The experimental data are described quite well by (7) and (8) with constant slopes $2A^2$ and B ($A^2 = 5,25 \cdot 10^{-3}$ MNm^{-2}K^{-2}, B = $3,48 \cdot 10^{-4}$ MNm^{-2}K^{-2}, T_k = 330 K). They give ($k_B T/2 \approx 0.01$ eV)

$$2H_k = 0.87 \text{ eV}; \qquad \alpha = 2.87 \cdot 10^{-24} \text{N}^{1/2}\text{m}^2; \qquad \ln(\dot{\varepsilon}_o/\dot{\varepsilon}) = 30. \qquad (11a,b,c)$$

According to generous estimates of the errors involved, $2H_k$ and $\ln(\dot{\varepsilon}_o/\dot{\varepsilon})$ should be correct within $\pm 5\%$ whereas the error limits of α may well be smaller.

With $\gamma_o = 1.27 \cdot 10^{-9}$N /8/ and $b = 3^{1/2} a_o/2$ ($a_o = 2,866 \cdot 10^{-10}$m room-temperature lattice parameter of α-Fe) we deduce from (3) and (11b)

$$(3/2)^{1/2} a/a_o = 1.60 . \qquad (12)$$

The right-hand side of (12) is definitely larger than the value unity expected from the separation of adjacent Peierls valleys on {110} planes. The experimental result shows clearly that in the temperature range 230 K to 330 K the motion of the screw dislocations involves kinks other than those of minimum height $a = (2/3)^{1/2} a_o$. The most likely candidates are kinks on {211} planes (shortest height $a = 2^{1/2} a_o = 1.73 (2/3)^{1/2} a_o$) or double kinks on {110} planes ($a = 2(2/3)^{1/2} a_o$). See also subsection III) and a forthcoming paper /10/.

II) In the stress regime $\tau^* > \hat{\tau}$ $H_{kp}(\tau^*)$ is calculated from the so-called line-tension model. In this model the interaction between adjacent parts of a dislocation is described by a line-tension γ_d.

The potential energy per unit length of a straight dislocation, $U(u)$, is assumed to be a unique function of the displacement u out of one of its Peierls valleys. In terms of $U(u)$ the Peierls stress τ_p is defined by ($U' = dU/du$, $U'' = d^2U/du^2$, etc.)

$$\tau_p = U'(u_p)/b, \qquad U''(u_p) = 0, \qquad U'''(u_p) < 0 , \qquad (13)$$

For $\tau \ll \tau_p$ we may write

$$H_{kp} = 2H_k - ab \left[\gamma_d/U''(0)\right]^{1/2} \tau^* \left[1 + \ln(\hat{\tau}/\tau^*)\right] + O(\tau^{*2}), \qquad (14)$$

where $\hat{\tau}$ may be expressed in terms of $U(u)$.

In the special case of a so-called Eshelby potential /11,3/

$$U(u) = 3^{3/2} \, ab \, \tau_p (u/a)^2 \left[1-(u/a)\right]^2 \qquad (15)$$

we have

$$ab \left[\gamma_d/U''(0)\right]^{1/2} = 3^{-1/2} H_k/\tau_p; \quad \hat{\tau} = 4 \cdot 3^{3/2} \tau_p \, . \qquad (16a,b)$$

Taking $2H_k$ from (11a) and $\ln(\dot{\varepsilon}_o/\dot{\varepsilon})$ from (11c), we may fit the effective shear stress between 130 K and 230 K quite well by (14). If for the remaining fit parameter the relationships (16) are used, one finds

$$\tau_p = 320 \text{ MN/m}^2 \, . \qquad (17)$$

The stress $\bar{\tau}$ separating the regimes of validity of the elastic-interaction and the line-tension model is defined by the requirement that the expressions (2) and (14) for $H_{kp}(\tau^*)$ shall agree, i.e. by

$$(\bar{\tau}/\hat{\tau}) \left[1+\ln(\hat{\tau}/\bar{\tau})\right]^2 = (2a \, U''(0)/b\hat{\tau}) \, (\gamma_o/\gamma_d) \, . \qquad (18)$$

Its numerical value in the present case is

$$\bar{\tau} \approx 75 \text{ MN/m}^2 \, . \qquad (19)$$

III) Several authors /2,5,12,13/ have noted that at effective stresses sufficiently close to the Peierls stress τ_p, i.e., for $(\tau_p - \tau^*) \ll \tau_p$, the functional dependence of the kink-pair formation enthalpy on τ^* becomes independent of the choice of $U(u)$. With the notations introduced above we have

$$H_{kp}(\tau^*) = (24/5)(b\gamma_d)^{1/2} \left[-2b/U'''(u_p)\right]^{3/4} (\tau_p-\tau^*)^{5/4} + O\left[(\tau_p-\tau^*)^{9/4}\right]. \qquad (20)$$

In the special case of the Eshelby potential (15) the proportionality factor in (20) may be expressed in terms of the kink-formation energy by means of the relationship

$$2H_k = 4(3/2)^{5/4} (b\gamma_d)^{1/2} \left[-2b/U'''(u_p)\right]^{3/4} \tau_p^{5/4} . \qquad (21)$$

Under the assumption of $\dot{\varepsilon}_o$=const. (which is justified according to the experimentally determined temperature variation of the activation enthalpy in this temperature range) the present data may be fitted quite well to (20) up to about 70 K (see Fig. 3). With $\ln(\dot{\varepsilon}_o/\dot{\varepsilon}) = 30$ the fit gives

$$\tau_P = 400 \text{ MN/m}^2, \tag{22a}$$

and, if use is made of (21),

$$2 H_k = 0.72 \text{ eV}. \tag{22b}$$

The temperature dependence of the effective stress calculated for the Eshelby potential according to /2/ can be fitted very well even up to 120 K with

$$\tau_P = 405 \text{ MN/m}^2; \quad 2 H_k = 0.64 \text{ eV}, \tag{23a,b}$$

which is shown in Fig. 2 as the dotted line denoted with III.

The following results appear to us particularly noteworthy:
(i) The Eshelby potential fits the experimental data quite well up to about 120 K.
(ii) The $\ln(\dot{\varepsilon}_o/\dot{\varepsilon})$ values deduced in the regimes I and III are about the same and thus compatible with the idea that the same dislocations determine the yield stress over the entire temperature interval investigated.
(iii) The Peierls stress τ_P and the kink-formation enthalpy H_k deduced from the measurements below 120 K (Eqs. 23a,b or 22a,b) do not agree with the τ_P value obtained in regime II (Eq.17) or with the H_k value obtained in regime I (Eq. 11a). It is thus not possible to account for the entire range of $H_{kp}(\tau^*)$ by an Eshelby potential (15) with fixed parameters. In itself, this is not surprising since we have seen that kinks other than the elementary kinks on {110} planes must be involved. We can hardly expect that a potential as simple as (15) describes such a situation well. The comparison between experiment and theory should therefore be based on more elaborate forms of U(u). The rather abrupt transition between the regimes II and III, each of which is quite well accounted for by the Eshelby potential, suggests another explanation: At low temperatures it is known that slip in α-Fe occurs exclusively in {110} planes /14/. It is natural to assume that in regime III the yield stress is controlled by elementary kinks on {110} planes. At high temperatures there is a strong tendency for α-Fe to slip on {211} planes /15,16/. The assumption that in the regimes I and II the yield stress is to a large extent determined by the kink-pair formation on {211} planes is supported by the numerical result (12) and by the observation

that the regimes I and II may be described by the same H_k value. Taken together, the two assumptions just made suggest that the $H_{kp}(\tau^*)$ curves for the two different types of kinks may cross at the stress level of the transition between II and III and that at about 130 K a rather abrupt transition in the kink mechanism of dislocation movement takes place.

Conclusions

In each of the three temperature regimes considered in this paper (I: T > 230 K, II: 130 K < T < 230 K, III: T < 130 K) the temperature dependence of the flow stress of pure α-Fe single crystals is well described by the theory of kink-pair formation and kink-kink interactions on screw dislocations. The transition between different laws around 230 K (sometimes called "the hump") is explained naturally as a change in the saddle-point interaction between two kinks of opposite sign.

The origin of the transition around 130 K is less clear yet. Our analysis shows that this transition cannot be explained in terms of an Eshelby potential with fixed parameters τ_p and $2 H_k$. A possible explanation is that the mode of motion of the screw dislocations changes from slip on a {110} plane at low temperatures to slip on {211}-planes at high temperatures. The quantitative investigation of this problem area is clearly a task for the future.

Acknowledgement

The support of Kernforschungszentrum Karlsruhe GmbH in the course of the experimental work is gratefully acknowledged.

References

/1/ J. Diehl, M. Schreiner, S. Staiger und S. Zwiesele, Scripta Met. 10, 949 (1976).
/2/ A. Seeger, Z. Metallkunde 72, 369 (1981).
/3/ A. Seeger and P. Schiller, Phys. Acoustics Vol. IIIA, Chapt. 8 (ed. by W.P. Mason) Academic Press, New York and London 1966.

/4/ A. Seeger and Ch. Wüthrich, Nuovo Cimento 33B, 38 (1976).
/5/ A. Seeger, J. Physique 42, C5-201 (1981).
/6/ S. Zwiesele and J. Diehl, in Proc. 5th Int. Conf. Strength of Metals and Alloys (ed. by P. Haasen, V. Gerold, and G. Kostorz) Vol. 1, p. 59, Pergamon Press, Oxford (1979).
/7/ F. Ackermann, H. Mughrabi, and A. Seeger, Acta Met. in press.
/8/ F. Ackermann, H. Mughrabi, and A. Seeger to be published.
/9/ J. Diehl, Ch. Leitz, and W. Decker, Z. Metallkunde, 61, 443 (1970).
/10/ A. Seeger, to be submitted to Krist. u. Techn.
/11/ J.D. Eshelby, Proc. Roy. Soc. A266, 222 (1962).
/12/ M. Büttiker and R. Landauer, Phys.Rev.Letters 43, 1453 (1979).
/13/ T. Mori and M. Kato, Phil.Mag.A, 43, 1315 (1981).
/14/ Y. Aono, E. Kuramoto, and K. Kitajima, Rep. Res. Inst. Appl. Mech., Kyushu Univ., Vol. XXIX, p. 127 (1981).
/15/ W.A. Spitzig and A.S. Keh, Met.Trans. 1, 2751 (1970).
/16/ M. Matsui, A. Kimura, and H. Kimura, in Proc. 5th Int. Conf. on the Strength of Metals and Alloys (ed. by P. Haasen, V. Gerold, and G. Kostorz) Vol. 1, p. 977, Pergamon Press, Oxford (1979).

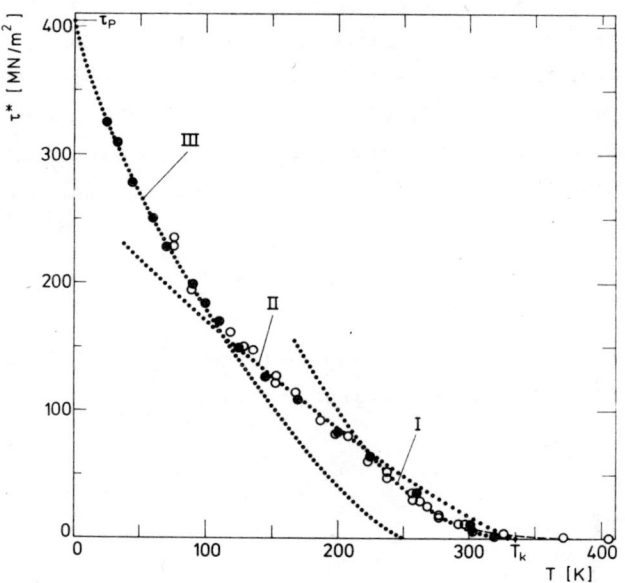

Fig. 1.

Temperature dependence of the effective resolved shear stress (macro-yield stress). ●New data, ○ Data of Zwiesele and Diehl /6/ corrected for $\dot{\varepsilon} = 8.5 \cdot 10^{-4} s^{-1}$.

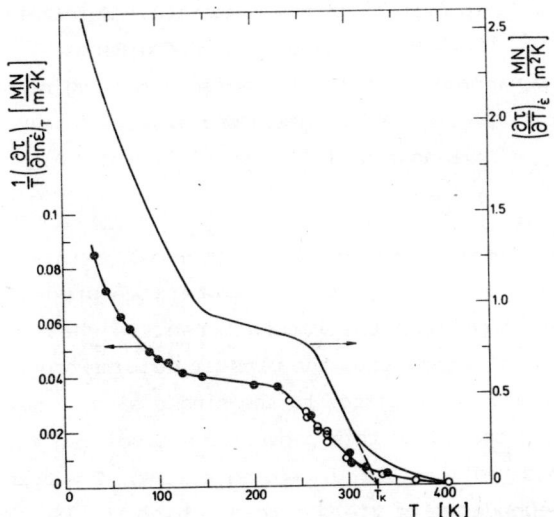

Fig. 2.

Temperature and strain-rate sensitivity of the resolved shear stress in dependence of the deformation temperature. ● New data, ○ Data of Zwiesele and Diehl /6/, corrected for $\dot{\varepsilon} = 8.5 \cdot 10^{-4} s^{-1}$.

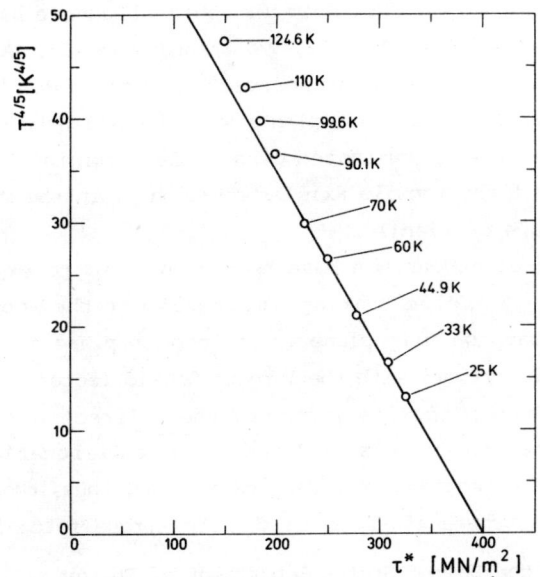

Fig. 3.

Resolved shear stress at low temperatures plotted versus $T^{4/5}$.

Selection of Slip Systems in Low Temperature Deformation of Niobium*
M. Meshii and Gun Woong Bang
Department of Materials Science and Engineering
Northwestern University
Evanston, Illinois 60201   U.S.A.

Abstract

The properties of plastic deformation of BCC metals at low temperatures depend strongly on what type of slips operates predominantly. The slip systems unpredicted from the largest resolved shear stress rule appear prominently and often control the plastic deformation. Considering the coplanar double slip in addition to the single slip, a new selection rule of slip system is proposed in this paper. The predicted slip systems and the experimental observations are in good agreement. The rule also predicts the orientation dependence of yield stress, which is also found to be in good agreement with the experimental results.

I. Introduction

The plastic deformation of BCC metals at low temperatures exhibits a number of unique properties/1/, one of which, the occurrence of anomalous slip is the main concern of this manuscript. Anomalous slip has been studied most extensively in Nb, however, this slip mode has been observed in other BCC metals such as Ta/2-5/, V/6-8/ and Mo/9,10/. As the term implies, the occurrence of this slip is unexpected as the anomalous slip plane observed belongs to one of {110} planes with a small Schmid factor/11-16/. In Nb, this mode of slip dominates plastic deformation at low temperatures below 113 K, if the tensile axis orientation is in the middle region of the unit stereographic triangle.

A number of mechanisms have been considered to explain the anomalous slip /14-16/. The clue linking a mechanism to the anomalous slip is the observation that the slip plane is the common plane to the slip directions of the two slip systems with the largest Schmid factors. The anomalous slip direction is the composite vector of these directions. It has been suggested/17/ that the stress field of a screw dislocation exerts a torque force on an intersecting screw dislocation and, thus, the double kink formation energy is substantially reduced. The torque force is exerted mutually

*Sponsored by the United States Department of Energy.

between the dislocations, and their motion takes place more readily on the common plane. Hence, the coplanar double slip, which was named anomalous slip in specimens with tensile axes in the middle of the unit stereographic triangle, takes place in spite of the fact that the resolved shear stresses are smaller on the common plane than on the initial slip planes of these dislocations.

The Criteria for the Operation of Anomalous Slip

For two screw dislocations with different Burgers vectors to interact, they must move. Therefore, the most probable combination of screw dislocations moving on the common plane with the assistance of the mutually exerted torque forces are those with the first and second highest Schmid factors (the primary and secondary dislocations). This leads us to the criterion for selection of the slip plane; the coplanar double slip plane is defined by the Burgers vectors of the two most highly stressed dislocations.

The anomalous slip plane observed in the specimens with the tensile axis oriented in the middle of the unit stereographic triangle, [100]-[110]-[111], is ($1\bar{1}0$) and is different from either of the initial slip planes, (101) or ($10\bar{1}$) for the two most highly stressed dislocations (Burgers vectors 1/2[$11\bar{1}$] and 1/2[111]). Hence, the slip plane observed is unexpected from the consideration of the Schmid factors for the single slip system. For any tensile axis orientation within the unit stereographic triangle, the most highly stressed slip system is unique, and is [$11\bar{1}$](101). On the other hand, the second highly stressed system is not unique. This can be seen in Table 1, in which the resolved shear stress for all <111>{110} slip systems are tabulated for several representative tensile axis orientations. It is, therefore, expected that the coplanar double slip plane is not unique within the unit triangle.

Although the Schmid factors for the primary and secondary dislocations on the common plane are considerably smaller than those on their respective initial slip planes, they are expected to move on the common plane because of the couple force. There should be, however, the lower limit in the resolved shear stress for this motion. Therefore, the second criterion for the operation of the coplanar double slip is that the resolved shear stresses for the primary and secondary dislocations on the common plane must be larger than the critical stress for the long distance motion of a screw dislocation under the influence of the couple force.

Examination of Possible Slip Systems

Referring to Table 1, the slip system [$11\bar{1}$](101) always has the highest

Table I. Schmid factors of tensile axis orientations within the [100]-[110]-[111] stereographic triangle.

Tensile axis	slip direction	Slip plane					
		(101)	(10$\bar{1}$)	(1$\bar{1}$0)	(110)	(011)	(01$\bar{1}$)
[100] A	[11$\bar{1}$] [111] [1$\bar{1}$1] [$\bar{1}$11]	0.408 0.408	0.408 0.408	0.408 0.408	0.408 0.408	0.0 0.0	0.0 0.0
[941] B	[11$\bar{1}$] [111] [1$\bar{1}$1] [$\bar{1}$11]	0.500 0.167	0.467 0.200	0.250 0.292 0.217	0.325	0.250 0.125	0.175 0.050
[210] B	[11$\bar{1}$] [111] [1$\bar{1}$1] [$\bar{1}$11]	0.490 0.163	0.490 0.163	0.245 0.245 0.245	0.245	0.245 0.082	0.245 0.082
[110] C	[11$\bar{1}$] [111] [1$\bar{1}$1] [$\bar{1}$11]	0.408 0.0	0.408 0.0	0.0 0.0	0.0 0.0	0.408 0.0	0.408 0.0
[441] C	[11$\bar{1}$] [111] [1$\bar{1}$1] [$\bar{1}$11]	0.433 0.062	0.334 0.037	0.0 0.0	0.433 0.099 0.099	0.062	0.334 0.037
[541] C	[11$\bar{1}$] [111] [1$\bar{1}$1] [$\bar{1}$11]	0.467 0.0	0.389 0.078	0.078 0.097	0.175 0.0	0.389 0.097	0.292 0.0
[332] D	[11$\bar{1}$] [111] [1$\bar{1}$1] [$\bar{1}$11]	0.371 0.186	0.148 0.037	0.0 0.0	0.371 0.223 0.223	0.186	0.148 0.037
[543] D	[11$\bar{1}$] [111] [1$\bar{1}$1] [$\bar{1}$11]	0.392 0.131	0.196 0.065	0.049 0.098	0.343 0.294 0.147	0.229	0.098 0.016
[111] E	[11$\bar{1}$] [111] [1$\bar{1}$1] [$\bar{1}$11]	0.272 0.272	0.0 0.0	0.0 0.0 0.272	0.272	0.272 0.272	0.0 0.0

Schmid factor. On the other hand, the second highest Schmid factor is either on the [111](10$\bar{1}$) slip system or on the [1$\bar{1}$1](110) slip system, depending on the tensile axis orientation. Therefore, the coplanar double slip plane will be (1$\bar{1}$0) or (011). These two cases are identified as B and D in Table 1 and Figure 1. The demarcation line between these two regions was established from the comparison of the Schmid factors of the competing slip systems as will be discussed in the following section.

The second criterion becomes the controlling factor for the tensile axis orientations in the region C. As can be seen in the table, the Schmid factors for the primary and secondary dislocations on the common plane become critically small. For example, in the case of the tensile axis orientation [541], the Schmid factors of the primary and secondary dislocations on the common plane is too small to sustain the coplanar double slip. Therefore, the continuation of the motion of the primary dislocations on the initial slip plane is preferred. For the tensile axis orientation in the region C of the unit stereographic triangle, the primary slip operates in the single slip mode.

The region A indicates a special region of high symmetry where four coplanar double slip systems are expected to operate actively. It can be seen in Table 1 that this orientation particularly favors the coplanar double slip mode as the Schmid factor for the coplanar double slip is equal to that for the single slips. The observation of abundant coplanar double slips has been reported for this orientation in Nb/16,19/.

The region E, represented by the [111] orientation, also possesses a high degree of symmetry. The three coplanar double slips have the same Schmid factor and are expected to operate, although the Schmid factor is significantly smaller than in Region A.

The slip plane for the coplanar double slip does not coincide with the primary or secondary slip plane in Region B. On the other hand, the situation in region D is different. The coplanar double slip plane predicted from the preceding consideration is (011), on which the primary dislocation possesses a relatively high Schmid factor (c.f. [543]); therefore, this plane can be regarded as the alternative primary slip plane. Direct evidence to ascertain if the single slip or the coplanar double slip has taken place, must be obtained to distinguish these two potential slip modes. This point will be further amplified in the discussion section.

Examination of Yield Stress

The yield stress of BCC single crystals is often reported in tensile stress instead of resolved shear stress, since the slip system to which the stress observed should be resolved, is not necessarily apparent. Then, the resolved shear stress can be computed for any slip system of interest.

It has been mentioned in the preceding section that the two critical stresses are involved for the coplanar double slip to produce the macroscopic deformation. The first critical stress is for dislocations to move sufficiently to interact with dislocations on another slip system. This critical stress for dislocation motion is defined on the initial slip plane on which the dislocations have the largest Schmid factor. The resolved shear stresses for both component dislocations must exceed this critical stress. The second critical stress is for the motion of both dislocations on the coplanar double slip plane under the influence of the couple force. For a given tensile axis orientation, if these critical stresses are surpassed before the third critical stress as the tensile stress increases, the coplanar double slip takes place (regions A, B, D and E). On the other hand, if the third critical stress is exceeded before the first or second critical stress, the macroscopic deformation will take place by the single slip mechanism (region C).

The plastic deformation of high purity niobium single crystals were examined extensively at tensile axis orientations [100], [941] and [441] at 77 K /16,18/. The tensile yield stresses were 215, 265 and 685 MPa, respectively, for the three orientations. The deformation took place by multiple coplanar double slips, by a unique coplanar double slip and by the single primary slip, respectively. For the [100] orientation, the eight single slip systems have the same Schmid factor, 0.408 for the initial dislocation motion and the combination of two out of the four slip directions gives four coplanar double slip planes, giving again the same Schmid factor, 0.408, because of its high symmetry; therefore, one of these systems can represent all the slip systems in this case. For the [941] orientation, four slip systems must be considered, while only one slip system needs to be considered for the [441] orientation. The computation is summarized in Table 2. The lowest resolved stresses (*) observed for each dislocation action in Table 2 are assumed to be the critical stresses, resulting in 124, 88 and 297 MPa, respectively for the critical stresses for single slip dislocation motion (SSDM), coplanar double slip (CPDS), single slip plastic deformation (SSPD).

The tensile stress necessary to give the critical stress for each dislocation reaction is calculated for various tensile axis orientations. Let us examine how these stresses change along the [100]-[110] line. The

Table 2   Resolved Shear Stress Comparison

Tensile axis	Tensile Yield Stress (MPa)	Slip System	Schmid factor	Resolved shear stress (MPa)	Dislocation action
[100]	215				
		[11$\bar{1}$] (101)	0.408	88*	SSDM
		[11$\bar{1}$] (1$\bar{1}$0)	0.408	88	CPDS
[941]	265				
		[11$\bar{1}$] (101)	0.500	133	SSDM
		[111] (10$\bar{1}$)	0.467	124	SSDM
		[11$\bar{1}$] (1$\bar{1}$0)	0.250	66*	CPDS
		[111] (1$\bar{1}$0)	0.292	77	CPDS
[441]	685				
		[11$\bar{1}$] (101)	0.433	297*	SSPD

results are plotted in Fig. 2, where M1, C1 and S1 lines represent the tensile yield stress corresponding to the first, second and third critical stress. The onset of the coplanar double slip, therefore, is controlled by the higher stress value of M1 or C1, the tensile stress necessary to start the primary single slip is represented by the S1 line. The figure indicates that the coplanar double slip on (1$\bar{1}$0) with [11$\bar{1}$] and [111] dominates over a wide range, except the region near [110] where the primary single slip, [11$\bar{1}$](101) controls the deformation. It also indicates that the initial dislocation motion is the control step for the coplanar double slip near [100], while the slip on the coplanar plane is the control process in the middle region.

Fig. 3 indicates the similar examination along the [110]-[111] line. The calculation predicts that the single primary slip dominates from [110] to 15° away, while the coplanar double slip dominates over the rest of the range. Similar examination can be carried out along any desired line. The boundary lines between two regions shown in Fig. 1 were determined by the intersection between S line and C or M line. Figs. 2 and 3 and similar plots along other lines can represent the tensile axis orientation dependence of yield stress of niobium single crystals at 77 K over the entire triangle.

Discussion

The coplanar double slip is the main slip mechanism for the macroscopic plastic deformation of Nb at low temperature for the majority of the tensile axis orientations as shown in Fig. 1 and in a number of experiments by various workers. The simple criteria for the occurrence of the coplanar double slip enables us to rationalize the phenomenon and to organize various observations systematically. The predictions based on the criteria are in good agreement with experimental observations.

For specimens with tensile axes in Region A, four sets of coplanar double slip were observed to operate /16,19/. A similar observation was also reported in V /8/. The largest number of experiments were carried out with specimens oriented in Region B. The appearance of the anomalous slip was most frequently reported for Nb /16,18/ and V /8/. For Region C orientations, the single slip has been reported to operate dominantly /16,18/. The slip lines observed for the single slip were fine and somewhat wavy as opposed to the distinct and straight slip lines usually observed for the coplanar double slips. The observations available for Region D are limited but indicate the appearance of the primary slip traces /12,16/. The analysis in the preceding section predicts these slips should be of coplanar double slip.

Recently, the present authors applied the strain analysis technique to resolve this question. The [332] oriented Nb single crystals were deformed in tension at 77 K. It was found that the UHV purified Nb specimens were deformed entirely in the coplanar double slip on (101) and (011). The oxygen doped specimens, however, deformed by the single slip mode on the same slip planes.

The orientation dependence of the computed yield stress of Nb is in good agreement with experimental observations, although the deviations among different reports make it difficult to compare the results in a general manner. The yield stresses measured along the [110]-[111] line by the present authors are indicated by the filled circles in Fig. 3. These yield stress values are generally in good agreement with results reported in literature by others./16,18,21/ The agreement in the orientation dependence of yield stress is excellent between the observed and calculated (solid lines) results. It is interesting to note that a similar orientation dependence study was carried out in pure Fe in which no coplanar double slip has been reported. The normalized yield stress of iron followed closely the S2 line beyond the intersection /20/.

The simple criteria assumed in this manuscript can be improved. The more accurate values for the critical stresses may become available in the future. Although these may shift the position of the boundaries between different regions, the general distribution of each region shown in Fig. 1 should remain unchanged. The effect of alloying on the appearance of the coplanar double slip may be an important agendum to be investigated further. The implication of the appearance of the coplanar double slip on solid solution softening/hardening effect has been pointed out previously./18,22/ It is believed that the role of the slip mode must be understood in comprehensive treatment of the low temperature plastic deformation of Nb and other BCC metals.

References:
/1/ Christian J. W.: The Proceedings of the Second International Conference on the Strength of Metals and Alloys (1970)I, ASM, p. 31.
/2/ Takeuchi S., Kuramoto E., and Suzuki T.: Acta Met. 20 (1972), 909.
/3/ Shields J. A., Goods S. H., Gibala R., Mitchell T. E.: Mat. Sci. Eng. 20 (1975) 71.
/4/ Webb G. L., Gibala R. and Mitchell T. E.: Proc. of the Third International Conference on the Strength of Metals and Alloys, Cambridge, Vol. 1 (1973) 515.
/5/ Nawaz M. H. A., Mordike B. L.: phys. stat. sol.(a) 32 (1975) 449; and Z. Metallk. 66 (1975) 644.
/6/ Taylor G., Bajaj R., Carlson O. N.: Phil. Mag. 28 (1973) 1035.
/7/ Bressers J., Creten R.: Scripta Met. 11 (1976) 33.
/8/ Creten R., Bressers J., DeMeester P.: Mat. Sci. & Eng. 29 (1977) 51.
/9/ Matsui H., Kimura H.: Mat. Sci. & Eng. 24 (1976) 247.
/10/ Jeffcoat P. J., Mordike B. L., Rogausch K. D.: Phil. Mag. 34 (1976) 583.
/11/ Reid C. N., Gilbert A., Hahn G. T.: Acta Met. 14 (1966) 975.
/12/ Foxall R. A., Duesbery M. A. and Hirsch P. B.: Can. J. Phys. 45 (1967) 607.
/13/ Duesbery M. A., Foxall R. A.: Phil. Mag. 20 (1969) 719.
/14/ Bolton C. J., Taylor G.: Phil. Mag. 26 (1972) 1359.
/15/ Bowen D. K., Taylor G.: Acta Met. 25 (1977) 417.
/16/ Garratt-Reed A. J., Taylor G.: Phil Mag. 33 (1976) 577, 39 (1979) 597.
/17/ Matsui H., Kimura H.: Scripta Met. 9 (1975) 971.
/18/ Nagakawa J., Meshii M.: Phil. Mag 45 (1982) 983.
/19/ Wasilewski R.J., Hutchings R., Loretto H. H.: Phil. Mag. 29 (1974) 521.
/20/ Sato A., Meshii M.: Proceedings of the International Conference on Fundamental Aspects of Radiation Damage in Metals, Gatlinburg, vol. 2 (1975) 984.
/21/ Ratka J. O., Sethi V. K., Gibala R.: Mechanical Properties of BCC Metals (1982) TMS-AIME, p. 103.
/22/ Meshii, M., Nagakawa J., Bang G. W.: Mechanical Properties of BCC Metals (1982) TMS-AIME, p. 95.

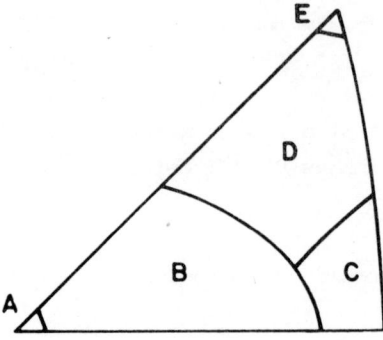

Fig. 1: Stereographic representation of tensile axis orientation vs. predicted slip systems.

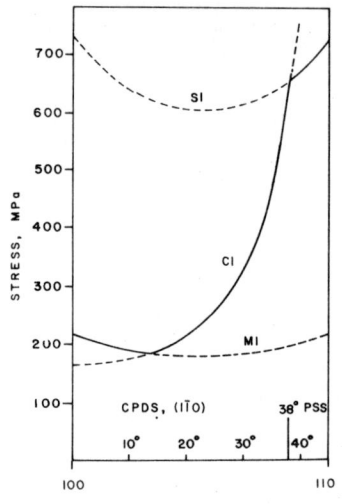

Figure 2

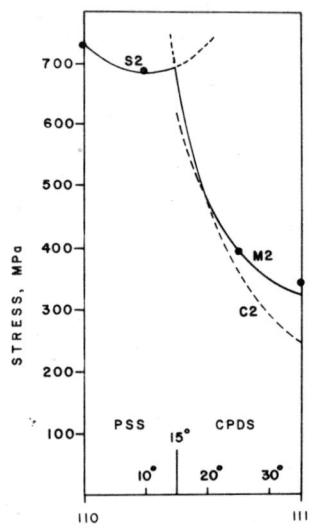

Figure 3

Fig. 2: The calculated orientation dependence of critical tensile stresses to activate three dislocation reactions along [100] to [110]. Single slip plastic deformation (S1), single slip dislocation motion (M1) and coplanar double slip (C1).

Fig. 3: The calculated orientation dependence of critical tensile stresses to activate three dislocation reactions along [110] to [111]. Single slip plastic deformation (S2), single slip dislocation motion (M2) and coplanar double slip (C2). Filled circles indicate yield stresses determined experimentally.

ELECTRON MICROSCOPE STUDIES OF CRYSTAL DISLOCATIONS

L.P. Kubin

Laboratoire de Métallurgie Physique. (L.A. 131 CNRS). Faculté des Sciences
40, Av. du Recteur Pineau. 86022 Poitiers Cedex. France.

INTRODUCTION

Since the first TEM observations of dislocations /1,2/, electron microscopy has considerably contributed to our understanding of the fundamental properties of dislocations, and hence of the plastic properties of crystalline materials. As in many other areas of physics, we can distinguish between -static properties, which have been widely investigated, with a constant improvement in resolution and which deal with an increasingly large variety of materials, and -dynamic properties, still difficult to approach, which are therefore much less well-documented. In both cases, either the properties of individual dislocations (i.e. their core properties or dissociation modes) or the properties of dislocation ensembles are searched for. For each of these specific purposes, one or several techniques of investigation are available, and a few of them will be accounted for and illustrated by recent examples of applications in which follows. For a more thorough overview, the reader is adressed to the general references given below, to the proceedings of recent electron microscopy conferences /3-5/, to recent monographs (e.g. /6,7/, among many others), or to a recent review by Hirsch in /4/ (I,p.146).

STATIC EXAMINATIONS OF DISLOCATIONS

The routine techniques for dislocation examination and identification make use of diffraction contrast as the dominant contrast mechanism. Diffracted or transmitted beams are intercepted by the objective aperture and prevented from contributing to the image. Bright and dark fields are easily obtained, since the microscope is operated far from its optimum resolution. In the classical two-beam dynamical conditions, the interaction between the electron beam and the displacement field of a dislocation produces a contrast of half-width $\xi_g/3$ (ξ_g is the extinction distance of the reflection used), i.e. $\geqslant 100\text{-}200$ Å.

For materials exhibiting strong departures from elastic isotropy (i.e. typically when the anisotropy ratio is outside the range 0.5-3), the simple extinction rules for defect identification do not hold any longer. Although symmetry considerations can be of some help, the nature of the defects is in general determined through a comparison between the micrographs and computer-simulated contrast maps, under various diffraction conditions (/7/,p.315, and /8/).

Improved resolution and high contrast can be obtained with use of the weak-beam (WB) technique, in which diffraction contrast originates from the highly distorted regions in the defect cores only. For a dislocation, the image width at half-peak height can be reduced to ~ 15Å, allowing dissociation widths of ~ 40Å to be separated, while other structural features down to 20Å in size can be resolved. Although some care should be taken in quantitatively analyzing the contrasts, the experimental procedures are relatively simple. The ultimate resolution of this method is somewhat below the values quoted above, but attaining it in practice requires an improvement in the experimental techniques and refined theoretical interpretations (/5/,p.79).

In 15 years, the WB technique has yielded a considerable amount of new results (see /9-11/ for reviews): dissociation widths and stacking-fault energies (γ) could be directly measured in several FCC and diamond-cubic crystals (e.g. $\gamma \sim 45$ mJ/m^2 for Cu, ~ 16 mJ/m^2 for Ag, ~ 30 mJ/m^2 for Au) and in HCP cobalt (~ 25 mJ/m^2, cf. /4/,I, p.198). The corresponding values of γ/Gb (G, shear modulus, b, Burgers vector of the partial dislocations) are between 3 and 7×10^{-3}, i.e. close to the limit of validity of linear elasticity for the calculation of dissociation widths. The developement of the WB technique has stimulated a renewal of interest in the properties of dissociated dislocations in FCC alloys and more especially in Cu-Al alloys, where constrictions, jogs, narrow dipoles.. were examined in detail /12-15/, in the dissociation modes of ordered alloys and in the measurement of antiphase boundary (APB) energies (e.g. /16/). Recently, a long-standing problem in the field of ordered alloys was solved with help of the WB technique applied to superlattice reflections /17/. The existence of APB tubes generated by glide of jogs on superdislocations, which are not aligned along the Burgers vector direction, had been postulated in order to explain the influence of ordering on work-hardening. These APB tubes could be identified in deformed Fe-Al crystals, in the B2 long-range ordered state; preliminary analysis of the faint contrasts observed suggest that the tubes were generated by elementary jogs of height ~ 5Å.

Figs. 1 and 2 reproduce WB illustrations of a particular mode of dissociation, the climb-dissociation, in which the fault plane is not a glide plane for the partial dislocations. The conditions for the existence of such configurations, and their consequences on plastic behaviour are not yet fully understood.

Finally, a large variety of dissociation modes could be analyzed in non-metallic materials, such as covalent and iono-covalent compounds, ceramics, minerals...(see /19/ for oxides).

For which concerns the investigations on two- and three-dimensional dislocation arrangements, several methods are available, which can be used in combination. High-voltage electron microscopy (in the MeV range) enables observations in foils 5 to 8 times thicker than in conventional 100 kV microscopy; it is particularly suited for the analysis of three-dimensional configurations, and for checking the reliability of the thin foil dislocation arrangements with respect to the bulk material /20/. By reducing the width of dislocation imeges, the WB technique allows the individual contrasts of dislocations to be resolved in dense arrays such as those formed after creep /21/, or cyclic deformation /22/. It has also been successfully applied to determine the dislocation periodicity and nature in interfaces, epitaxial layers or low-angle grainboundaries (see e.g. /23/). The stereo. technique /24/, and coherent optical methods (/3/,p.95, cf. also fig.3) can also yield useful information on the dislocation substructures.

Phase contrast is the dominant contrast mechanism for object detail $\leqslant 10$-15Å, i.e. when the microscope is operated near its optimum resolution. Some of the electron beams leaving the specimen are recombined, so that the phase differences at the exit surface of the crystal can interfere and produce intensity variations on the image (which is then nothing else but an on-line hologram). HREM (High Resolution Electron Microscopy) thus allows a projection of the crystal potential or of the charge density to be imaged. The method requires considerable care, however, when a detrmination of the exact positions of atomic rows or columns is attempted. This is because of the strong electron-matter interaction, which cannot be treated simply, and because of the influence of the microscope itself, which alters the phases and does not identically transmit all the spatial frequencies. Thus, the unique advantage of HREM with respect to conventional diffraction techniques (using X-rays, neutrons...) lies in its ability to retain information about the phases while allowing local crystallographic examinations.

Since the diffraction pattern displays the spectrum of spatial frequencies present in the crystal, the resolution attained is dictated by the largest diffraction vector allowed to contribute the image, provided that this frequency is not filtered by the microscope transfer function. Using commercial 100-200 kV microscopes, the point resolution obtained is ~ 3Å, close to the theoretical limit of ~ 2.5Å, and the fringe resolution ~ 1.5Å. The foil thicknesses are usually of the order of 100Å. An account of the state of the art, of the experimental techniques and of the interpretation procedures will be found in /3-5/ and in the reviews /25,26/. It should be emphasized that the reading of these "electron interferograms" is never straightforward and requires a carefully controlled experimentation and a step-by-step fitting with computer-simulated images.

HREM has been successfully applied to crystallographic structure analysis in materials with large unit cells, for instance complex oxides formed by a stacking of elementary polyhedral assemblies, or ordered alloys with commensurate or non-commensurate superstructures. A typical example will be found in the study by Van Tendeloo and coworkers of ordering in the gold-manganese system (/4/,I,p.226).

For which concerns crystal defects examinations, a reliable analysis can only be performed when the atomic columns, parallel to the electron beam are not distorted. This implies, for instance, that dislocations must be observed end-on, and that the screw component of their displacement is lost. The method, thus, applies well to planar defects which involve no lattice distortion such as coherent twins (as illustrated by fig.4) and interfaces. To investigate the atomic configurations of dislocation cores, or to discriminate between several theoretical proposals, a resolution somewhat smaller than the lattice spacing is needed. This is why results bearing on metals (lattice spacings ~ 3Å) are scarce for the moment; for instance, in the dislocation core images obtained in BCC Mo, or in HCP Ti, no deviation from the elastic solutions could, up to now, be detected /27/.

Lattice fringe imaging (i.e. the interference between the transmitted and one strong reflected beam) usually brings little information since the first Fourier component of the crystal potential only is retained, but this method can also be useful for investigations in metals as illustrated by fig.5 : a set of $\{111\}$ planes has been imaged in aluminium, showing that 60° dislocations are dissociated (with a width of splitting 8Å), while pure edges are not (/3/,I, p.294).

For crystals with lattice parameters $\geqslant 5$Å, and particularly tetrahedrally-coordinated crystals and compounds, HREM yielded many significant results about dislocation cores. In germanium and silicon, for instance, the 30° partial was shown to be of the "glide" type rather than of the "shuffle" type, while an unexpected core structure was evidenced for the Lomer dislocation /28-30/.

The distortions in the vicinity of low- and medium-angle boundaries, the nature of the dislocations and their periodicity were also investigated. Typical examples of applications to metals are concerned with molybdenum (fig.6). and gold (/3/,I,p.284). In gold, tilt boundaries could be analyzed in terms of dislocations by Scholtz and Bethge up to a misorientation of 20° (/4/,I,p.238).

Studies on the core structure of defects and interfaces will possibly benefit in the near future from the fast-growing capacities of the dedicated Scanning Transmission Electron Microscope (STEM), which combines the high spatial resolution of the TEM with the analytical facilities of the microprobe analyzer.

In such apparatus, operating at 100kV, the electron beam (current: 10^{-9}-10^{-10} A) is focussed into a probe 5-15Å in diameter, which scans areas of side 20-50Å in specimens ∼100Å thick. A volume element typically containing one or a few thousand atoms can be analyzed in a number of operating modes. The few examples listed below aim at showing that, as for HREM, the continuous improvement provided by this technique gradually opens a new and fascinating field of investigation.

In the Convergent Beam Electron Diffraction (CBED) mode, the point- and space-groups of perfect or defected crystals can be investigated at a scale 10-50Å. This method was used to determine the crystallographic nature of twins (in Au), of antiphase boundaries (in partially ordered Cu_3-Au), through the spot splitting induced by these defects in the microdiffraction pattern, by Cowley and coworkers (/5/,I,p.633). By considering the symmetry of the pattern, it is also possible to determine the point symmetry of a defect core. In a preliminary investigation, the CBED pattern associated with the star-shaped core of a screw dislocation in α-iron was simulated, showing that a mirror <101> line disappears as a result of dissociation. It was, however, concluded that the resolution needed to distinguish such features is presently beyond the limits of the STEM (/3/p.554).

The analytical possibilities of the STEM are best illustrated by a recent experiment on impurity segregation in the cores of non-screw dislocations in Ge and Si /31,32/: HREM observations showed that precipitates of crystalline nature (3.5Å interplanar spacing) are formed along a continuous cylinder parallel to the dislocation lines and lying along the dilated areas. These precipitates were assumed to contain ∼1000 foreign atoms per 100Å of dislocation line. X-ray microanalysis performed in the STEM revealed no metallic impurity of atomic number larger than 9, so that Electron Energy Loss Spectroscopy (EELS) was attempted. A significant oxygen K-edge could be detected in the following conditions : beam size 5Å, scanned area 45x30Å, recording times 25 to 150 s. Under electron doses of ∼10^{10} C/m^2, however, irradiation-induced desorption of the impurity took place. A tentative interpretation of these experiments is that a dense high-pressure phase (coesite) of SiO_2 is formed as a result of oxygen segregation in the dislocation cores.

In conclusion for this part, electron microscope studies of static dislocations are still in progress, and gradually approach the resolution needed for core structure investigations. As conventional TEMs are now close to their optimal resolution, further progress is expected to arise from the STEMs, till in evolution, and from a new generation of TEMs operating at intermediate voltages, i.e. between 300 and 500 kV.

DYNAMIC EXAMINATIONS OF DISLOCATIONS

The technique of in situ straining in the electron microscope yields a direct insight into the dynamical properties of dislocations. Its achievements, limits and potentialities have been reviewed several times (/33,34,20/, and /4/, IV,p280). As a result of the contradictory requirements of reducing thin foil effects by going to high voltages, and of avoiding radiation damage, the optimum experimental conditions are, again, in favour of intermediate voltages /35/. For most materials of low or medium atomic number, and provided that their flow-stress is $\geqslant 10^{-3}G$, reliable in situ experiments can be performed using conventional 100, or better 200kV microscopes. This will be illustrated below by two examples. (The corresponding instrumentation has been described in /36/). In both cases, an attempt has been made to draw quantitative conclusions as regards macroscopic plastic properties.

<u>Cyclic deformation of pure copper single crystals.</u> Fatigue properties of copper and nickel have already been investigated by in situ HVEM by several authors /34/. In the present case, cyclic deformation was performed in pure shear on specimens extracted from prefatigued single crystals supplied by H. Mughrabi (MPI, Stuttgart). A central feature in the cyclic deformation of FCC crystals is, for plastic strain amplitudes between 10^{-4} and 10^{-2}, the localization of the strain in Persistent Slip Bands (PSBs). PSBs are characterized by a state of dynamical equilibrium, involving a balance between multiplication and annihilation of screw and non-screw dislocations. The aim of the present work was to directly determine numerical values for some of the microstructural parameters entering the models of dynamical equilibrium /37,38/.

Fig. 7 shows the developement of a dislocation loop originating from a wall in the PSB structure, which produces two screw segments in the dislocation-free channel. This process is responsible for the multiplication of screw dislocations; their subsequent annihilation takes place by mutual cross-slip. Fig.8 illustrates the local stress distribution in a channel, obtained by measuring the local curvature radii of such loops; these results are in good agreement with those of Mughrabi /39/, based on static TEM axamination of dislocations pinned under load by neutron irradiation.

The model of dynamical equilibrium developed by Lépinoux /40/, makes use of the following observations: i) in the channels, screw dislocations move as individuals rather than by groups of the same sign. ii) The motion of screw dislocations contributes to one half of the total plastic strains in PSBs; the other half arises from the developement of loops between the two walls (cf. fig.7). iii) The values of the local stresses are consistent with a critical distance for the annihilation of two screw dislocations by cross-slip of ∼600Å, in agreement with previous determinations /37/. In consequence, the lifetime of a screw dislocation inside a channel is estimated to $1/7^{th}$ of cycle, under the conditions of dynamic equilibrium. A calculation of the irreversibility of slip, i.e. of the ratio of irreversible to total plastic flow yields a value of 0.85 in the PSBs.

Pseudoelasticity in DO_3-ordered Fe-Al alloys. Pseudoelasticity (PE) and Shape-Memory Effects (SME) by transformation are usually associated with the reversible nucleation and growth of thermoelastic martensite. The corresponding mechanical properties are characterized by a recovery of the applied strain, either during unloading (PE), or during a temperature rise following the deformation test (SME). These effects were found in single crystals of Fe-Al alloys, deformed by single glide in the DO_3 long-range ordered state, and for aluminium concentrations, x, between 0.2 and 0.25. However, no martensitic transformation could be detected. In addition, PE, which took place at room temperature, appeared to be promoted by orientations favouring {110} slip /41/, as confirmed by optical examinations under load. In situ tests were performed in foils oriented for single slip, for five different concentrations and for two orientations of the tensile axis, one in the twinning sense, the other in the antitwinning sense /42/. Fig.9 shows that, under stress, the superlattice dislocations of Burgers vector $4 \times \frac{1}{4}\langle 111 \rangle$ do not move as a whole. Rather, the superpartial dislocations ($b = \frac{1}{2}\langle 111 \rangle$) move as individuals, leaving APBs behind them. Fig.10 is extracted from a sequence of in situ loading-unloading cycles in superlattice dark-field: it appears that PE results from the reversible motion of the superpartial dislocations, under the surface tension of the APBs developed during their forward motion.

The mechanism proposed to explain these observations numerically accounts for the mechanical properties of these alloys, and their dependance on temperature and concentration. It is based on the following inequality, valid at zero applied stress:

(1) $$\gamma(x) > \tau_f(T,x) \, b \quad ,$$

where γ is an APB energy, and τ_f includes all the stresses opposing the backwards motion of dislocations. When eq.(1) is fulfilled, PE is obtained. If the temperature is decreased, τ_f increases, as the main contribution to this term is a lattice friction stress. Below a critical temperature T_o, such that $\gamma = \tau_f(T_o) b$, PE disappears and "true" plastic strains are obtained. However, if the specimen is subsequently heated above T_o, backwards motion of the dislocations will take place; this is typically a shape-memory effect.

Since the recovered strains can be as large as 0.1, these alloys seem to be the only example known of reversible dislocation motion over long distances.

REFERENCES

/1/ Bollmann W.: Electron Microscopy.(Stockholm Conference. 1956).Almquist and Viksell. Stockholm 1957, p.136.
/2/ Hirsch P.B., Horne R.W., Whelan M.J.: Phil. Mag. 1 (1956) 677.
/3/ Electron Microscopy 1978. Ed. J.M. Sturgess. The Microscopical Society of Canada 1978.
/4/ Electron Microscopy 1980. 7th Eur. Congress on El. Microscopy and 6th Int. Conf. on HVEM. Ed. P. Brederoo et al. Laboratory for Electron Microscopy, Leiden 1980.
/5/ Electron Microscopy 1982. 10th Int. Congress Hamburg. Deutsche Gesellschaft für Elektronenmikroskopie e.V. Frankfurt 1982.
/6/ Edington J.W.:Monographs in Practical Electron Microscopy in Materials Science. Macmillan Philips technical library 1975.
/7/ Diffraction and Imaging Techniques in Material Science. Ed. S. Amelinckx R. Gevers, J. Van Landuyt (2nd edition). North-Holland Amsterdam 1978.
/8/ Head A.K., Humble P., Clarebrough L.M., Morton A.J., Forwood C.T.: Computed electron micrographs and defect identification. North-Holland Amsterdam 1973.
/9/ Howie A.: J. of Microsc. 117 (1979) 11.
/10/ Stobbs W.M.: Electron Microscopy in Materials Science. Ed. U. Valdrè, E. Ruedl. Comm. of the Eur. Communities Brussels Vol.II 1975, 593.
/11/ Cockayne D.J.H.: Ann. Rev. Mater. Sci. 11 (1981) 75.
/12/ Carter C.B.: Phil. Mag. 36 (1977) 147.
/13/ Wintner E., Karnthaler H.P.: Phil. Mag. 36 (1977) 1317.
/14/ Carter C.B.: Phys. Stat. Sol. a 54 (1979) 395.
/15/ Carter C.B.: Phil. Mag. A 41 (1980) 619.
/16/ Crawford R.C., Ray I.L.F.: Phil. Mag. 35 (1977) 549.
/17/ Chou C.T., Hirsch P.B.: Phil. Mag. A 44 (1981) 1415.
/18/ Rivière J.P., Cadoz J.: J. Microc. et Spectr. Electroniques 7 (1982) 183.
/19/ Bretheau T., Castaing J., Rabier J.R., Veyssière P.: Adv. in Physics 28 (1979) 835.
/20/ Kubin L.P.: Impact de la Microscopie Electronique sur les Sciences Fondamentales. Ed. Ph. Buffat E.P.F.L. Lausanne 1979 p.253.
/21/ Caillard D., Martin J.L.: Acta Met. 30 (1982) 437.
/22/ Antonopoulos J.G., Winter A.T.: Phil. Mag. 33 (1976) 87.
/23/ Carter C.B., Kohlstedt D.L., Sass S.L.: J. of the Amer. Cer. Soc. 63 (1980) 623.
/24/ Diepers H.: Phys. Stat. Sol. 24 (1967) 235,623.
/25/ Nobel Symposium 47. Direct Imaging of Atoms in Crystals and Molecules

Chem. Scripta 14 (1978-79) 7-293.

/26/ Spence J.: Experimental High Resolution Electron Microscopy. Oxford Science Publishers 1980.

/27/ Bourret A.: Private communication 1982.

/28/ Bourret A., Desseaux J., D'Anterroches C.: Microscopy of Semiconducting Materials. Conf. series 60. The Inst. of Physics Bristol London 1981 p.9.

/29/ Anstis G.R. and coworkers: Microscopy of Semiconducting Materials. Conf. series 60. The Inst. of Physics Bristol London 1981 p.15.

/30/ Bourret A., Desseaux J., Renault A.: Phil. Mag. A 45 (1982) 1.

/31/ Bourret A., Colliex C.: Ultramicroscopy 9 (1982) 182.

/32/ Bourret A., Colliex C., Trebbia P.: J. de Physique Lettres 44 (1983) L-33.

/33/ Kubin L.P., Martin J.L.: Strengh of Metals and Alloys (ICSMA 5). Ed. P. Haasen, V. Gerold, G. Kostorz. Pergamon Press 1979, III, 1639.

/34/ Proc. of the Int. Symposium In Situ HVEM. Halle. Crystal Res. and Technol. 14 (1979) n° 10, 11.

/35/ Martin J.L., Kubin L.P.: Phys. Stat. Sol. a 56 (1979) 487.

/36/ Kubin L.P., Lépinoux J., Rabier J.R., Veyssière P., Fourdeux A.,: Strength of Metals and Alloys (ICSMA 6) Ed. R.C. Gifkins Pergamon Press 1982, II, 953.

/37/ Mughrabi H.: Strength of Metals and Alloys (ICSMA 5). Ed. P. Haasen, V. Gerold, G. Kostorz. Pergamon Press 1979, III, 1615.

/38/ Essmann U.: Phil. Mag. A 45 (1982) 171.

/39/ Mughrabi H.: Continuum Models of Discrete Systems 4. Ed. O. Brulin, R.K.T. Hsieh. North-Holland 1981, 241.

/40/ Lépinoux J.: Thèse 3° Cycle. University of Poitiers 1983.

/41/ Guédou J.Y.: Thesis. University of Grenoble.

/42/ Kubin L.P., Fourdeux A., Guédou J.Y., Rieu J.: Phil. Mag. A 46(1982) 357.

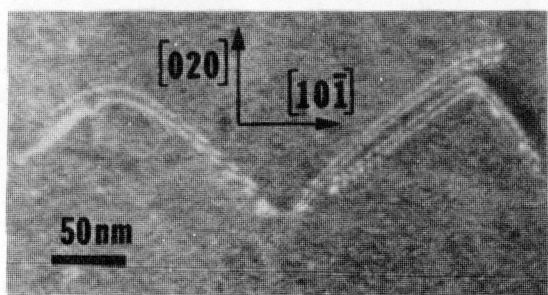

Fig.1 Climb-dissociated dislocation in $L1_2$ long-range ordered Ni_3Al. g: 020. The dissociation reaction is: $\langle 110 \rangle \rightarrow 2 \times \frac{1}{2} \langle 110 \rangle$. Detailed analysis reveals that all the non-screw segments are dissociated in planes which do not contain the Burgers vector of the superpartials (courtesy P. Veyssière).

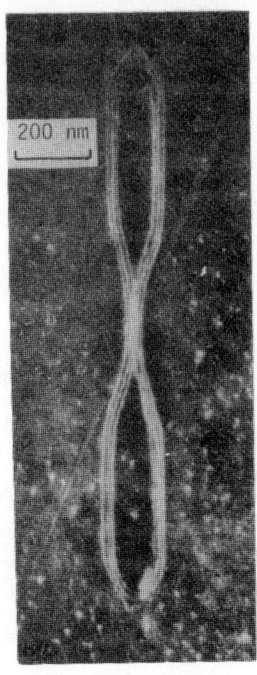

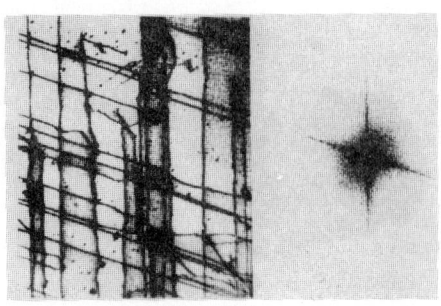

Fig.3 Screw dislocations (two systems) in niobium after straining at 50 K, and the corresponding laser diffractogram.

Fig.2 Climb-dissociation of an edge dislocation in Al_2O_3. g: $0\bar{3}30$. The three partials have the same Burgers vector, $\frac{1}{3}[\bar{1}010]$, which is perpendicular to the fault plane (Courtesy J.P. Rivière and J. Cadoz, after /18/).

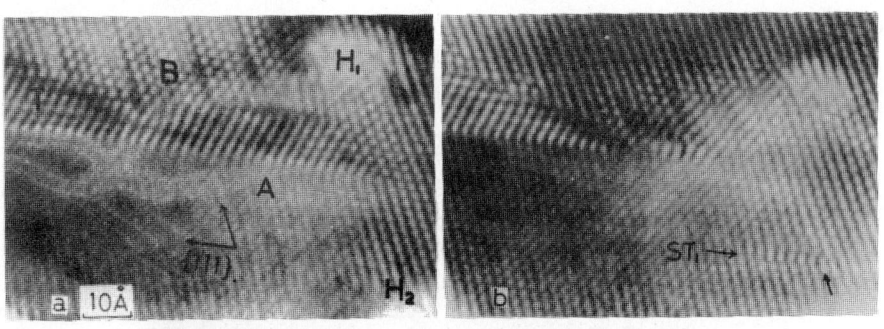

Fig.4 A twin boundary in gold and its migration under observation. The boundary is sharp in A, and curved in B. ST is a thin twin plate. (Courtesy H. Hashimoto and coworkers, after /3/).

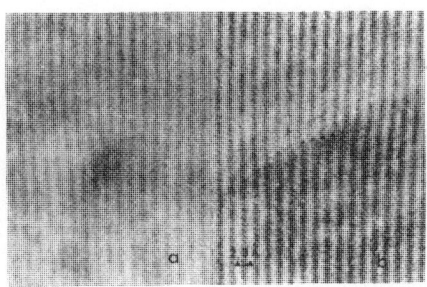

Fig.5 {111} fringes in Al (2.3 Å spacing). a) non-dissociated adge dislocation
b) dissociated 60° dislocation (Courtesy A. Bourret and J.M. Pénisson, after /3/).

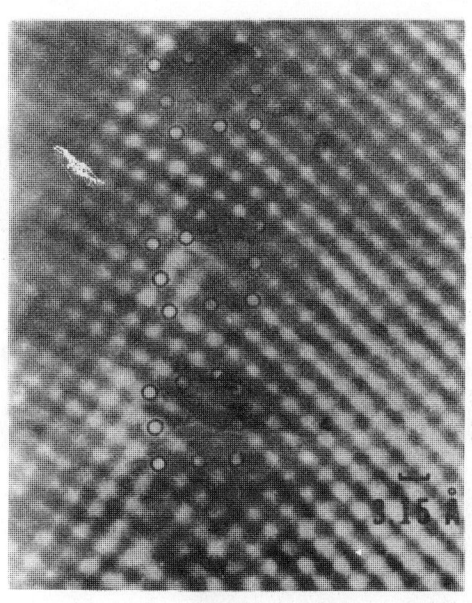

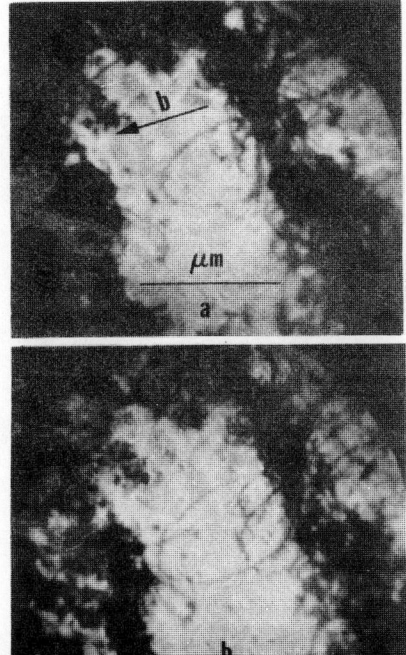

Fig.6 Dislocation structure of a $\Sigma 41$ boundary in Mo. The Burgers vectors are indicated by arrows. (Courtesy J.M. Pénisson and R. Gronski, after /5/).

Fig.7 Development of a dislocation loop originating from a wall of the PSB structure in fatigued copper. $\bar{2}02$ dark field, foil plane: (101).

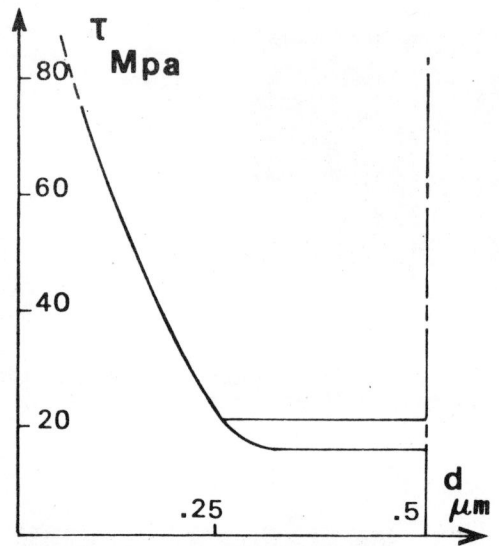

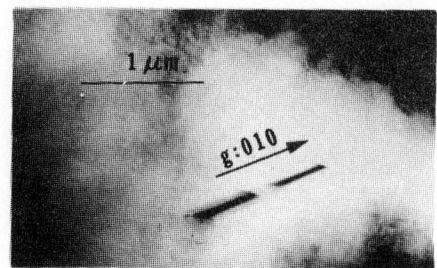

Fig.9 010 superlattice **dark field** under load in Fe$_3$Al (DO$_3$ order). The superlattice dislocation is extended by the motion of the superpartials which leave APBs behind them.

Fig.8 Stress distribution in the channel of a PSB (Width 1µm), as determined from the local curvatures of 28 loops such as the one of Fig.7.

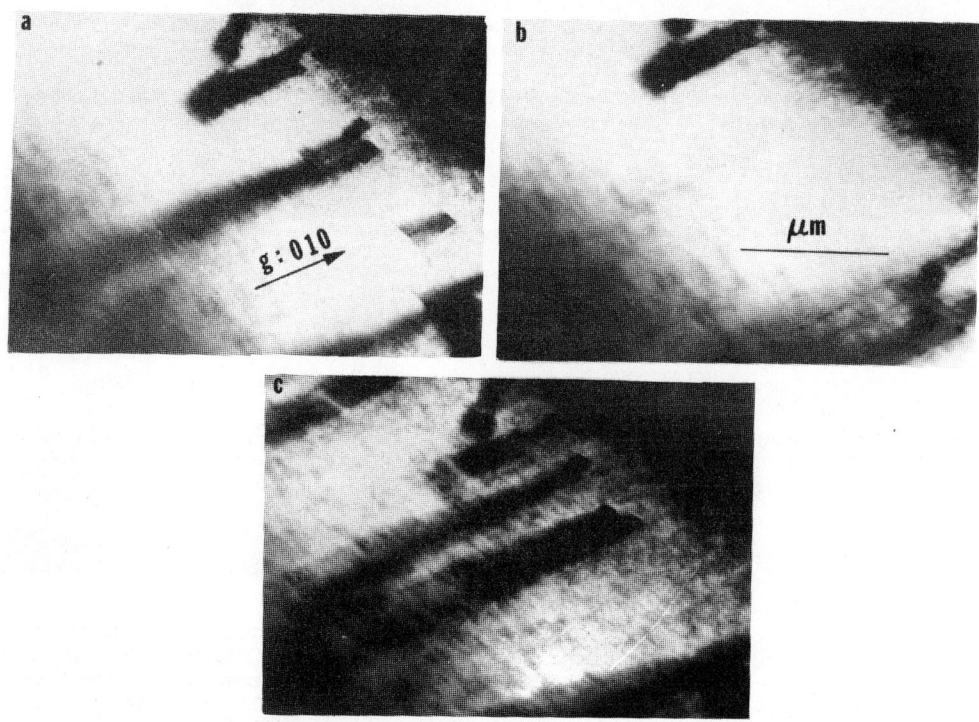

Fig.10 Loading-unloading **sequence** in Fe$_3$Al. 010 superlattice dark field. a)c): under load, b): under zero stress. The dark contrasts originate from the APBs trailed by the superpartial dislocations.

THEORY OF YIELD STRESS OF DILUTE BCC ALLOYS

Hideji Suzuki

Department of Physics, Faculty of Science, University of Tokyo, Bunkyo-ku, Tokyo 113, Japan

1. Introduction

   The characteristics of solution hardening of bcc alloy crystals differ considerably from that of fcc alloys owing to the high Peierls-Nabarro stress to move a screw dislocation in a bcc crystal. The present author discussed the solution hardening of bcc alloys in terms of the resistance to move a kink and the change in the energy of the kink pair nucleation [1-3]. The yield stress calculated by the theory shows good agreement with the experiments on high concentration alloys. However, the calculation gives too large solution softening at low temperatures in dilute alloys compared with observations. Kitajima, Aono, Abe and Kuramoto [4] found that Fe-N alloy crystals show rapid solution hardening below 30 K and solution softening at temperatures between 150 and 200 K, while the yield stress of Fe-Si alloy crystals is nearly independent of the concentration of silicon up to 1.3 at% below 77 K.

   The previous theory treated the kink velocity controlled by a barrier due to a large number of solute atoms, and was formulated for a continuous number of solute atoms. Therefore, a barrier in a dilute alloy becomes that of a fraction of a solute atom, which is nonsense. Besides the previous theory did not discuss the effect of solute atoms on the kink pair formation in detail. Therefore in this paper the interaction between a kink and a solute atom is discussed in detail, and also the effect of solute atoms on the activation enthalpy for the kink pair formation is calculated. The yield stress of bcc dilute alloys is then discussed on the basis of these results.

2. Interaction between a solute atom and a screw dislocation

   Computer simulations [6] have demonstrated that the atomic position at the core of a screw dislocation in a bcc crystal is quite different from the elasticity solution. Suzuki [1] showed that the interaction between a solute atom and the screw dislocation is strong and nearly the same as far as the solute atom is in one of the six atomic rows at the core of the screw dislocation, while it is negligibly weak for solute atoms in the outside of the core. The most important is the change in the interaction energy as a solute atom enters or leaves the core of the dislocation.

The absolute values of the difference in the interaction energy between a solute atom at the core and that in the outside of the core of the dislocation was given by

(1) $$E = 0.122(\varepsilon_\mu' + 1.52\varepsilon_a) \text{ eV}$$

for iron alloys [1], where ε_μ' is the Takeuchi's modulus misfit parameter [7], which is given by

(2) $$\varepsilon_\mu' = (\varepsilon_\mu + A\varepsilon_a)/[1 - \beta(\varepsilon_\mu + A\varepsilon_a)]$$

and ε_a the size misfit parameter. Here

$$\varepsilon_a = (1/a)(da/dc), \quad \varepsilon_\mu = (1/\mu)(d\mu/dc),$$

$$A = -\frac{2(1-2\nu)}{(1-\nu)} \frac{\Delta\mu/\mu}{\Delta V/V}, \quad \beta = \frac{2(4-5\nu)}{15(1-\nu)}$$

a is the lattice parameter, μ the shear modulus, c the concentration of the solute, ν Poisson's ratio and V the molar volume. The values of A and β for iron are about 4.3 and 0.5 respectively. The interaction energy E is of the order of 0.1 eV for various substitutional solute atoms and it is -0.108 eV for a silicon atom in iron.

It must be mentioned that the position dependence of the interaction energy of an interstitial solute atom with a screw dislocation is rather similar to that of a substitutional solute atom though its magnitude is considerably larger in the case of interstitial solute atoms than that of substitutional solute atoms. The configuration of surrounding solvent atoms differs significantly from the elasticity solution at the core of a screw dislocation, so that the interaction differs completely from the calculation based on the elasticity theory for solute atoms at the core of dislocation. Sato and Meshii [8] avoided this difficulty considering solute atoms in the outside of the core, but they used a large misfit strain center with a radius of 2b for an interstitial solute atom in order to obtain appropriate magnitudes of interaction to fit the experiments by Nakada and Keh [9] with their theory. It is obvious that the radius of the misfit strain center should be smaller than b in the case of dilute interstitial solute alloys. As mentioned elsewhere [3] the solution hardenings in Fe-N alloys measured by Nakada and Keh are explained approximately by the same interaction as the substitutional alloys if we assume $|E| = 0.40$ eV.

3. Activation enthalpy required to nucleate a kink pair

The saddle point configuration in the process of a kink pair nucleation is affected by solute atoms. However the interaction energy of a substitutional solute atom with a screw dislocation is of the order of 0.1 eV. The bending of the dislocation by the interaction with a solute atom is usually smaller than that by the Peierls potential. Hence we neglect the local bending by each solute atom, and average the interaction energy along the direction of the screw dislocation over the distance Λ_p, which is the kink pair width at the saddle point configuration.

Then the potential energy to the motion of a straight dislocation parallel to the z-axis is given by

$$(3) \qquad V(x) = V_P(x) + V_S(x)$$

where $V_P(x)$ is the Peierls potential and assumed to be

$$(4) \qquad V_P(x) = (\tau_p bd/2\pi)[1-\cos(2\pi x/d)]$$

Here d is the distance between neighbouring Peierls potential valleys. The potential $V_S(x)$ is the average interaction energy with solute atoms and approximated by a "well" potential which has the value Eb/Λ_p when a solute atom is in one of the six atomic rows at the core of the dislocation, or else it vanishes. The potential is caused by the core structure peculier to a screw dislocation in a bcc crystal, and the energy change occurs rather abruptly as the solute atom enters or leaves the core of the dislocation. We assume

$$V_S(x) = 0 \quad \text{for } x \leq (1-1/n)d/2$$

(5)
$$V_S(x) = \frac{iEb}{2\Lambda_P}[1-\cos\{2n\pi(\frac{x}{d} - \frac{1}{2} - \frac{1}{2n})\}]$$
$$\text{for } (1-1/n)d/2 \leq x \leq (1+1/n)d/2$$

$$V_S(x) = iEb/\Lambda_P \quad \text{for } (1+1/n)d/2 \leq x \leq (3-1/n)d/2$$

where $n > 2$ and i is the increase of the number of solute atoms at the core of the dislocation segment with the length Λ_P.

The activation enthalpy for the nucleation of a kink pair is then written as

(6)
$$H(\tau,i,E) = 2(2W_0)^{1/2} \int_{x_0}^{x_m} [V(x) - \tau bx]^{1/2} dx$$

by the method of Celli et al. [10], where W_0 is the line tension of the dislocation, and x_0 and x_m are the positions of the dislocation before the thermal activation under the shear stress τ and of the most advanced part at the saddle point configuration, respectively.

Figure 1 shows the calculated relation between $H(\tau,i,E)$ and τ/τ_P for $n = 3$. It is easily seen that $H(\tau,i,E)$ decreases as iE increases. The frequency of the nucleation of a kink pair on the dislocation line of the length Λ_P is given by

(7)
$$p = (\nu L/\Lambda_P) \sum_{i=0}^{N} g(i,c,\Lambda_P) \exp[-H(\tau,i,E)/kT]$$

where $g(i,c,\Lambda_P)$ is the probability of increasing by i the number of solute atoms at the core of a dislocation during the motion of the dislocation segment with the length of Λ_P and is given by [1]

(8)
$$g(i,c,\Lambda_P) = \exp(-2n) \sum_{k=m}^{N} \frac{n^{2k-m}}{k!(k-m)!}$$

In dilute alloys the approximation by the gaussian distribution function causes serious error.

When the dislocation velocity is controlled by the frequency of the kink pair nucleation, the dislocation velocity is given by

(9)
$$v = pd$$

If the yield stress is given by the force required to move a dislocation at a definite velocity v_0, we obtain the flow stress from eqs.(6), (7) and (9), putting $v = v_0$. An approximate solution may be obtained by using the largest term in the summation in eq.(7) instead of the summation itself. Then the problem is now reduced to solve the equation

(10) $\qquad H(\tau,i,E)/kT - \ln g(i,c,\Lambda_p) = H(\tau_1,0)/kT$

where τ_1 is the shear stress required to move a screw dislocation in the bcc crystal at a definite velocity. The following relation is well established by experiments [11-13]

(11) $\qquad H(\tau_1,0)/kT = 25$

approximately, except the measurements at very low temperatures. Figure 2 shows the calculation for Fe-Si alloys, which shows that the solution softening decreases at low temperatures, though the concentration dependence of the yield stress does not agree with the experiments [4].

4. Force required to move a kink in a dilute alloy

A kink on a screw dislocation may be hidered from moving at the strongest barrier. In a dilute alloy the barrier must be a single solute atom. The stress required to overcome the barrier without the thermal activation is given by

(12) $\qquad \tau_0 = |E|/\Lambda_k ab$

if the kink does not change its shape under the stress, where Λ_k is the width of a kink.

However, if the interaction energy is very large, we cannot neglect the change in the kink width under a large applied stress. The kink width decreases and the force to move the kink increases. The kink tends to shrink under the applied stress when its effective end reaches the potential barrier due to the solute atom as shown by the curve 1 and 2 in Fig.3. The force required to initiate the translational motion of the narrowed kink is the maximum one required to pass through the barrier, and this force is equal to that required to shrink the kink to the narrowest width. Using this condition we have the narrowest kink width to be

(13) $$\Lambda_k' = \frac{2W_0 d^2}{E + (E^2 + 4W_0^2 d^2 \Lambda_k^2)^{1/2}}$$

where W_0 is the line tention of the dislocation. This kink width is obtained under the assumption that there is no thermal activation.

If the force required to move a kink without the thermal activation is higher than the Peierls-Nabarro stress, the yield stress at very low temperatures increases rapidly by small amounts of solute atoms and reaches a plateau at the force required to move a kink passing through a solute atom. Aono et al. [5] observed such a relation between the yield stress and the concentration of solute in Fe-N dilute alloys at 4.2 K. Using their data we estimated the interaction energy E for nitrogen in iron at 0.48 eV. This value is larger than that previously estimated from the high temperature solution hardening in Fe-N alloys [3]. The previous value, 0.40 eV, corresponds to the average change of the energy, while the present estimation is for the largest change in the energy.

The interaction energy E for a carbon atom is slightly larger than that of nitrogen atom, while those of substitutional solute atoms are of the order of 0.1 eV or smaller than this value. Therefore the force required to move a kink overcoming the barrier due to an interstitial solute atom is always higher than Peierls-Nabarro stress, while the situation is the reverse in substitutional alloys. Then the addition of small amounts of interstitial solute atoms causes significant hardening at very low temperatures, while substitutional solute atoms causes no hardening.

The solution softening by interstitial solute atoms takes place at higher temperatures than substitutional solute atoms. This is easily seen in Fig.4, which shows the activation enthalpy vs applied stress relations for the kink pair nucleation process and for the kink motion overcoming the barrier due to a solute atom. From this figure we may say that the solution softening takes place above 100 K in Fe-N alloys. Meanwhile, the solution softening may take place above 10 K in substitutional alloys though the magnitude of softening is much smaller than the observation at low temperatures.

When two kink pairs are formed succesively at nearly the

same position, two kinks of the same sign move. We call this kind of two kinks as a double kink. A double kink can pass through the barrier due to a single interstitial solute atom at very low temperatures. However when a kink is prevented from moving by a barrier the next kink pair is nucleated preferentially at the opposit side of the barrier by the help of the stress field of the previous kink. The independent formation of kink pairs on both sides of the barrier may form a superjog, which resist the kink nucleation by the back stress of piled-up kinks, as discussed in previous papers [1-3]. The resisting force is given by

(14) $$\tau_j = \mu b^2 / 2L$$

where L is the distance between neighbouring superjogs. This stress is additive to nucleate a kink pair without any back stress. The probability of the superjog formation may be proportional to the concentration of solute atoms. The observed results by Aono et al. are explained if we assume $L = b/6c$.

5. Discussions

The calculated solution softening in Fe-Si alloy crystals at 35 K is very small and cannot explain the significant softening around 3 at% Si observed by Kitajima et al [4]. They observed similar softening around 2.5 at% Si at 77 K. It must be noticed that at higher concentrations than those the force to move a kink exceeds that to nucleate a kink pair. As already mentioned when the force to move a kink increases many superjogs are formed. Pairs of edge dislocations are formed at the superjogs and each edge dislocation can move if the applied force exceeds the interaction with the opposite dislocation. At low concentrations superjogs cannot grow to a sufficiently large size, because kinks move over long distances. Therefore the softening by the motion of edge dislocations in the trail of a superjog is observed when the resistance to the motion of a kink becomes significant.

The solution softening was clearly observed by Kataoka et al. [14] in KCl-KBr solid solutions at 4.2 K. In these crystals the Peierls-Nabarro stress does not differ markedly between an edge dislocation and a screw dislocation. The size interaction of a solute atom with an edge dislocation is significant in this system due to the difference in ionic radii between Cl- and Br-. The size interaction energy varies over a distance longer than an atomic spacing in its effective region, because the core of a dislocation does not extend in these crystals. Therefore the Peierls-Nabarro stress for an edge dislocation changes locally by the stress field caused by solute ions. Moving edge dislocations intersect with screw dislocations of various slip systems and assist the formation of kink pairs. Thus solution softening in this system is observed at very low temperatures. The peculiar interaction between a solute atom with a screw dislocation in bcc alloys is the reason why there is no solution softening in these alloys at very low temperatures.

References

/1/ Suzuki H.: Nachrichten der Akademie der Wissenschaften in Gottingen II. Mathematisch-Physikalische Klasse (1971) No.6 p.113.
/2/ Suzuki H.: Rate Process in Plastic Deformation of Materials, ed. by J.C.M. Li and A.K. Mukherjee, ASM (1975) p.47.
/3/ Suzuki H.: Dislocations in Solids, Vol.4, ed. by F.R.N. Nabarro, North-Holland, Amsterdam (1979) p.191.
/4/ Kitajima K., Aono Y., Abe H. and Kuramoto E.: Strength of Metals and Alloys, ed. by P. Haasen, V. Gerold and G. Kostorz, Pergamon, Oxford (1979) p.965.
/5/ Aono Y., Kitajima K. and Kuramoto E.: Scripta Met. 14 (1980) 321.
/6/ Vitek V.: Crystal Lattice Defects 5 (1974) 1.
/7/ Takeuchi S.: Scripta Met. 2 (1968) 481.
/8/ Sato A. and Meshii M.: Acta Met. 21 (1973) 753.
/9/ Nakada Y. and Keh A.S.: Acta Met. 16 (1969) 903.
/10/ Celli V., Kabler M., Ninomiya T. and Thomson R.: Phys. Rev. 131 (1963) 58.
/11/ Takeuchi S. and Maeda K.: Acta Met. 25 (1977) 1485.
/12/ Kuramoto E., Aono Y., Kitajima K., Maeda K. and Takeuchi S.: Phil. Mag. 39 (1979) 717.
/13/ Aono Y., Kitajima K. and Kuramoto E.: Scripta Met. 15 (1981) 275.
/14/ Kataoka T., Uematsu T. and Yamada T.: Jpn. J. Appl. Phys. 17 (1978) 271.

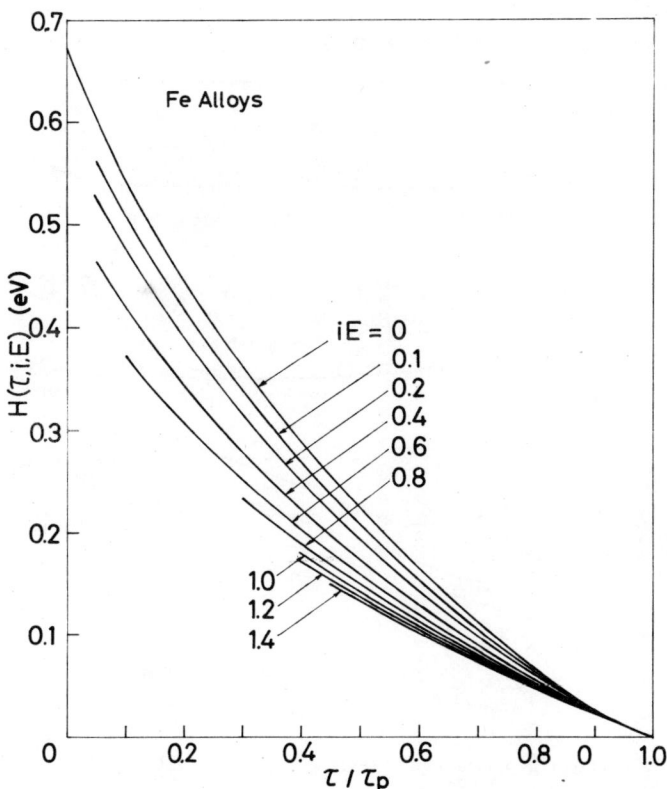

Fig.1 Effect of solute atoms on the activation enthalpy for a kink pair formation in iron alloys

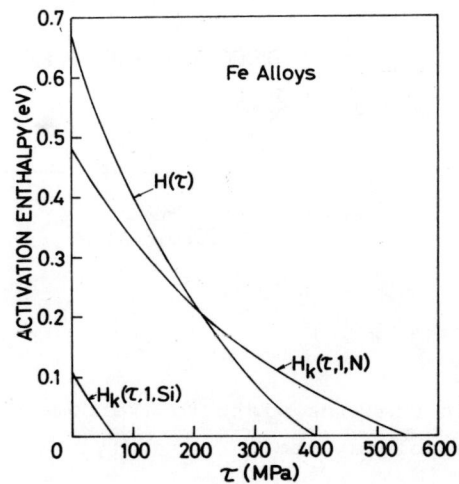

Fig.4 Comparison of activation enthalpies for different processes.

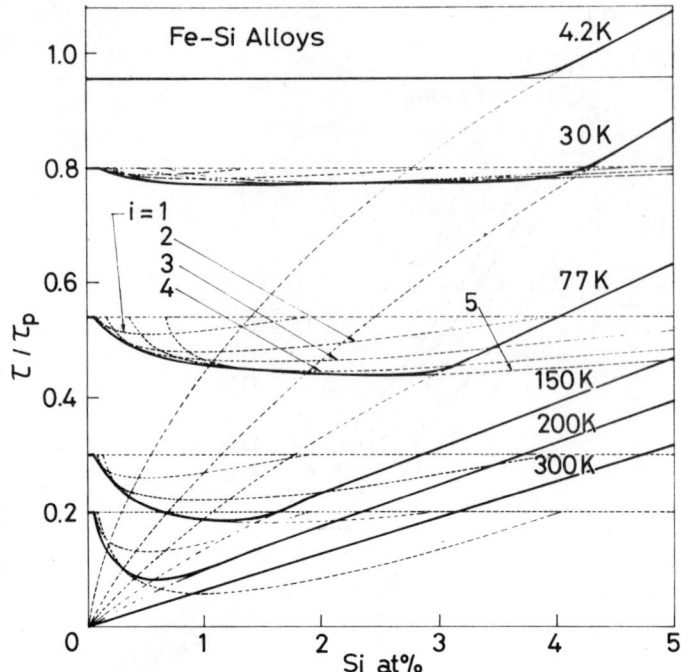

Fig.2 Calculated yield stress of Fe-Si alloy crystals plotted against the solute concentration.

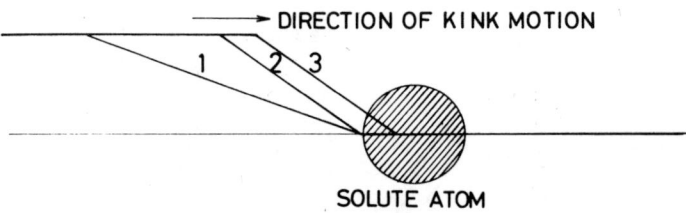

Fig.3 Change in the kink width to overcome the barrier caused by a single solute atom.

THE SNOEK-KÖSTER RELAXATION IN BODY-CENTRED CUBIC METALS

M. Weller, M. Tietze, J. Diehl, and A. Seeger

Max-Planck-Institut für Metallforschung, Stuttgart, Germany (F.R.)

It has been known for some time that internal friction (IF) of b.c.c. metals shows maxima as a function of measuring temperature that appear only after cold working of the samples and that are associated with the presence of interstitially dissolved foreign atoms (ISA).

Following Nowick and Berry /1/, in appreciation of Snoek's /2/ discovery of the effect and of Köster's /3/ systematic investigation of the origin of the phenomenon, which subsequently became known as "cold-work peak", the relaxation process causing the above mentioned IF maximum is now called Snoek-Köster (SK) relaxation. Inspite of numerous experimental investigations and several theoretical approaches essential questions regarding the experimental evidence for and the physical interpretation of the SK relaxation remained unclear until recently (see /4,5/). E.g., for the systems Nb-O and Ta-O peak temperatures reported by different authors lay several hundred K apart. A general difficulty was to account for the experimentally determined activation enthalpies, which are appreciably higher than those of the corresponding Snoek relaxation (reorientation of ISA in otherwise undisturbed b.c.c. crystals).

The present paper summarizes our state of knowledge, making use of recent work on Nb-O and Ta-O /5/ and the kink model of the SK relaxation /6/, and presents new data on Fe-N. It will be seen that the Fe-N results support an important conclusion of /5/, namely that a given type of foreign interstitials (e.g. C,N,O, or H) may give rise to two distinct SK peaks in the same material. Furthermore, the Fe-N measurements give additional information on the variation of the SK relaxation with the amount of plastic deformation and clarify the relationship of the SK relaxation to Kê's grain-boundary peak /7/.

Results on Niobium and Tantalum

Cold-worked Nb-O shows in one and the same sample two well separated IF maxima at temperatures above the Snoek relaxation (at concentrations $c_O = 10^{-3}$-10^{-4}). Analogous results not to be discussed here were obtained on Ta-O /5,8/. In Nb-O these two peaks, denoted by SK1 and SK2, are located at approximately 550 K and 730 K (for measuring frequency $f \simeq 1$ Hz).

SK2 is much larger than SK1 and rather stable against annealing (up to temperatures exceeding the peak temperature by about 100 K). By contrast SK1 is less stable and more sensitive against annealing. A startling observation is that in Nb-O the activation enthalpy of relaxation of the high-temperature peak SK2 is lower than that of SK1. As explained in detail in /5/, the existence of two SK maxima resolves a number of apparent contradictions in the literature on the temperature of the SK relaxation.

Measurements on α-Iron

A specific aim of our measurements on Fe-N was to investigate whether the existence of two distinct SK relaxations is a more general phenomenon and whether the high-temperature peak (if existing) is really of Snoek-Köster type.

Iron monocrystals of high purity were doped with nitrogen between $C_N = 5 \cdot 10^{-5}$ and $6 \cdot 10^{-4}$. The IF of undeformed and plastically deformed samples was studied at temperatures up to 950 K. **Fig. 1** shows the results on two samples of the same crystallographic orientation. Curve 1 was measured on crystal A ($C_N = 4.5 \cdot 10^{-4}$) before deformation, curve 5 after a quite heavy deformation by swaging (25% reduction in area). Curves 2a,b, 3a,b and 4a,b were obtained on crystal B ($C_N = 6 \cdot 10^{-4}$) after successive degrees of smaller deformations in tension and torsion. The deformed crystals show two peaks at 550 - 630 K (1) and at 800-850 K (2) with peak heights increasing with the degree of deformation. Peak (1) is slightly reduced after the second runs (curves b). Both peaks are shifted to lower temperatures with increasing degree of deformation.

The influence of annealing is brought out more clearly by **Fig. 2** for the second deformation stage of crystal B. Curves $\alpha, \beta, \gamma, \delta$, were obtained in subsequent runs. After annealing to 710 K or 880 K peak (1) is decreased and shifted slightly to higher temperatures. Peak (2) remains unchanged after annealing to 880 K.

The preceeding experiments verify the existence of two SK peaks in α-Fe. We shall henceforth denote them by SK1 and SK2. We identify the low-temperature peak SK1 with the "classical" SK peak in

α-Fe /2,7,3/.

To our knowledge the present measurements are the first that observe the high-temperature peak SK2 on α-Fe monocrystals. Whereas there do not appear to exist previous monocrystal measurements in the temperature range in question, IF peaks at about 800 K had been previously reported on deformed α-Fe polycrystals containing ISA's /10,11/ (comp. also /1,9/). The identification of these peaks with Kê's grain-boundary sliding peak /7/ appears highly questionable in view of the present single-crystal results.

Discussion and Conclusions

We shall first discuss the question whether the available experimental evidence supports the viewpoint that the SK relaxation is due to a dislocation - ISA interaction. Both Schöck's theory /12/ and the kink-model /4,6/ to be considered below are based on the concept that dislocation segments of average length $\bar{L}$ bow out under the action of the applied shear stress, and that the presence of ISA enhances the energy loss associated with the dislocation movement.

A first test of the validity of such dislocation models is that the relaxation strength Δ (or the height of the IF peak) should be independent of the temperature. The study of the relaxation strength of SK2 in Nb-O has shown that Δ is indeed temperature-independent over a fairly wide temperature range /5/.

The relaxation strength is expected to increase proportional to the number of dislocation segments participating in the relaxation process and to the third power of their length, or, equivalently, to the product of the density of the participating dislocations and the square of the segment length. Unless $\bar{L}$ is reduced very drastically with increasing deformation (overcompensating the increase in dislocation density) one expects an increase of Δ with increasing plastic deformation that is, however, weaker than that of the total dislocation density. This appears to be in qualitative agreement with Fig. 1 (and the results in /5/).

The relaxation time, whose temperature dependence may usually be described by an Arrhenius law

$$\tau = \tau_o \exp(H^{SK}/kT), \qquad (1)$$

reflects variations of the dislocation segment length L more directly since the dislocation - ISA-interaction theories predict it to be independent of the number of dislocation segments participating in the relaxation process but to increase with L ($\tau_o \propto L$ or $\propto L^2$, see below). Since in an IF measurement at frequency f the peak temperature T_p is determined by

$$2\pi f \; \tau(T_p) = 1, \qquad (2)$$

a decrease or increase of L leads via (1) to a decrease or increase of T_p.

The slight reduction of the peak temperatures of both SK peaks with increasing deformation may thus be understood in terms of the shrinkage of the distances of nodes etc. in the dislocation arrangement with increasing plastic deformation. As one would expect, annealing treatments result in opposite variations of T_p (comp. T_p (SK1) in Fig. 2).

The existence of two distinct SK peaks may be attributed to L distributions peaking at two $\bar{L}$ values that differ by at least one order of magnitude. The origin of two strongly differing $\bar{L}$ values is a task for future clarification. It has been suggested /5/ that small precipitates may subdivide long dislocations into smaller segments which then would give rise to the SK1 relaxation. An alternative interpretation is offered by observations of dislocation arrangements in deformed metals indicating a partitioning into wide regions with a low density of long dislocation segments and narrow regions of densely packed and presumabely much shorter dislocation segments (e.g. dislocation walls, glide-zones, cell- or subboundaries). The two groups of L values required in order to account for the two SK peaks may be tentatively associated with the length of free dislocation segments within these two structural components of the dislocation arrangement of deformed metals.

While it may be stated that the preceding qualitative discussion is in satisfactory agreement with the dislocation - ISA-interaction model, quantitative interpretations of the SK relaxation requires a much more detailed model. This is especially true with respect to the magnitude of the <u>activation enthalpy</u> H^{SK} of the relaxation process, which we have so far left out of our consideration

In Seeger's model /4,6/ it is the bowing out of <u>screw</u> dislocations that is involved in the Snoek-Köster relaxation of b.c.c. metals. The mobility of these dislocations is controlled by the stress-assisted thermally activated formation of pairs of kinks of opposite sign and the migration of the kinks along the dislocation lines. The kink motion is impeded by the ISA in the neighbourhood of the screw dislocations. The "dragging force" exerted by the ISA on the kinks results from the reorientation of the ISA (i.e., the Snoek-effect mechanism) under the influence of the stress field of a moving kink.

With regard to the ultimate fate of the kinks generated on the screw dislocations the theory makes an important distinction /6,13/. If the temperature is low enough for the kinks present in thermal equilibrium to be negligible (the criterion is that $x_K \gg L$, where x_K is the average separation of kinks along an otherwise straight dislocation in thermal equilibrium) the recombination of kinks of opposite sign may be disregarded. Then the distance travelled by the two members of a newly generated kink pair is about L. In the opposite case, $x_k \ll L$, the recombination of kinks on the same dislocation line plays a very important rôle. This results in a stronger dependence of the relaxation time on L, viz. $\tau_o \propto L^2$ (instead of $\tau_o \propto L$ for $x_k \gg L$). In the first case ($x_k \gg L$) the activation enthalpy H^{SK} of the SK relaxation is given by the sum of the activation enthalpy H^S of the Snoek effect and of the formation enthalpy $2 H_k$ of a kink pair. In the second case the activation enthalpy is $H^{SK} = H^S + H_k$, since the density of "kink sinks" increases with temperature, leading to a reduction of the activation enthalpy H^{SK}.

In a simplified manner the situation is outlined in the <u>Arrhenius-type diagramm</u> $\ln \tau$ vs. $(kT)^{-1}$ of <u>Fig. 3.</u> Two discrete dislocation segment lengths L_1 and L_2 have been assumed. At the change-over from $x_k \gg L$ to $x_k \ll L$ the slope of $\ln \tau$ vs. $(kT)^{-1}$ and thus H^{SK} is reduced. The temperature at which this change over occurs varies with L in the manner indicated. The diagramm demonstrates on the one hand that in IF experiments at a fixed frequency f and hence constant τ (exemplified by the dashed line), two peaks should appear if two sufficiently widely separated L distributions exist in the sample. On the other hand it can be seen that under these conditions a frequency (or τ) interval exists (marke by dotted lines) in which the IF peak at the lower temperature (SK1) should show the higher activation enthalpy of the case $x_k \gg L$ and the peak at higher temperatures (SK2) should show the lower activation enthalpy of the case $x_k \ll L$. Such an unusual behaviour of the activation enthalpy has been observed on Nb-O /5/. We conclude from this that the Nb-O measurements /5/ fall indeed in the interval just mentioned.

The preceding considerations implied that the ISA concentration C_d in the surroundings of the dislocation is independent of temperature. As discussed in /4,13/, C_d may vary with temperature (especially at high temperatures and low ISA concentration) if the binding energy H^B between ISA and dislocation is positive. This introduces an additional contribution to H^{SK} which, in the limiting case of high temperatures and low ISA concentration, is equal to H^B. A detailed discussion of this point lies beyond the scope of the present paper.

The main results of the present paper may be summarized as follows. The experiments on the Snoek-Köster relaxation in dilute Fe-N alloy single crystals agree well with the viewpoint that the SK-relaxation process is due to dislocation-ISA interactions. It has been shown that the existence of two SK peaks is not confined to the Group-V transition metals. In addition a possible relationship has been found of the high temperature IF peak SK2 to what was hitherto considered as the "grain-boundary sliding" relaxation peak.

References

/1/ A.S. Nowick and B.S. Berry, Anelastic Relaxation in Crystalline Solids, Academic Press, New York and London (1972).
/2/ J.L. Snoek, Physica (Utrecht) 8, 711 (1941).
/3/ W. Köster, L. Bangert und R. Hahn, Archiv f. Eisenhüttenw. 25, 569 (1954).
/4/ A. Seeger, phys.stat.sol.(a) 55, 457 (1979).
/5/ A. Seeger, M. Weller, J. Diehl, Z.L. Pan, J.X. Zhang, and T.S. Kê, Zeitschr. f. Metallk. 73, 1 (1982).
/6/ A. Seeger, J. de Physique 42, C5-201 (1981).
/7/ T.S. Kê, Trans. AIME 176, 448 (1948).
/8/ U. Rodrian and H. Schultz, Zeitschr. f. Metallk. 73, 21 (1982).
/9/ R. De Batist, Internal Friction of Structural Defects in Crystalline Solids, North-Holland, Amsterdam (1972).

/10/ K. Bungardt und H. Preisendanz, Archiv f. Eisenhüttenw. **29**, 241 (1958).

/11/ M.L. Bernshtein und E.S. Tikhomirova, Relaxation Phenomena in Metals and Alloys (B.N. Finkelshtein,ed.), Consultants Bureau, New York, 1963, p. 211.

/12/ G. Schöck, Acta Met. **11**, 617 (1963).

/13/ A. Seeger, Scripta Met. **16**, 241 (1982).

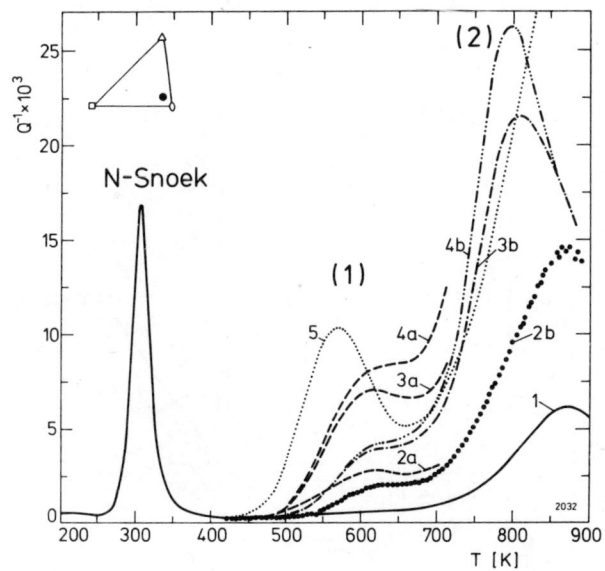

Fig. 1.

Temperature dependence of the IF of Fe monocrystals A ($C_N=4.5\cdot10^{-4}$) and B ($C_N=6\cdot10^{-4}$), $f \simeq 2$ Hz. Curves 1 and 5 from crystal A before and after swagging (25% reduction in area). Curves 2 to 4 from crystal B after successive plastic deformation. 2a,b after 5% in tension, 3a,b after additional 2.5% in torsion, 4a,b after additional 2.5% in torsion. All curves measured with increasing temperature, curves b after the corresponding curves a and cooling down. (For crystal orientations see stereographic triangle.)

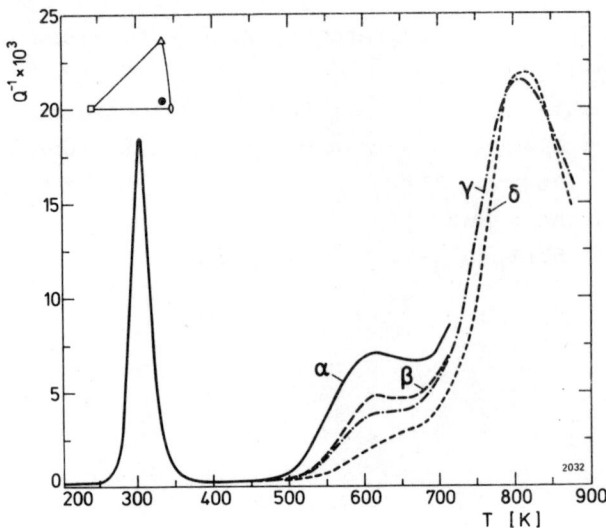

Fig. 2.

Influence of annealing on the IF of crystal B ($C_N = 6 \cdot 10^{-4}$) after 5% plastic deformation in tension and 2.5% in torsion ($f \simeq 2$ Hz, heating rate 2 K s^{-1}) α: first run, β: after annealing by run α to $T_A = 710$ K, γ: after additional annealing to $T_A = 710$ K, δ: after $T_A = 880$ K.

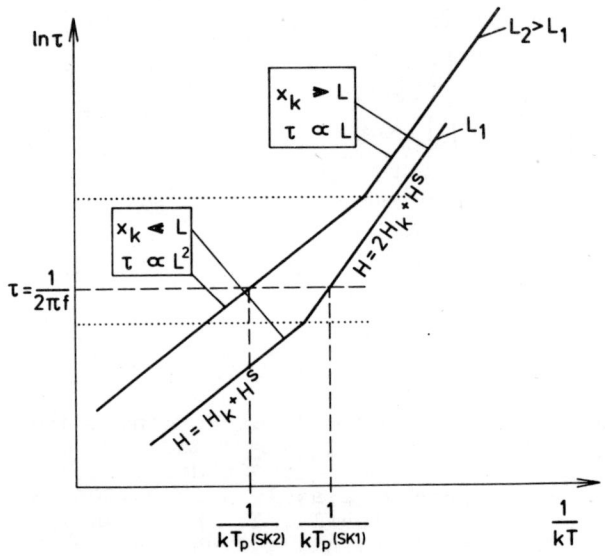

Fig. 3.

Schematic Arrhenius-type diagramm for the kink model and for two discrete dislocation segment lengths L_1 and L_2.

- 222 -

ON THE DISLOCATION ARRANGEMENT IN Fe-3wt%Si SINGLE CRYSTALS
AFTER DEFORMATION IN TENSION BETWEEN 113 AND 573 K

B. Šesták and M. Bucki

Institute of Physics, Czechoslovak Academy of Sciences
Na Slovance 2, 180 40 Prague 8, Czechoslovakia

1. Introduction

Plastic deformation of single crystals of iron- 3wt.% silicon alloy has been investigated in detail using macroscopic tests and observation of slip traces /1-4/. It was found that addition of silicon to iron significantly incereases the critical resolved shear stress (from 10 MPa for iron to 150 MPa for Fe-3%Si alloy at room temperature) and substantially changes the work-hardening behaviour. Stages II and III of the work-hardening curves are absent for Fe-3%Si alloy single crystals deformed to necking in the range from 113 K to 573 K. A characteristic feature of the beginning of plastic deformation of this alloy is localization of slip in slip bands separated by undeformed crystal regions. During increasing deformation the old bands broaden and new ones appear. The average shear strain γ_B concentrated in the slip bands was found to be relatively independent of the total specimen strain γ as long as the whole specimen is filled up with the bands, i.e. up to $\gamma \simeq \gamma_B$ (values of γ_B are given in Table 1 /4/). Deformation $\gamma > \gamma_B$, till necking of the specimens, realizes by slip distributed homogeneously along the whole specimen gauge length.

In addition to these studies a systematic investigation was made, by electron transmission microscopy (TEM), of the dislocation arrangements which develop in Fe-3%Si single crystals during deformation in tension at temperatures in the range from 113 to 573 K /5/. In this paper a part of the results, namely the dislocation arrangement in the slip bands, is presented and discussed.

2. Experimental procedure

The specimens investigated were in all respects similar to the specimens used in papers /2, 3/. They were prepared from large Fe-3±0.1wt.%Si single crystals grown by floating zone melting. The specimens oriented for single slip on $(\bar{1}01)$ $[111]$ - slip system were deformed at 113, 295, 403, 473 and 573 K in tension at a nominal strain rate $\dot{\varepsilon} = 5.5 \times 10^{-5} \mathrm{sec}^{-1}$. Sections parallel to $(\bar{1}01)$ primary slip plane, (101) secondary slip plane and (001) plane were cut from deformed specimens. Thin foils suitable for TEM were prepared by the method described in /6/ and examined in JEM 6A microscope operating at 100 kV. Some of them also in JEM 1000 microscope operating at 1000 kV.

Dislocation densities were measured mostly in (001) foils because the thickness of these foils was simply determined from the length of straight primary dislocations parallel to $[111]$ direction. In addition, variations of the dislocation density perpendicularly to the primary slip plane were averaged using these foils.

3. Experimental results

Examples of shear stress-shear strain curves of the crystals deformed at various temperatures are shown in Fig. 1.

Basic features of the dislocation arrangement observed in the slip bands after deformation at various temperatures were qualitatively similar. Examples of this arrangement as observed in foils parallel to $(\bar{1}01)$ primary slip plane are shown in Figs. 2 and 3. It consists of large primary glide loops elongated parallel to the primary $[111]$ Burgers vector and small prismatic loop debris of various sizes elongated approximately in $[1\bar{1}1]$ direction. Secondary dislocations were observed only on a very few isolated places in the foils.

AT 473 K (Fig. 2) the primary glide loops are highly elongated. Their parts parallel to $[111]$ direction, "screw parts", are long, relatively straight and arranged in groups. The edge segments are up to a few microns long and their density is low. The density of the small prismatic loop debris is very small. At 113 K (Fig. 3) the primary glide loops are less elongated. The transition between the screw and edge parts is smooth so that the loops are of an elliptical shape. The density of loop debris is high and at some places they start to form clusters.

The dislocation arrangement observed in (001) foils which intersect the primary slip plane under 45° corresponds well to that in $(\bar{1}01)$ foils.

Table 1 summarizes the dislocation density measurements. It is seen that density ρ_B^l of dislocations forming the primary loops significantly decreases with increasing temperature. At 473 K ρ_B^l is in fact equal to the density of screw parts of the loops. Density ρ_B^t of all dislocations was also determined. The difference between ρ_B^l and ρ_B^t results mainly from the loop debris.

After deformation $\gamma > \gamma_B$ at all temperatures the main component of the dislocation arrangements are clusters or bundles of edge dipoles, multipoles and prismatic loops. With increasing deformation beyond γ_B the bundles join together forming long irregular braids along the primary slip plane. Their overall direction coincides with that of 71° - dislocations.

4. Discussion

The main components of the dislocation arrangement observed in the slip bands at all temperatures are large primary dislocation loops elongated parallel to their Burgers vector and a distribution of small loop debris. During proceeding deformation behind $\gamma \simeq \gamma_B$ this arrangement characterized by long dislocation segments of approximately screw orientation is gradually transformed into arrangement where dense clusters of edge dipoles, multipoles and small elongated loops dominate /5/.

According to surface observations /1, 4/ the glide of dislocations in the isolated bands is predominantly concentrated to their periphery. It is manifested by broadening of the bands at the expense of undeformed crystal volume and by a relatively constant shear strain concentrated in the bands. It suggests that inside the bands the primary glide dislocations are immobilized by mutual interactions and an equilibrium dislocation density is adjusted. At $\gamma \simeq \gamma_B$ the whole crystal is filled up by the bands so that the imposed strain rate cannot be accommodated by expanding of the slip in to the virgin crystal parts, and the dislocation loops in the temporarily hardened interior of the bands start to glide again under an increasing stress. Their screw part annihilate while the edge parts are mutually captured and forme stable dipoles which together with the loop debris accumulate in the crystal forming clusters. As a result the density of long curved dislocations of approximately screw character does not change remarkably with increasing deformation. On the other hand, the density of edge dislocations increases, their clusters join together forming dense wavy braids which before necking of specimens occupy a large volume fraction.

The observed dislocation arrangements prove that the plastic deformation of the studied crystals in the temperature range under investigation is entirely due to glide of primary dislocations and up to the necking clearly corresponds to stage I-hardening which is typical of pure b.c.c. metals at intermediate temperatures, where interactions of primary dislocations are responsible for work-hardening. This conclusion corroborates the previous observations of slip traces and work-hardening characteristics /2/.

In the following, effect of temperature on the dislocation arrangement in the slip bands will be discussed and explained on the basis of dislocation interactions.

A striking feature of the dislocation arrangement as observed at 473 K in foils parallel to the primary slip plane are very long and straight dislocations of [111] direction. They are parts of primary dislocation loops highly elongated in this direction. The edge segments are almost completely absent in the micrographs. On the other hand at 113 K and 295 K the primary loops are less elongated. As a result their arms approximately parallel to [111] are more curved and the density of their edge parts is larger in comparison to 473 K. In addition, the density of debris loops is significantly higher at 113 K with respect to 473 K. It witnesses to much larger activity of screw dislocations during the deformation process at 113 K.

At the first sight these results seem to contradict to observations in pure b.c.c. metals where quite the reverse is found in accordance with the high Peierls stress of screw dislocations in comparison to non-screw ones. On second thought, however, we recognize that there is a strong hardening by solute atoms in Fe-3%Si alloy and some evidence exists for believing that this hardening reduces mobility of non-screw dislocations approximately to that of screw dislocations. In the first place, early measurements of edge dislocation velocities in Fe-3%Si single crystals led to this conclusion /7/. The second evidence comes from the fact that work-hardening of these crystals in the range from 113 to 573 K is similar to stage I hardening of pure b.c.c. metals at intermediate temperatures. It is accepted that comparable mobilities of screw and non-screw dislocations are a necessary prerequisite for this type of work-hardening. From these facts it follows that in Fe-3%Si alloy, in contradistinction to pure b.c.c. metals, the ratio of screw and non-screw mobilities should remain close to one with decreasing temperature, at least up to 113 K. As a result in the whole temperature range the isolated dislocation loops should be ellipses with not to large ratio of the axes. At 473 K the observed dislocation arrangements contradict, however, to this conclusion. Instead of the elliptical loops long, straight "screw" dislocations are seen and their low slip activity is obvious. In order to explain this inconsistency interactions of primary dislocations have to be considered.

For the discussion of this temperature effect in terms of dislocation interactions it is convenient <u>to divide the flow stress</u> τ (in the case, when the slip bands occur $\tau \cong \tau_0$ the critical resolved shear stress) <u>into components</u> /2, 3/

$$\tau(\gamma, T) = \tau^*(T) + \tau_G^c + \tau_G^i (\gamma, T)$$

where τ^* is the effective stress (the dynamic friction stress), $\tau_G^c \cong 90$ MPa for Fe-3%Si alloy is the static friction stress due to solution hardening by silicon atoms, (its temperature dependence is supposed to be equal to that of shear modulus G) and $\tau_G^i \cong \alpha Gb\sqrt{\rho}$ is the internal stress (α is a constant smaller than 1, b is the Burgers vector and ρ is the dislocation density). The temperature dependence of τ_G^i results from the temperature dependence of both the dislocation arrangement and the shear modulus.

<u>The dislocation densities</u> ρ_B^l given in Table 1 were used for an estimation of τ_G^i. The density of dislocations at the CRSS can be in principle determined from the condition that at a constant strain rate the macroscopic yielding of crystals occurs at a minimum applied stress /8, 9/. A homogeneous distribution of mobile and accumulated dislocations in the whole specimen is assumed in this model. A corresponding calculation cannot be performed for our case because the plastic deformation during yielding is localized in the slip bands. In this case the dislocation density is rather controlled by dynamics of the slip bands formation where cooperative motion of dislocations emitted from a source is important /10-12/. Therefore, it appears

that a comparison of the measured dislocation densities with the calculated ones is not yet possible.

Our results show that the density ρ_B^1 increases with decreasing temperature, i.e. when the flow stress increases. There are not enough experimental data to establish a reliable relation between these quantities. Our measurements at three temperatures may be well fitted by

$$\rho_B^1 = 3.5\,(\tau - 85.1)\,10^{11}\,m^{-2}, \qquad 1)$$

which can be considered as a linear dependence of dislocation density ρ_B^1 on $(\tau - \tau_G^c)$ (a small temperature dependence of τ_G^c is neglected).

According to interferometric measurements on the surface /4/ the shear strain γ_B localized in the glide bands can be well expressed as

$$\gamma_B = 0.183\,(\tau - 92.8) \qquad 2)$$

(the measurements admit a dependence on $(\tau^2 - \text{const.})$ as well /4/). The last two equations indicate an approximately linear relationship between ρ_B^1 and γ_B, which suggests that the average slip distance

$$l = \gamma_B / \rho_B^1 \times b \simeq 2.1 \times 10^{-3}\,m \qquad 3)$$

$(b = 2.48 \cdot 10^{-10}\,m)$

is nearly independent on the deformation temperature and of the order of the specimen diameter.

<u>Internal stress</u> which develops inside the glide bands was calculated according to

$$\tau_G^i = \alpha\,G\,b\,\sqrt{\rho_B^1}$$

with $\alpha = 0.22$. This α - value was determined using a simple model of elastic interaction between one moving and two symmetrically located screw dislocations. The values of internal stress τ_G^i calculated in this way are given in Table 1, together with τ_G^c and τ^*. This division of the critical resolved shear stress, which is also shown in Fig. 5, is based on the calculated values of τ_G^i and on measurements by Zárubová /3/.

An inspection of Table 1 and Fig. 5 shows that at 473 K values of τ_G^i and τ^* are approximately equal. It suggests that dislocations inside the slip bands are, in comparison to the periphery of the bands easily stopped by elastic interaction when passing on parallel slip planes. Then the originaly elliptical loops can be transformed into array of long "screw" dislocations by movement of edge segments as illustrated in Fig. 6. This is well possible when the applied stress is smaller than the passing stress of screw dislocations $\tau_p \simeq \tau_G^i$ and larger than the corresponding drag stress τ_d. The drag stress is the stress necessary to cover the increment in the energy due to the increase in the length of the screw segments. At $\tau > \tau_d$ infinite extension of the loops in the direction of their Burgers vector is ensured. For the drag stress τ_d = 6 MPa ($\lesssim \tau^*$) the upper limit of the loop width necessary for their extension was estimated to be $\simeq 2 \mu$m. Such loop widths agree with observations. Thus, it may be concluded that at 473 K the applied stress adjusts itself so that $\tau^* > \tau_d, \tau_p^* \lesssim \tau \simeq \tau_G^i$ and the plastic deformation occurs mainly by slip of edge dislocations on large distances, whereas the temporarily immobilized long dislocation segments of [111] orientation accumulate in crystals. This mechanism works till $\gamma \simeq \gamma_B$, when the crystal volume is filled up by the glide bands.

At 113 K the adjusted effective stress $\tau^* \simeq 94$ MPa is large in comparison to the calculated internal stress $\tau_G^i \simeq 20$ MPa. The effect of elastic interactions between the passing screw dislocations can be therefore considered smaller than at 473 K. As a result one can expect that at 113 K the dislocation loops remain elliptical, which is actually observed. Consequently both edge and screw dislocations will contribute to plastic deformation in a comparable way. This is witnessed by high density of prismatic loops which are produced at large jogs during glide of screw dislocations. In this picture screw dislocations inside the glide band at 113 K are, in comparison to 473 K, relatively mobile. Although during proceeding deformation the plastic strain is accommodated mainly by broadening of the existing bands and formation of new ones, a restricted slip inside the bands cannot be excluded. It is probably one of the reason of the scatter in measurements of γ_B at 113 K, which is significantly larger than the accuracy of the measurements.

5. Conclusion

Dislocation arrangement in slip bands in Fe-3wt%Si single

crystals has been investigated by TEM. In the slip bands the plastic shear strain γ_B is localized at the beginning of plastic deformation. In the temperature range from 113 to 573 K following results were obtained:

1) In the slip bands only primary dislocations were found. Their density significantly increases with decreasing deformation temperature. For the total specimen strain $\gamma \lesssim \gamma_B$ this density is relatively independent of γ.
2) Density ρ_B^1 of the primary dislocation loops depends on the applied stress similarly as γ_B so that an approximately linear relation exists between ρ_B^1 and γ_B.
3) The average slip distance is of the order of specimen diameter, independently of temperature.
4) At 473 K arrays of relatively straight dislocations of $[111]$ direction dominate in the slip bands and the calculated internal stress is about of the same value as the effective stress. At 113 K elliptical dislocation loops elongated in $[111]$ direction together with large density of small prismatic debris loops are seen in the micrographs. The calculated internal stress is 5 times smaller than the effective stress.
An explanation of this difference based on dislocation interactions is suggested. In comparison to 113 K where $\tau_G^i \ll \tau^*$, at 473 K screw parts of the expanding dislocation loops are immobilized by mutual interactions and mainly slip of edge dislocation segments takes place. As a result loops highly elongated in $[111]$ direction are produced and the long $[111]$ arms accumulate in the slip bands.
5) Formation of the slip bands where relatively high plastic deformation is localized is undoubtedly a consequence of the large static friction stress τ_G^c. This stress stabilizes groups of screw dislocations against attraction and repulsion, i.e. it screens effects of dislocation interaction stresses. As a result high local equilibrium densities of moving dislocations may occur soon after activation of a source. The dislocations remain close together and follow closely their slip plane. Consequently, the slip traces on Fe-3%Si crystals are less wavy than on iron and people working on fatigue takes Fe-3%Si alloy for a material with planar slip and put it in line with such materials as α - brass and austenitic steels, which is from microscopic point of view not too

felicitous association.

References

/1/ Zárubová N., Kadečková S.: Czech. J. Phys. B 22 (1972) 215.
/2/ Zárubová N., Šesták B.: phys. stat. sol. (a) 30 (1975) 365; 479.
/3/ Zárubová N., Kadečková S.: Proc. 5th Int. Conf. Strength of Metals and Alloys (edit. P. Haasen, V. Gerold and G. Kostorz) Vol. 2, p. 1031, Pergamon Press, Oxford 1979.
/4/ Šesták B., Novák V.: phys. stat. sol. (a)23 (1974) 703.
/5/ Bucki M.: Thesis, Institute of Physics, Czech. Acad. Sciences, Prague 1974.
/6/ Bucki M., Gemperle A.: Czech. J. Phys. B23 (1973) 1273.
/7/ Stein D.F., Low J.R., Jr.: J. Appl. Phys. 31 (1960) 362.
/8/ Takeuchi S.: Journ. Phys. Soc. Japan 27 (1969) 929.
/9/ Raghuraman S., Arsenault R.J.: Scripta Met. 12 (1978) 753.
/10/ Loh B.T.M.: Supplement to Trans. Japan Inst. Metals 9 (1968) 13.
/11/ Arsenault R.J., Kuo C.T.K.: Metallurgical Trans. 9A (1978) 459.
/12/ Blahovec J.: Unpublished results.

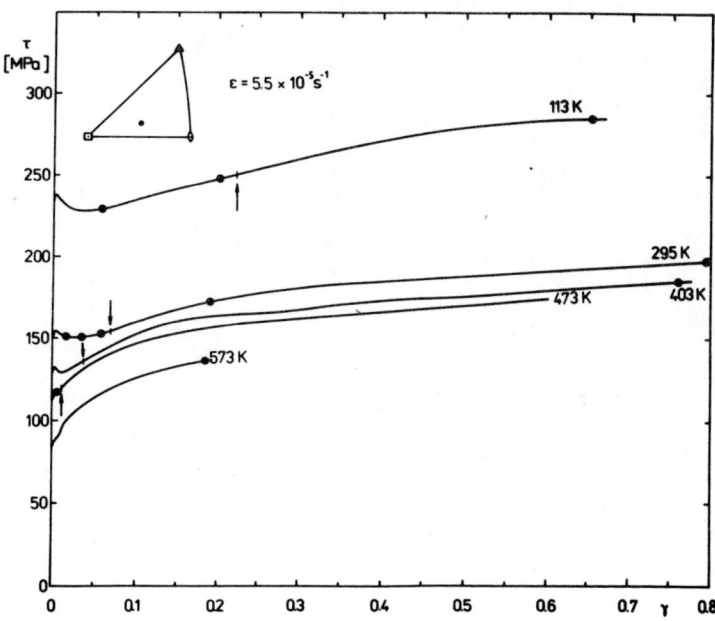

Fig. 1 Shear stress-shear strain curves of Fe-3wt%Si crystals deformed at various temperatures showing the strains (o) at which the dislocation structures were analysed. The shear strain $\gamma = \gamma_B$ at which the specimen surface is just covered by slip bands is indicated by arrows. The initial orientation of the specimens is also shown.

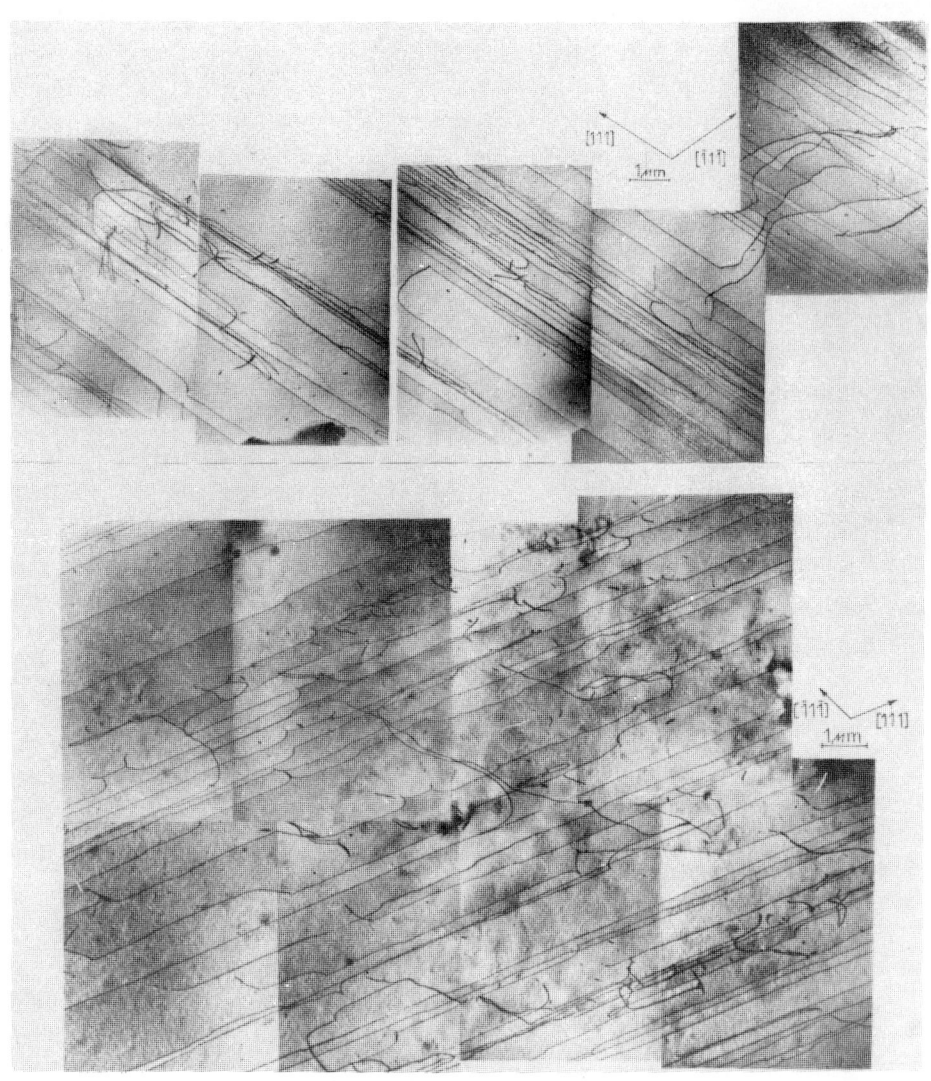

Fig. 2 Examples of the dislocation arrangement observed in slip bands after deformation at 473 K ($\gamma = 0.7$ %). Foil parallel to ($\bar{1}01$) primary slip plane.

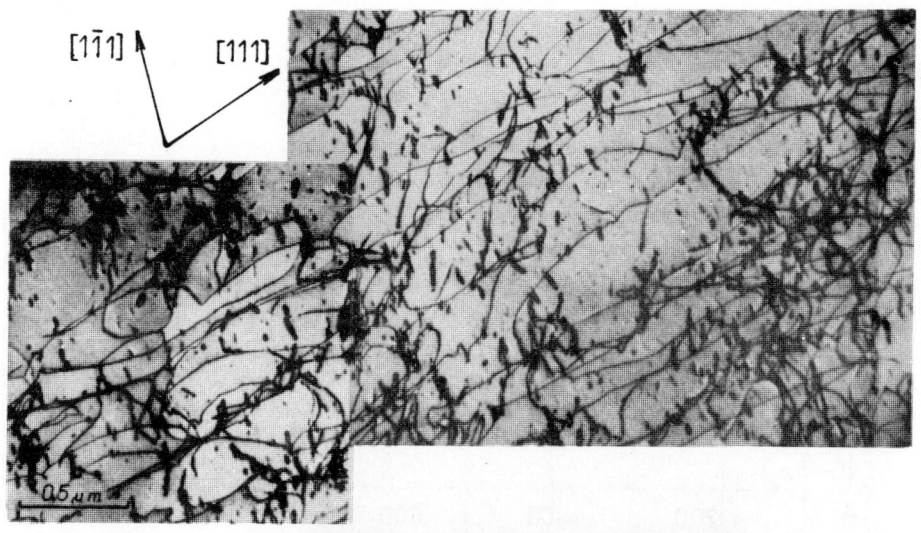
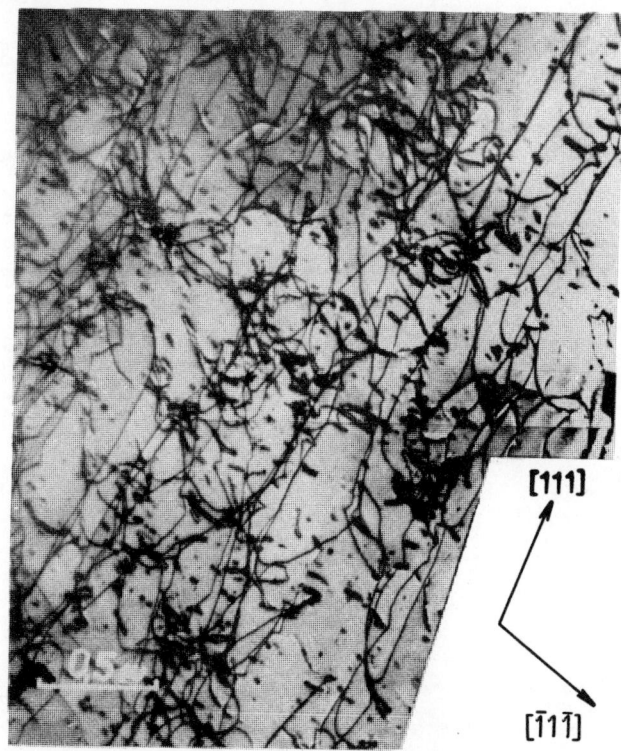

Fig. 3 Examples of the dislocation arrangement observed in slip bands after deformation at 113 K (γ = 5.8 %). Foil parallel to ($\bar{1}$01) primary slip plane.

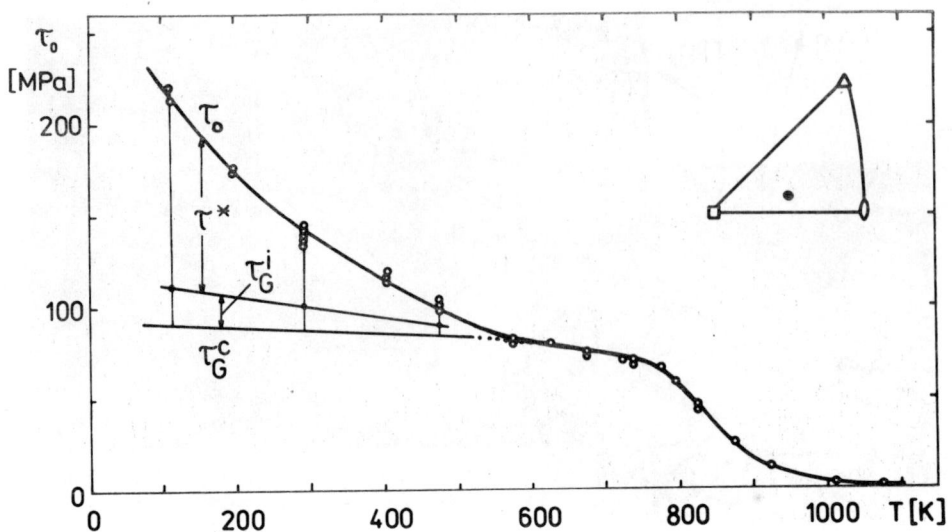

Fig. 4 Division of the critical resolved shear stress of Fe-3wt.%Si single crystals into three stress components τ_G^c, τ_G^i and τ^*.

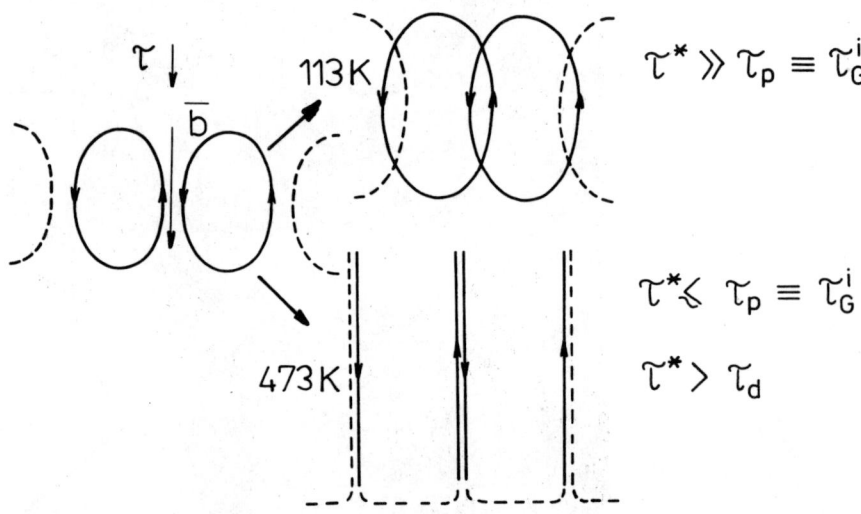

Fig. 5 Schematic illustration of dislocation loops passing on parallel slip planes at 113 and 473 K in Fe-3%Si single crystals.

Table 1.

T /K/	γ /%/	τ /MPa/	τ_0 /MPa/	γ_B %	γ/γ_B	$\rho_B^l \cdot 10^{-13} \text{m}^{-2}$	$\rho_B^t \cdot 10^{-13} \text{m}^{-2}$	$\tau_p \equiv \tau_G^i$ /MPa/	τ_G^c /MPa/	τ^* /MPa/
113	5.8	215	215± 5	22± 4	0.26	4.7	9.0	20	90	104
	20	240			0.90	4.6	10.3			
295	1.6	140	140± 5	7±1.2	0.22	2.3	3.5	14	87	38
	3.5				0.50	1.6	3.8			
	5.8				0.82	2.6	5.0			
473	0.5	100	100± 5	1.2±0.5	0.41	0.27	0.3	1) 7	84	9
	0.8				0.66	0.34	0.4			

1) Calculated with $\rho_B^l = 0.5 \times 10^{13} \text{m}^{-2}$, which is local density of screw dislocations arranged in groups.

DISLOCATION MOBILITY AND OVERCOMING OF LOCAL BARRIERS AT LOW TEMPERATURE AS DEDUCED FROM INTERNAL FRICTION DATA

V.I. Startsev, V.Ya. Platkov

Physico-Technical Institute of Low Temperatures, Acad. Sci. Ukrain. SSR, 47 Lenin Ave., Kharkov 310164, USSR.

An overview is presented of the available data on the dynamic behaviour of dislocations obtained by internal friction measurements. Theoretical concepts and experimental data are considered concerning the amplitude-dependent and -independent internal friction and its connection with quasi-viscous motion of dislocations, as well as with the motion involving thermally activated and athermal overcoming of local obstacles.

Special attention is paid to low-temperature peculiarities of the dislocation mobility. The results of investigations of the electron drag of dislocations are presented together with the role of this drag in overcoming the obstacles by the inertia mechanism. The dynamics of local obstacle overcoming changes due to a sharp decrease in the electron drag at the superconducting transition.

The dislocation motion is quasi-viscous between or over barriers and thermally activated, when barriers are overcome by thermal fluctuations. Barriers can also be overcome by either inertial or quantum mechanisms. The latter are, however, realized at low temperatures only. In a real case, we deal with a complex combination of all the mechanisms of dislocation motion.

In all the cases, the dynamic dislocation behaviour may be studied with using data on the internal friction. Data on the quasiviscous motion with its principal characteristic, the damping coefficient B, are obtained from investigations of the amplitude-independent internal friction δ_i. The frequence dependence of δ_i is of a resonance nature /1/, different resonance curve sections being related to dislocation structure parameters, including B, in a different way. The amplitude-independent internal friction and the related modulus defect ($\Delta M/M$); for the resonance curve ascending branch are given by equations /1/:

(1) $\quad \delta_i = (\Omega \Delta_0 / \pi^2 C) N L^4 B \omega$

(2) $\quad (\Delta M/M)_i = (6 \Omega \Delta_0 / \pi) N L^2$

where N is the dislocation density, L the dislocation segment average length, $\Delta_o = 4(1-\nu)/\pi^2$ (ν being the Poisson coefficient); $C = 2Gb^2/\pi(1-\nu)$ (G being the shear modulus in the slip direction), ω the vibration frequency, and Ω the orientation multiplier. The two above equations contain three independent variables: B, N and L. Therefore, if we are to know B from measurements in this section of the resonance curve, we have to measure independently the dislocation density or to determine the dislocation segment average length.

The descending branch sound absorption is

(3) $$\delta_i = 8\Omega G b^2 N / \pi B \omega$$

The maximum frequency usually lies in the mHz range (Fig.1). Determination of the modulus defect for frequencies over ω_m involves considerable difficulties; therefore the experimental data are treated only with eq. (3) containing two variables, N and B, to be found. The frequency corresponding to the maximum of the frequeny dependence of the decrement and its magnitude are given by relations /1/:

(4) $$\omega_m = 0.084 \pi^2 C / L^2 B$$

(5) $$\delta_m = 2.2 \Omega \Delta_o N L^2$$

Equations (4) and (5) also contain three independent variables: B, L and N. The maximum of the frequency dependence of δ_i is broadened, and the curve covers several orders of the frequency magnitude. Therefore, a single measurement method is not sufficient for the two resonance curve branches, and the absolute value of B cannot be determined without independently measured dislocation density.

Among the first works involving determination of B by the ultrasound dislocation resonance absorption study were those reported in refs. 2-4. Even these early afforts brought interesting results on the temperature dependence of B for LiF, copper and Cu-Mn alloy, on the absolute value for KCl and KBr, etc. Subsequently the method was gradually improved and much attention was given in particular to the important problem of separating the background losses /5-7/.

The dislocation drag is a consequence of the interaction with various elementary excitations of the crystal lattice (phonons, electrons, magnons) and also with impurity atoms and other dislocations. The contributions of the mechanisms vary with the temperature ranges. For this reason, the temperature dependence of B is of a paramount importance for the identification of the dislocation drag mechanisms.

The principal contribution to the dislocation drag in metals is the interaction with phonons and electrons. There is a large variety of phonon drag mechanisms /9/, but they are all characterized by a strong temperature dependence. It may vary from T^5 (in the low temperature range) to T (above the Debye temperature). As consequence, at temperatures just above 0 K the phonon mechanism contributions to the drag are negligibly small and it may be dominated by the electron drag contribution, which is not dependent on temperature. The electron drag is directly proportional to the conduction electron density and naturally is not the case with insulators. In metals the electron and phonon drag contributions become equal at about 10 K. There is no temperature dependence of the radiation drag either. Its contribution is, however, small and comparable with the phonon drag at still lower temperatures.

It was of interest to investigate B as a function of temperature on antimony single crystals, since the normal electron density is low there and thus, the electron drag contributuon was small. Measurement results of refs. 7, 8 are shown in fig. 2. In a 100-300 K temperature range a pulse method was used in the measurements, while at 4.2 K the measurements were carried out by means of the composite oscillator. In the former case the resonance absorption of dislocation segments was studied in the frequency range of 7.5 to 122.5 mHz. The dislocation-related component was separated by two procedures: by subtracting the pre-deformation internal friction and analytically. The dislocation density was determined by etch pits. It was revealed that the frequency dependence of the dislocation internal friction was in agreement with the predictions of the Granato-Lücke theory /1/. The damping coefficient B decreased monotonically with temperature from 9×10^{-5} dyne.s/cm^2 at 300 K to 1×10^{-5} dyne.s/cm^2 at 6 K. The B(T) dependence that resulted was easy to describe in terms of superposition of the "slow" phonon relaxation and phonon wind mechanisms.

An unusual behaviour of B in the range 77-500 K was found in LiF single crystals /10/. The absorption coefficient was measured in a way similar to that described above. In this crystal, throughout the temperature range studied, B remained constant. A comparison with the phonon drag theory /9/ suggests that this behaviour of B was due to an anomalously significant role of the "slow" phonon relaxation mechanism among all the other dislocation drag phonon mechanisms. This experimental result agrees with data of ref. 3 that B was the same at 78 and 300 K. The study of the coefficient B for LiF by measuring dislocation displacement as displayed by etch pits /11/ also suggests that B was independent of T in a range of 77-300 K.

The temperature dependence of B for such a typical metal as copper was studied in refs 12 and 13. The B (T) curves of ref. 12 were for Cu single crystals with minor impurities in the temperature range 4.2-300 K and had, as usual, maxima between 70 and 130 K. These were probably due to losses induced by thermally activated dislocation relacation processes responsible for so-called Bordoni peaks. The contributions of the relaxation and viscous components within the dislocation ultrasound absorption in copper were separated in ref. 13. The B(T) dependence obtained by the authors of ref. 13 disregarding the relaxation component of ultrasound absorption also included a broad maximum near 90 K; however, the separation of the viscous component resulted in the true B(T) dependence. It can be subdivided into two characteristic section: the lower-temperature one (4.2-20 K), where B is practically independent of T, and the higher-temperature one (20-300 K), where B rises monotonically with T (fig. 3). The former section is dominated by the electron dislocation drag, independent of T, while the latter by the phonon one, which may be well described by the "slow" phonon relaxation and phonon wind mechanisms.

Electron and phonon dislocation drag was also investigated

in Al /14/. The dislocation component of the ultrasound absorption was separated by the "dynamic" bias-stress method. The dependence B(T) was obtained for a range of 10-250 K, where B changed from 1.5×10^{-5} to 4.5×10^{-5} dyne.s/cm^2. There was a surprising fact as follows: the T-independent electron drag dominated in dislocation drag in a very wide temperature range, up to 50 K. Above 50 K the coefficient B monotonically increased with T, as is implied by the phonon drag mechanisms.

The electron dislocation drag is directly proportional to the conduction electron density. When a metal transits into the superconducting state, electrons make up Cooper pairs, which do not interact with dislocations, and electron drag should sharply decrease. To know whether this is so, temperature dependences of B were measured in normal (n-) and superconducting (s-) states /14/. Figure 4 shows temperature dependences of the dislocation part of the absorption coefficient for lead in n- and s-states. The s-n transition was induced by application of a magnetic field above critical. Since in a small temperature range, N and L remain essentially constant, the dislocation part of the ultrasound absorption coefficient δ_d is proportional to B and therefore, the $\delta_d(T)$ curves in fig. 4 reflect the temperature dependence of B. In the n-state, as is seen from fig. 4, B does not depend on T. Here B is due to the electron drag, independent on temperature, as was once predicted by the theory /16, 17/. In the s-state, δ_d decreases with T, which corresponds to reducing the electron drag B. The latter fact is due to a decreasing normal electron density.

Those are the basic mechanisms that were found by the investigation of the dislocation amplitude-independent internal friction in crystals at low temperatures.

The dislocation motion in crystals is due not only to the viscous drag, but also to overcoming various obstacles. Information on the dislocation dynamic behaviour, when it completely depends on obstacle overcoming, may be obtained by studying the amplitude-dependent internal friction. As during the quasi-viscous motion of dislocations, in the case where the dislocation motion dynamics is governed by local obstacle overcoming, each of the mechanisms involved is prevalent in a certain temperature range. In the lower temperature range, essential contributions may come from inertial and quantum mechanisms. Therefore the amplitude-dependent internal friction is important to study over a very wide range of temperatures, down to the lowest ones.

Such studies were carried out in the kHz range on impure cooper single crystals /18/ and KCl single crystals /19/. With lowering temperature, the amplitude dependence curves were displaced into a region of larger vibration amplitudes ε_o, thus suggesting the thermally activated nature of overcoming of pinning centres by dislocations. Treatment of experimental results is terms on the reaction rate theory yielded enthalpy values for the activation of thermally activated overcoming of impurity atoms by dislocations. The enthalpy appeared to be so small (0.07-0.1 eV) that the very existence of the dislocation hysteresis responsible for the amplitude dependence of δ could not be explained. The situation was helped by Indenbom and Chernov /20/ who considered the role of thermal fluctuations in hysteresis loss and proposed a method to determine the characteristics of the dislocation interaction with local pinning centres. The experimental data of refs. 18 and 19 and those of ref. 21 on the temperature effect on the amplitude dependence of the internal friction in NaF in the range 4.2 to 300 K were treated in ref. 20 and reasonable activation parameter values were obtained, which are also consistent with dislocation mobility data resulting from the dislocation motion observation by etch pits.

The dynamic dislocation behaviour dominated by pinning centre overcoming was investigated by measuring the amplitude dependent internal friction and the modulus defect in unstrained and plastically strained bismuth single crystals /22/ at temperatures between 110 and 205 K, in high purity molybdenum single crystals /23/ and antiminy single crystals /24/ of various purity in a range 6.5-300 K. Dependences of the activation energy and the activation volume of pinning centre overcoming by dislocations on the applied stress, length distribution function of dislocation segments, which proved to be power dependence, as well as the dislocation-defect interaction force law were thus studied.

As mentioned, B of antimony, because of low normal electron density and therefore weak electron drag of the damping coefficient, decreases at lowering T down to the helium temperature (see fig. 2.) Therefore, at low temperature, where B is small, the character of pinning centre overcoming by dislocations may be altered and, accordingly, there may be singularities in the low temperature amplitude-dependent internal friction behaviour. The first experimental observation of the amplitude-dependent internal friction behaviour in antimony was reported in ref. 24 at temperatures below 30 K. Unlike at higher temperatures, where decreasing T causes the amplitude dependences to displace towards larger amplitudes (fig. 5), at $T < 30$ K there is a reverse displacement and increased curve slope (fig. 6). An analysis showed that this feature of the internal friction versus temperature was due to easier unpinning of dislocation segments at $T < 30$ K because of action of the internal mechanism suggested in ref. 25. The authors of ref. 28 came to a similar conclusion in a discussion of their results which were that in a lead single crystal, at a temperature slightly lower than T_c (superconducting transition temperature), the stress amplitude required for the internal friction to be constant coincided in the s- and n-states, and in a Pb + 0.3 at. % Sn single crystal this occurred essentially at T_c. In both cases the action of the internal mechanism involved a significant decrease in B (in antimony, featuring small electron drag, it was by lowering T, while in lead by transferring the sample into the s-state). In molybdenum the conduction electron density is large and so is naturally the T-independent electron drag; therefore, in a temperature range used in ref. 23, B could not decrease so much, as to meet the coditions required for the inertial mechanism action. This is the reason for the absence in molybdenum of the singularities of the temperature dependence of the internal friction which were observed in antimony.

In a low temperature range some interesting effects can also be observed different from the above described features of the dislocation dynamics. Thus, the theory /27, 28/ predicts that at low temperatures the quantum mechanism of pinning centre overcoming by dislocations may be manifested. However, there were no experimental investigations of the dislocation dynamics involving the internal friction under conditions with strong quantum effects.

The study of the amplitude-dependent internal friction in the n- and s-states provides information on the mechanisms of pinning centre overcoming by dislocations under these conditions. The measurement of the dislocation internal friction in the course of repeated transitions between the s- and n-states suggested that its magnitude did not change in the process. Hence, an important conclusion was drawn that during the superconducting transition there is no dislocation multiplication /29/. The study of the effect of various valence impurities on the amplitude-dependent internal friction in the s- and n-states found that dislocation interaction with impurity atoms may range from essentially elastic to almost completely electrostatic. However, the stress for dislocation unpinning from various impurities at the superconducting transition changes but little. This means that the quasistatic mechanism of changing screening of differently valent atoms during the n-s transition plays no essential role in the alteration of the conditions of pinning centre overcoming as against the dynamic mechanisms due to changing electron drag /30/.

In type II superconductors, in the mixed state, the dislocation dynamics may largely depend on the dislocation interaction with Abrikosov vortices (fluxoids). In Pb-In single crystals the character of the displacement of the amplitude dependence vs. magnetic field curves varies markedly, according to the particular dislocation pinning centre type. The monotonic evolution shown in fig. 7 suggests that Abrikosov vortices may change the damping coefficient and thereby affect the pinning centre overcoming dynamics. As the local barrier height becomes smaller in response to increased indium concentration and ordering, the dependence of the internal friction on the magnetic field becomes nonmonotonic (fig. 8), suggesting that Abrikosov vortices may also be regions restricting the dislocation motion /31/.

The results presented here demonstrate the efficiency of the internal friction method, particularly for studying the dislocation dynamic behaviour, at low temperature.

References

/1/ Granato A.V., Lücke K.: J. Appl. Phys. 27 (1956) 583.
/2/ Suzuki T., Ikushima A., Aoki M.: Acta Metall. 12 (1964) 1231.
/3/ Mraček Mitchell O.M.: J. Appl. Phys.: 36 (1965) 2083.
/4/ Platkov V.Ya., Efimenko V.P., Startsev V.I.: Fiz. Tverd. Tela 9 (1967) 2799.
/5/ Mason W.P., MacDonald D.E.: J. Appl Phys. 42 (1971) 1836.
/6/ Kaufmann H.R., Lenz D., Lücke K.: Intern. Conf. Internal Friction and Ultrasonic Attenuation in Crystalline Solids, vol. 2, p. 177, 1973.
/7/ Pal-Val P.P., Platkov V.Ya., Startsev V.I.: Phys. Stat. Sol. (a) 38 (1976) 383.
/8/ Pal-Val P.P.: Thesis, Physico-Technical Institute of Low

Temperatures, Kharkov, 1982.
/9/ Al´shitz V.I., Indenbom V.L.: Uspechi Fiz. Nauk 115 (1975) 3.
/10/ Petchenko A.M., Startsev V.I.: Fiz. Tverd. Tela 16 (1974) 3655.
/11/ Darinskaya E.V., Urusovskaya A.A., Opekunov V.I., Abramchuk G.A., Alekhin V.A.: Fiz. Tverd. Tela 20 (1978) 1240.
/12/ Kaneda T.: J. Phys. Soc. Japan. 28 (1970) 1205.
/13/ Kobelev N.P., Soifer Ya.M., Al´shits V.I.: Fiz. Tverd. Tela 21 (1979) 1172.
/14/ Hikata A., Johnson R.A., Elbaum C.: Phys. Rev. B2 (1970) 4856.
/15/ Kobelev N.P., Soifer Ya.M.: Fiz. Tverd. Tela 21 (1979) 1362.
/16/ Kravchenko V.Ya.: Fiz. Tverd. Tela 8 (1966) 927.
/17/ Holstein T.: Appendix to the papr Tittman B., Bömmel H.: Phys. Rev. 151 (1966) 178.
/18/ Saul R.H., Bauer Ch.L.: J. Appl. Phys. 39 (1968) 1469.
/19/ Platkov V.Ya., Ledneva N.N., Startsev V.I.: Fiz. Tverd. Tela 11 (1969) 3659.
/20/ Indenbom V.L., Chernov V.M.: Phys. Status Solidi (a) 14 (1972) 347.
/21/ Kardashov B.K., Nikanorov S.P., Voinova O.A.: Phys. Status Solidi (a) 12 (1972) 375.
/22/ Nikanorov S.P., Romanov A.D., Tsinman E.A.: Fiz. Tverd. Tela 16 (1974) 2984.
/23/ Kaufmann H.-J., Pal-Val P.P.: Phys. Status Solidi (a) 62 (1980) 569.
/24/ Pal-Val P.P., Platkov V.Ya., Startsev V.L.: Fiz. Nizk. Temp. 7 (1981) 361.
/25/ Granato A.V.: Phys. Rev. B4 (1971) 2196.
/26/ Isaac R.D., Schwarz R.B., Granato A.V.: Phys. Rev. B18 (1978) 4143.
/27/ Natsik V.D.: Zh. Eksp. T$_e$or. Fiz. 61 (1971) 2540.
/28/ Natsik V.D.: Fiz. Tverd. Tela 16 (1974) 526.
/29/ Platkov V.Ya., Polunina L.N., Startsev V.I.: Fiz. Tverd. Tela 13 (1971) 1881.
/30/ Pal-Val L.N., Platkov V.Ya., Roshchupkin A.M.: Fiz. Nizk. Temp. 6 (1980) 1980.
/31/ Beloshapka V.Ya., Platkov V.Ya.: Fiz. Nizk. Temp. 8 (1982) 1217.

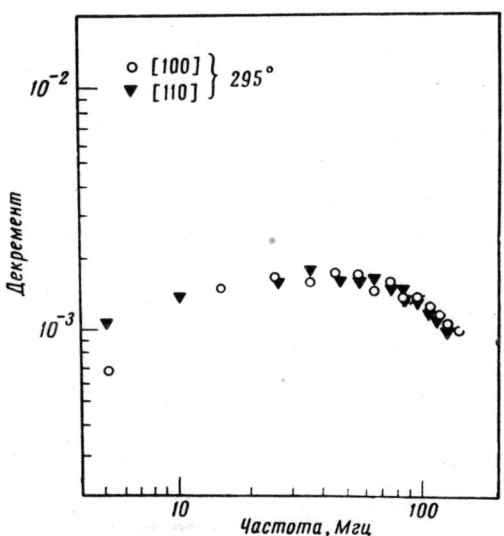

Fig. 1 Frequence dependence of dislocation damping in copper at 295 K for longitudinal vibrations.
    ○ data points for the sound propagation direction /100/,
    ▼ for the sound propagation direction /110/.

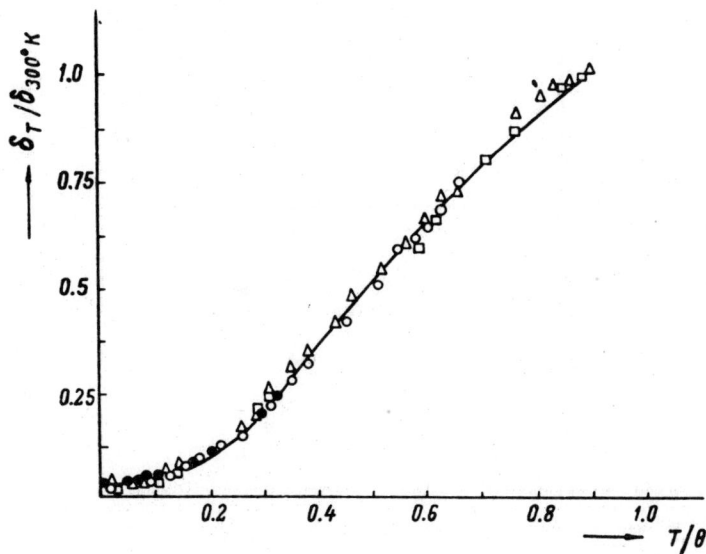

Fig. 2 Reduced temperature dependence of B for copper /13/.

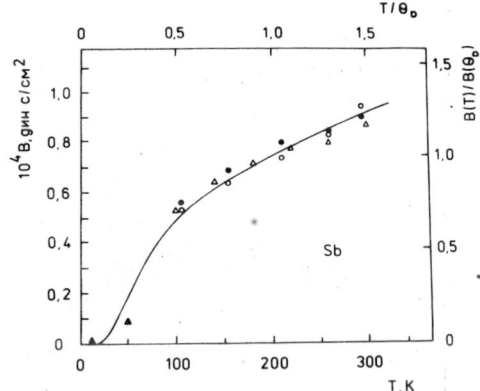

Fig. 3 Temperature dependence of the damping coefficient B in antimony /8/.

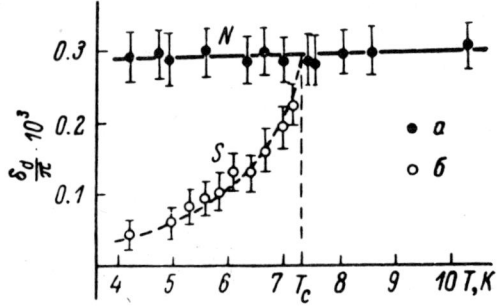

Fig. 4 Temperature dependence of the dislocation part of the decrement δ_d proportional to the damping coefficient B /15/.
a) normal state;
b) superconducting state.

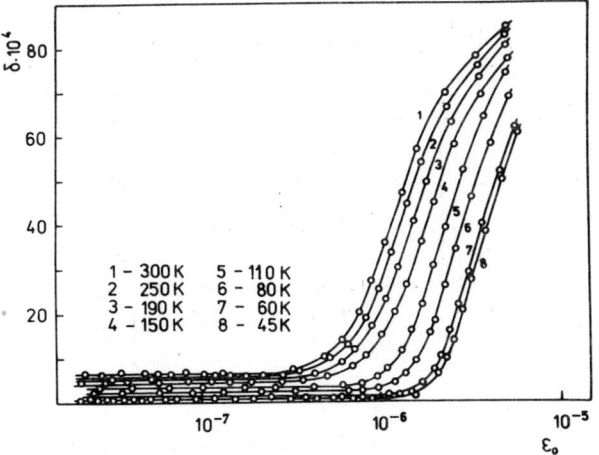

Fig. 5 Effect of temperature on the amplitude-dependent internal friction due to thermally activated pinning centre overcoming by dislocations in antimony /24/.

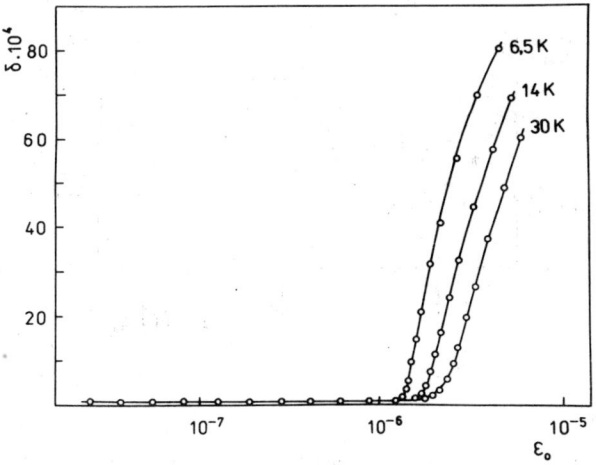

Fig. 6 Anomalous displacement of the amplitude-dependent internal friction with temperature chaning below 30 K, due to the inertial mechanism of pinning centre overcoming by dislocations /24/.

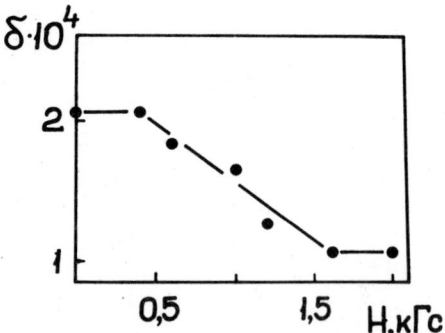

Fig. 7 Dependence of the decrement dislocation part on the magnetic field magnitude for a Pb+3 at. % in single crystal, $\varepsilon_o = 6.8 \times 10^{-5}$ /31/.

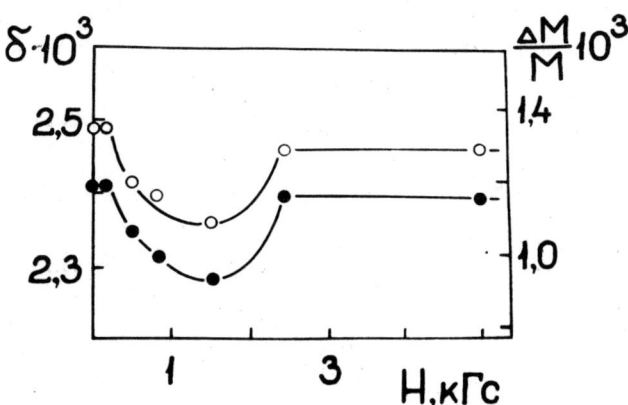

Fig. 8 Dependence of the decrement dislocation part and of the modulus defect on the magnetic field for Pb + 12 at. % In single crystals, $\varepsilon_o = 2 \times 10^{-6}$.
  data points for the decrement,
  data points for the modulus defect /31/.

SECTION 3

THE STRUCTURE AND PROPERTIES
OF DEFECTS
IN NON-METALLIC MATERIALS

DEFECTS IN IONIC CRYSTALS AND OXIDES.

J.PHILIBERT

Université Paris-Sud, F-91405 - ORSAY.
Laboratoire de Physique des Matériaux, C.N.R.S., Bellevue, F-92190 - MEUDON.

Abstract.

Main properties of point defects and dislocations in ionic crystals are reviewed. Emphasis is put on dislocations in relation with plastic properties : slip systems, slip anisotropy. Some peculiarities of stacking faults and dissociation of dislocations in oxides are discussed, particularly the meaning of the climb dissociation, rather than glide dissociation, observed in materials which only show plasticity at high temperatures.

I. INTRODUCTION.

Under the heading of "Ionic Crstals" may be classified a rather large number of materials from the alkali and alkaline earth halides to oxides and chalcogenides, whose "ionicity" is high (Table I). Actually in many compounds the covalent part of the bonds cannot be entirely ignored, because in most oxides bonding has some intermediate character (iono-covalent bonding). But so far atomistic calculations of defects have always been based on a purely ionic bonding. The present paper will be mainly dealing with oxides.

Some oxides are often considered as "good" ionic crystals, comparable to alkali halides, because they are insulators. With a purely ionic conductivity, as MgO, $Al_2O_3 - \alpha$, or Y_2O_3, they only suffer very tiny deviations from stoichiometry. A majority of oxides display large or very large deviations from stoichiometry and they behave like semi-conductors with a p or a n-type : examples are transition metal oxides $M_{1-x}O$ with NaCl structure (M = Ni, Co, Mn or Fe) and $Cu_{2-x}O$, which are p-type, $UO_{2\pm x}$ (fluorite structure), TiO_{2-x} of n-type,... The deviation x may range from 10^{-5} to 10^{-1} or more, according to compounds and depends on temperature and oxygen partial pressure [2]. More complex oxides have also been studied : spinel $Mg Al_2 O_4$ or more exactly $MgO, (Al_2O_3)_n$ with $1 \leqslant n \leqslant 3,5$ and ferrites with spinel structure, forsterite Mg_2SiO_4, garnets, etc... without forgetting a "covalent" oxide like SiO_2.

In many cases the crystal structure can be described on the basis of an oxygen close-packed lattice : FCC for MgO, NiO,... and for spinels, HCP for $Al_2O_3-\alpha$, distorted hexagonal for TiO_2,... Cations occupy defined interstitial positions in this lattice. But this description is not a universal one, and a cation lattice based description is probably more relevant in some compounds.

For detailed references about defects the reader is invited to refer to some books [2][3] or review papers [1] [4] [5] [6] [7].

II. POINT DEFECTS.

Besides the SCHOTTKY or FRENKEL defects common to all ionic compounds in thermal equilibrium, point defects in oxides have two other origins:

- Structural or constitutive vacancies. In Al_2O_3-α for instance, two thirds of octahedral interstices are occupied, the other one-third are vacant in an ordered way. The latter are highly energetic and they are considered as "interstitial" sites. In MgO, cations occupy all the octahedral sites and the tetrahedral sites behave like interstitials for cations. In several cases, the distinction between vacancy and interstitial becomes ambiguous, as it depends on the reference structure. With large concentrations of dopant, charge compensating defects are so many that long range order can occur on the corresponding sublattice (example : anion sublattice in ZrO_2 or CeO_2 doped by di- or tri-valent cations).

- Deviations from stoichiometry, which are obtained thanks to vacancies or interstitials of one species (or both, cations and anions as in TiO). The defects behave as neutral or charged entities, depending on the binding of electrons or holes with the lattice defect.

Point defect production may be described in a quasi-chemical way:

$$1/2\, O_2 \rightleftarrows O_o + V_M$$
$$\rightleftarrows O_o + V'_M + h^\bullet$$
$$\rightleftarrows O_o + V''_M + 2h^\bullet$$

In this example incorporation of oxygen in the lattice (O_o) from the gas phase ($1/2\, O_2$) requires a cation vacancy V_M either neutral, singly or doubly charged. Electron holes ($h^\bullet$) are produced accordingly. The KROGER-VINK notation, as used above, may be somehow delusive : electrons or holes are not strictly trapped at the defect site. In a divalent metal oxide, a vacancy with a double charge means two delocalized holes, whilst a neutral vacancy corresponds to holes bound to nearest neighbour ions (i.e. M^{3+} instead of M^{2+}). In other words, they correspond to several acceptor levels in the band gap.

The concentration of defects of a given charge state depends on temperature and oxygen partial pressure. For large deviations of stoichiometry, defects aggregate in clusters or form complexes (1 vacancy + 1 FRENKEL defect in FeO, or even larger aggregates). The state of aggregation is still in most cases poorly characterized, at the exception of alkaline earth oxides (thanks to spectroscopic techniques) [5].

In other oxides, typified by TiO_2, point defect concentration remains low, and composition changes are obtained with the help of planar defects, known as "shear faults" : they can be described as missing oxygen planes in an oxygen deficient crystal.

Little is known about minority defects, i.e. defects in the oxygen sublattice for a metal deficient oxide. Their nature (vacancies, interstitials, or molecular defects) remains an open question in most cases. As their concentration is very low, there are very few methods available for their study. A better knowledge of their nature and their diffusivity in the bulk and along extended defects (dislocations, grain boundaries) would be appreciated, as these minority defects are controlling high temperature plasticity [1][8].

III. DISLOCATIONS.

Dislocations in ionic crystal disclose special features, partly because of their electric charge. This problem will not be discussed in the present paper, and the reader is referred to some review papers [3][9]. We shall restrict ourselves to the atomic structure of dislocations.

1°) Burgers vector (table 2).

When both sublattices (cations and anions) coincide, like in NaCl or MgO, one is left with a situation identical with metals : $\vec{b}$ lies along the more close-packed row and its length is equal to the smallest repeat distance. Example : $\vec{b} = \frac{a}{2} <110>$ in NaCl structure (NaCl, MgO, NiO,...)

When sublattices are different, $\vec{b}$ lies along a close-packed direction, but not necessarily along the more close-packed, and its length is not always the shortest repeat distance. In spinel, $\vec{b}$ is just the shortest of possible vectors. But in Cu_2O for instance the easiest slip direction is $<110>$, $\vec{b} = a<110>$, whilst the shortest repeat distance is $a<100>$. A similar result is observed in TiO_2. In sapphire $Al_2O_3\alpha$ (fig.1), for prismatic glide, a very long Burgers Vector (8.22 Å) is preferred to shorter ones (4.75 Å or 5.12 Å) which could have been expected (fig.2). Table 2 gives the elastic energy of dislocations for different Burgers vectors.

2°) Glide plane (Table 3).

Glide plane is always a close-packed plane - at least when such planes exist in the structure ! - but not always the more close-packed. In NaCl structure, {110} is the easiest glide plane, although {100} is the densest plane consisting of cations and anions, or {111} the densest one, but consisting of cations or anions (alternate charge planes). In spinel both {111} and {110} glide planes are frequently observed. The second seems to be the easiest according to the latest experiments {10}. In many cases glide occurs along "planes" which have a corrugated atomic structure (prism plane in $Al_2O_3-\alpha$). In garnets, no close-packed plane exists, and plastic deformation proceeds by climb at temperatures higher than 0.78 T_M [11] (where T_M is the melting point).

All these results are difficult to rationalize on a simple basis, and usual criteria fail [1][5]. Several factors are interplaying : core structure, possible dissociation in partials, electrostatic charge effects, elastic energy, Peierls force,... But the actual glide system cannot always be predicted, as these factors may lead to contradictory results. The anisotropy of glide - i.e. the existence of several glide systems - is generally poorly understood, and its temperature dependence still less understood (see below § VI).

IV. STACKING FAULTS.

Possible stacking faults can be more or less described by simple considerations based on geometrical arguments (hard sphere model) or electrostatic ones.

In alkali halides, earliest calculations were carried out by FONTAINE [12] through a planewise lattice summation and for an unrelaxed configuration, for S.F. on {100}, {111} and {110} planes. More recent calculations [13] are atomistic type calculations : they include ion relaxation, and are based on potentials derived from point defect studies. It is found that $\frac{a}{2}$ [001] (100) faults are unstable. Intrinsic faults on {111} (typical of FCC) are stable (minima of energy) with little crystal relaxation. On the other hand $\frac{a}{4}$ {110} ($1\bar{1}0$) have comparable or lowest energy, but they present local maxima of energy, so no stable semi-infinite fault exists. After a rather strong relaxation there is a net dilatation of the crystal. The values of γ are highest than found by Fontaine (0.29 J/m^2 instead of 0.19 for NaCl).

Fontaine's method has been extended to several oxides : taking in account only coulombic energy, and neglecting relaxation, and small lattice distorsions (i.e. a simplified crystal structure has been used [11][24]): polarization energy is eventually included by dividing the energies by the high frequency dielectric constant. The degree of confidence one can give to these computations remains questionable. A distinction can be made between two types of faults, according as the S.F. affects only one sublattice (cation sublattice where the structure is described on the basis of interstitial sites in an oxygen close-packed lattice) or both sublattices.

In $Al_2O_3 - \alpha$ a low S.F. energy is predicted in the basal plane for the cationic fault ($\gamma = 0.54$ J.m^{-2}), a quite higher one for a cationic + anionic fault - which would be bounded by a Shockley partial - ($\gamma = 1.86$ J. m^{-2}). But the cations faults in the prism planes are found to be very energetic (4 to 5 J.m^{-2} [24]. All these results are only partially in agreement with TEM observation (see below).

Similar results are found for <u>spinels</u>, an FCC crystal with 56 ions per unit cell. Computations have been performed for normal, inverse and disordered structures (these adjectives refer to the occupancy of tetrahedral and octahedral sites by divalent and trivalent cations). Computed S.F. energies are of the order of 1 J.m^{-2} [24], values leading to dissociation widths of a few b's, that is not observable - contrarily to TEM observations. Configuration 1/4 [110] {110} with the translation perpendicular to the fault plane is found to be the less energetic (0.76 J.m^{-2} for disordered structure).

In Y_2O_3 (a complex structure with 80 ions per unit cell), a rather low energy SF (80 m J.m^{-2}) has been predicted on {001}. It is produced by removing four successive planes or by a shear $\frac{a}{2}$<110> [16]. In garnets, a still more complex structure (160 ions per unit cell), SF also affects both sublattices, and different faults have been considered and their energy calculated. These S.F. introduce either lattice disorder or electrostatic defects [11].

V. DISSOCIATION.

When $\vec{b}$ is equal to the shortest repeat period of the lattice, no dissociation has ever been observed in alkali halides or simple oxides, contrarily to some predictions based on S.F. energy [12][14]. A possible dissociation along :

$$\frac{a}{2} <110> \rightarrow \frac{a}{4} <110> + \frac{a}{4} <110>$$

was expected, the repulsion between partiale stabilizing the S.F. However, since the S.F. configuration is not a local minimum of energy, the dissociation would be analogous to that in BCC metals, and described as a distribution of fractional dislocations rather than two well defined partials. Thereby Fontaine and Haasen [17] predicted a d/b value from 6 to 18. But more recent calculations do not find any evidence for dissociation. In NaCl atomistic computations show a core spread on about 2b [15].

When $\vec{b}$ is large or very large, the stability of such dislocations is questionable. On the basis of elastic energy considerations (see table 2), these dislocations should decompose in perfect dislocations with smaller Burgers vectors or dissociate into partials. This assumed structure of dislocations has to be in agreement with the observed glide. In these materials, plastic deformation requires temperature higher than $T_M/2$ and they behave in a brittle manner at room temperature. However some plasticity is observed at room temperature around indentations [18], and at medium temperatures under hydrostatic pressure [19][20].

At low temperature dislocations are found undissociated by TEM ($1/2<110>$ dislocations in spinel [21]), or glide dissociated ($<110>$ dislocation in Y_2O_3 [16]).

After high temperature deformation, dislocations appear frequently climb dissociated [21][22][23], i.e. the S.F. ribbon does not lie in the glide plane, a process which involves some climb of the partial dislocations, and thereby point defect diffusion (diffusion limited on small distances as the climb process may be conservative thanks to the exchange of matter between the partials).

Let us give a few examples of climb dissociation. In spinel structure crystals climb dissociation has been observed in nickel ferrites [25] and in spinel mineral MgO, n Al_2O_3 with various values of n [21]. For n = 1.1, dissociation of $<110>$ edge dislocations in two colinear partials is observed : $1/2 <110> \rightarrow 1/4 <110> + 1/4 <110>$ (cf.fig.4). It occurs in a $\{110\}$ plane perpendicular to the Burgers vector, but for n = 1.8, dissociation is observed in other planes : $\{001\}$, $\{113\}$. In both n = 1.8 and n = 3.5 spinels, some flexibility of the S.F. ribbon is observed : bend or twisted ribbon, without constrictions where the orientation is changing.

In $Al_2O_3 - \alpha$, dissociation of basal glide dislocations is only observed when they form faulted dipoles, in which case they are climb dissociated [27]. Dislocations responsible for prismatic glide, which have a long Burgers vector (8.22 Å) are found to be climb dissociated in three partials according to (cf. fig.1) :

$$<10\bar{1}0> \rightarrow 1/3 <10\bar{1}0> + 1/3 <10\bar{1}0> + 1/3 <10\bar{1}0>$$

The S.F. plane is found to be any one of the prism planes $\{11\bar{2}0\}$ or $\{10\bar{1}0\}$, or even pyramidal planes, which also expresses some flexibility of the S.F. ribbon [22][26][28]. This observation shows the S.F. energy is rather isotropic [29]. The same S.F. observed for prism plane climb dissociation is also observed for basal dislocations dissociated according to :

$$1/3 [11\bar{2}0] \rightarrow 1/3 [10\bar{1}0] + 1/3 [01\bar{1}0]$$

by climb in a prism plane.

Besides dissociation of partials there is another way of reducing the energy of prism dislocations : decomposition into basal dislocations :

$$<10\bar{1}0> \rightarrow 1/3 <11\bar{2}0> + 1/3 <21\bar{1}0>$$

a very easy process for screw dislocations, but involving some climb for edges [22]. Such decomposition occurs with profusion so that a basal dislocation network is build up, which opposes the glide of prism dislocations [28] . Both configurations, decomposed and dissociated, have been simultaneously observed, which allows a determination of S.F. energy, in good agreement with other determinations [29] .

In Y_2O_3, after high temperature deformation, $\vec{b}$ = a <100> dislocations are climb dissociated. Interestingly the same S.F. is involved in this case and in the glide dissociation observed at low temperature [16] .

Climb dissociation clearly corresponds to a lower energy state than glide dissociation [29] , but it is naturally expected only at temperatures high enough for the occurence of climb. A point which remains unclear is the mechanism which allows the glide of such dissociated dislocations. In near stoichiometric spinel, pure climb is preferred, after some limited glide at the very beginning of the deformation [10][21] . For non-stoechiometric spinel, as well as for Al_2O_3, well defined slip lines are observed [10][31] .

Actually there is no definite evidence that dislocations are really climb dissociated during deformation. There are many contradictory evidences. In spinel undissociated dislocations produced by room temperature indentation do dissociate after annealing at 1000°C [21]. In spinel, climb dissociated dislocations are observed after rather fast quench of the specimen [21] . The S.F. ribbon width is determined by a static equilibrium between 3 different forces : applied stress, elastic interaction between partials, S.F. tension, and the first one varies during cooling : observed configuration do vary with cooling rate and with anneal treatment [26] (e.g. broadening due to point defect diffusion). TEM observations of Al_2O_3 deformed by prism glide at low temperature ($\sim$ 400°C) under hydrostatic pressure [19] are expected to give further insight on the structure of the gliding dislocation. There is strong evidence than diffusion helps the broadening of the S.F. ribbon - which favours a core structure presenting at least some incipient dissociation of the climb type. Internal stresses would strongly affect the partial configuration. In these conditions, comparison with computed values of the S.F. energy is not straight forward. However in $Al_2O_3-\alpha$ many independent determinations converge towards a well defined range of S.F. energy (0.1 - 0.25 Jm^{-2}, [29]).

VI. GLIDE ANISOTROPY.

Glide anisotropy remains most of the time very intriguing and poorly understood.

In alkali and silver halides, the CRSS has been measured for {110} and {100} glide planes versus temperature, for pure and doped crystals [32] . The anisotropy is very pronounced, as {100} planes are quite harder than {110}

At lower temperatures this anisotropy probably reflects differences in the Peierls force, as it varies systematically along the series of halides [32] . However it is only partly explained by differences in ion polarizability. At higher temperatures, anisotropy is related to the interactions of dislocations with point defects - mainly dimers (foreign cation + charge compensating vacancy) [33] . In cuprite Cu_2O, three different slip systems have been observed [34] with two different Burgers vectors (Table 3). The shortest Burgers vector {100} is only observed if the temperature is high enough, whilst at low temperatures {110} glide direction prevails, perhaps because of an incipient dissociation in (110) planes, which seems favoured on the basis of simple geometric arguments. But no dissociation has ever been demonstrated by T.E.M.

In spinels, two glide planes seem more favourable on the basis of dissociation criteria : {111} and {110} . Experimental evidence has been for a long time contradictory [5] , partly due to a bad choice of crystal orientation (the Schmid factor systematically favouring one glide system). Nowadays, whatever the molecular composition of MgO, $(Al_2O_3)_n$ with $1 \leq n \leq 3.5$, {110} plane seems to be the easiest glide plane. At high temperatures [10][27][35] $<1/2>\{110\}$ $\{1\bar{1}0\}$ dislocations can climb dissociate on a {110} plane, which would have the lower S.F. energy. At low temperatures, the situation is more confuse. Around room temperature indentations,{111} , {110}, and {100} glide planes have been observed in ferrites and chromites [21] . In $Mg Al_2O_4$ however, {111} is preponderant over {110} . But by compression tests under hydrostatic pressure, {110} has been observed to be the easiest glide plane, between room-temperature and 800°C . In this range no evidence for climb dissociation has been claimed [20]. Let us remind the {111} plane was predicted to be the favoured glide plane a long time ago by HONSTRA [36] , on the basis of a dissociation process in this plane. The two partials 1/4 <110> would dissociate further in a similar way to Shockley partials in FCC metals (cf. fig.4) :

$$1/4 <110> \rightarrow 1/12 <211> + 1/12 [12\bar{1}]$$

a dissociation confined to the {111} plane. This dissociation involves a fault in the oxygen sublattice. It is apparently energetically too costly - and it has only been exceptionally observed, probably thanks to local stresses (e.g. network in ferrites [25]).

A similar situation prevails in Al_2O_3-α . Glide was predicted by KRONBERG [37] to be the easiest on the basal plane, because the dissociation of the basal dislocation according to :

$$1/3 <11\bar{2}0> \rightarrow 1/3 <10\bar{1}0> + 1/3 <01\bar{1}0>$$

would proceed further, in the basal plane

$$1/3 <10\bar{1}0> \to 1/9 <2\bar{1}\bar{1}0> + 1/9 <11\bar{2}0>.$$

The last dissociation which involves a fault in the oxygen sublattice has been exceptionnaly observed [26]. Common S.F. faults only involve the cation sublattice.

Nevertheless prism glide is expected to be harder than basal one, as the dislocation structure is probalby simple in the second case. This is actually observed at high temperature. But new results obtained down to low temperatures (200°C) with the help of a confining pressure to avoid fracture show that below 700°C prism glide becomes easier [19]. This change in glide anisotropy still remains unexplained. Room temperature indentation is not very useful in this respect, as twinning occurs profusely [18].

A topics related to glide anisotropy is the occurence of cross-slip. Cross-slip in alkali halides and silver halides is observed to be easier from $\{100\}$ to $\{110\}$ than the inverse (for a review, see [33]).

Cross-slip has also been observed in spinels at high temperature between $\{110\}$ and $\{111\}$ planes [21] by optical microscopy. Its mechanism is related to the evolution of the climb dissociation in an unclear way.

Generally cross-slip has not yet received very much attention in oxides, and its role in medium temperature range remains to be investigated.

VII. INTERACTIONS BETWEEN DISLOCATIONS AND POINT DEFECTS.

Both elastic and electrostatic interactions are expected and atomistic computations are necessary for a correct computation, as shown by a paper in this symposium [33].

In non-stoichiometric oxides, one can wonder whether the relative concentrations of single defects and complexes are similar in the bulk and in the vicinity or in the core of dislocations. There is some evidence from diffusion studies that majority point defects are similar in the bulk and in dislocation core, at least for NiO, an oxide where deviation of stoichiometry remains low ($< 10^{-3}$) : self-diffusivity in the bulk and along dislocation lines ("pipe diffusion") practically follows the same pO_2 dependence [38].

Low temperature mechanical properties do not seem to be very sensitive to point defects [39], their concentration is generally larger than the impurity concentration, and these materials present an intrinsic behaviour. But at high temperature, these point defects have a very strong effect, as demonstrated by the creep rate law [1] :

$$\dot{\varepsilon} = \dot{\varepsilon}_0 \ (pO_2)^m \ \sigma^n \ \exp(-\Delta H/kT)$$

The pO_2 dependence reflects the variation of composition, i.e. the point defect concentration. The latter affects the self-diffusivity, thereby the climb rate and the above equation is derived on this sample basis [1]. Along the same lines, impurities affect creep rate as far as they affect the diffusivity by a doping effect with aliovalent solutes, eg. doped Al_2O_3 [41]. Thorough investigations have been performed in several oxides: Cu_2O [34][40], CoO [41] and NiO [42] and succeeded in assessing the nature of oxygen defects.

The case of water as an impurity deserves a special attention. It has been known for a long time that water strongly softens SiO_2 [44]. A phenomenon which has received several explanations, due to the strongly covalent bonding of this structure [45][46]. There is no evidence of similar effect in other oxides. In this symposium LiF crystals are shown to present some hardening due to the pressure of OH^- anions.

VIII. CONCLUSIONS.

Ionic crystals and oxides disclose many similarities because of identical crystal structures and a predominant type of bonding. But oxides have some problems of their own due to deviation from stoichiometry which can take large values. Better atomistic computations would be helpful in order to improve our knowledge of the dislocation core structure, the Peierls force and the interaction with point defects. The effect of doping has probably been not sufficiently studied. A similar remark applies for the role of cross-slip in plastic deformation. In-situ experiments by straining the specimens in the electron microscope have been impeded by the high required values of stress and temperature : they will probably bring new insight on the behaviour of dislocations in these materials [47].

REFERENCES.

[1] T.BRETHEAU, J.CASTAING, J.RABIER, P.VEYSSIERE.
Adv. Physics (1979) 28, 835-1014.

[2] P.KOFSTAD. Non stoichiometry, diffusion, and electrical conductivity of binary metal oxides. Wiley Interscience (1972).

[3] M.T.SPRACKLING. The plastic deformation of simple ionic crystals. Academic Press. London (1976).

[4] J.CASTAING. Annales de Phys.Fr.(1981)6,195-221.

[5] T.E.MITCHELL, L.W.HOBBS, A.H.HEUER, J.CASTAING, J.CADOZ, J.PHILIBERT. Acta Metal.(1979)27,1677-1691.

[6] M.G.BLANCHIN, J.CASTAING, G.FONTAINE, A.H.HEUER, L.W.HOBBS, T.E.MITCHELL. J.Physique, colloque C3, (1981)42,C3-1-11.

[7] J.PHILIBERT. J.Micros.Spetrosc.Electr.(1976)1,641-670.
     "   "   "   (1980)5,499-514.

[8] A.DOMINGUEZ-RODRIGUEZ, J.CASTAING. Radiation Effects (1983)77.

[9] R.W.WHITWORTH. Adv.Physics (1975)24,203.

[10] R.DUCLOS, N.DOUKHAN, B.ESCAIG. Acta Met.(1982)30,1381-1388.

[11] J.RABIER.Thesis,Université de Poitiers (1979).

[12] G.FONTAINE. J.Physique (1966)27,201-323.

[13] P.W.TASKER, T.J.BULLOUGH. Philos.Mag.(1981) A43,313-324.

[14] F.GRANZER, V.BELZNER, M.BUCHER, P.PETRASCH. J.Physique (1973),34,C9,359.

[15] M.P.PULS, C.B.SO. Phys.Stat.Solidi (1980)b,98,87-98.

[16] R.J.GABORIAUD, M.BOISSON. J.de Physique(1980),41, C6, 171-174.

[17] G.FONTAINE, P.HAASEN. J.Phys.Chem.Solids (1967), 28, 25-53.

[18] B.J.HOCKEY. J.Am.Ceram.Soc.(1971), 54, 223-231.

[19] J.CASTAING, J.CADOZ, S.H.KIRBY. J. de Physique (1981), 42, C3, 43-47.
                J.Amer.Ceram.Soc.(1981), 64, 504-511.

[20] S.H.KIRBY, P.VEYSSIERE. Philos.Mag.(1980),A41, 129-136.

[21] N.DOUKHAN. Doctor thesis, Université de Lille (1980).

[22] J.CADOZ, J.CASTAING, J.PHILIBERT. 9th Int.Conf.Electron.Microsc. TORONTO (1978), 1, 606-607.

[23] J.B.BILDE-SÖRENSEN, A.R.THÖLEN, J.J.GOOCH, G.M.GROVES. Philos.Mag.(1976), 33, 877.

[24] J.RABIER, P.VEYSSIERE, J.GRILHE. J.Physique (1973), 34, C9, 373-377.

[25] P.VEYSSIERE, J.RABIER, H.GAREM, J.GRILHE. Philos.Mag.(1976),33,143-163.

[26] J.P.RIVIERE, J.CADOZ. J.Microsc.Spectros.Electron.(1982),7, 183-211.

[27] W.T.DONLON, T.E.MITCHELL, A.H.HEUER. Philos.Mag.(1979), A40, 351.

[28] D.S.PHILLIPS, J.CADOZ. Philos.Mag.(1982), A46, 583-595.

[29] P.LAGERLOF, T.E.MITCHELL, A.H.HEUER, J.P.RIVIERE, J.CADOZ, J.CASTAING, D.S.PHILLIPS. To be published.

[30] J.CADOZ, J.CASTAING, D.S.PHILLIPS, A.H.HEUER, T.E.MITCHELL. Acta Metall. (1982), 30, 2205-2218.

[31] J.CADOZ, D. HO KIM, M.MEYER, J.P.RIVIERE. Rev.Phys.Appl.(1977)12, 473-481.

[32] W.SKROTZKI, P.HAASEN. J.Physique (1981), 42, C3, 119-148.

[33] M.P.PULS, This Symposium.

[34] A.AUDOUARD, J.CASTAING, J.P.RIVIERE, B.SIEBER. Acta Metall.(1981),29, 1385-1400.

[35] M.H.LEWIS. Philos. Mag.(1968), 17, 481.

[36] J.HONSTRA. J.Phys.Chem.Sol.(1960), 15, 311.

[37] M.L.KRONBERG.Acta Metall.(1957), 5, 507. (1979) A39, 581.

[38] A. ATKINSON, A.TAYLOR. Philos.Mag.(1979)A39,581.

[39] A.DOMINGUEZ-RODRIGUEZ, J.CASTAING, J.PHILIBERT. Mat.Sci.Engin.(1977),27, 217-223.

[40] T.BRETHEAU, C.MARHIC, M.SPENDEL, J.CASTAING. Philos.Mag.(1977),35,1473-1487.

[41] A.DOMINGUEZ-RODRIGUEZ, R.MARQUEZ, J.CASTAING, J.PHILIBERT. Philos.Mag.(1982), A46, 411-418.

[42] J.CABRERA-CANO, A.DOMINGUEZ-RODRIGUEZ, R.MARQUEZ, J.CASTAING, J.PHILIBERT. Philos.Mag.(1982), A46, 397-407.

[43] B.J.PLETKA, T.E.MITCHELL, A.H.HEUER. Phys.Stat.Solidi (1977), a39, 301.

[44] D.GRIGGS. Geophys.J.Roy.Astr.Soc.(1967), 14, 19.

[45] D. GRIGGS, J.Geophys.Res.(1974), 79, 1653.

[46] P.B.HIRSCH. J.Physique (1981), 42, C3, 149-160.

47 J.CADOZ, D.HO KIM, J.PELISSIER, R.VALLE. J.Mat.Sc.(1982), 17, 211-214.

TABLE 1

Ionicity factors, after Ref [1]

R = NaCl structure
W = Wurtzite
Q = Tetragonal
PH = Pseudo-Hegaxonal

	Crystal structure	Phillips	Levine	Hübner Leonhardt
NaCl	R	0.935	0.936	
MgO	R	0.841	0.839	
TiO	R			0.41
MnO	R		0.887	
FeO	R		0.873	
CoO	R		0.858	0.80
NiO	R		0.841	0.79
BeO	W	0.602	0.62	
ZnO	W	0.616	0.653	0.63
Al_2O_3	PH		0.796	
Cr_2O_3	Al_2O_3		0.772	0.72
Fe_2O_3	Al_2O_3		0.677	0.67
TiO_2	Q		0.686	
Cu_2O	cubic		0.56	

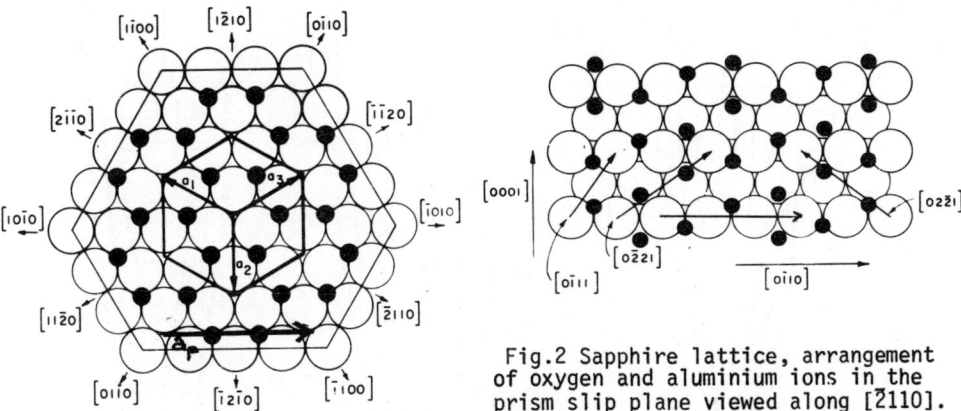

Fig.1 Sapphire lattice, projection on basal (0001) plane. Large circles are oxygen ions. Small circles are Al ions (filled). Only one layer of oxygen ions is shown - together with the basal hexagonal cell vectors and some Burgers vectors.

Fig.2 Sapphire lattice, arrangement of oxygen and aluminium ions in the prism slip plane viewed along [$\bar{2}$110]. Several possible Burgers vectors are shown.

TABLE II

Dislocation characteristics in oxides as compared to Aluminium. After Ref [1].

	Oxygen sub-lattice	Burgers vector $\vec{b}$	$\|b\|$ (Å)	Modulus μ (Pa)	μb^3 eV	μb^2 eV/Å
Al		1/2 <110>	2.86	2.7×10^{10}	4	1.4
MgO	cfc	1/2 <110>	2.98	1.25×10^{11}	21	6.9
CoO	cfc	1/2 <110>	3.01	0.7×10^{11}	12	4
NiO	cfc	1/2 <110>	2.96	1.35×10^{11}	22	7.4
$MgAl_2O_4$	cfc	1/2 <110>	5.7	1.2×10^{11}	135	24.4
BeO	hcp	1/3 <11$\bar{2}$0>	2.7	1.6×10^{11}	20	7.3
Al_2O_3-α	hcp	1/3 <11$\bar{2}$0>	4.76	2×10^{11}	135	28.3
		<10$\bar{1}$0>	8.22		555	67.5
TiO_2	hcp (distorded)	<001>	2.96	1×10^{11}	16	5.5
		<101>	5.46		102	18.6
Cu_2O	bcc	<001>	4.27	1×10^{10}	5	1.1
		<011>	6.04		14	2.3
UO_2	cubic	1/2 <110>	3.86	9.4×10^{10}	33.8	8.75
Y_2O_3	vacant	1/2 <111>	9.18	6.5×10^{10}	314	34.2
	cubic	<100>	10.6		484	45.7
$Y_3Fe_5O_{12}$	/	1/2 <111>	10.72	7.8×10^{10}	600	56
		<100>	12.38		925	75

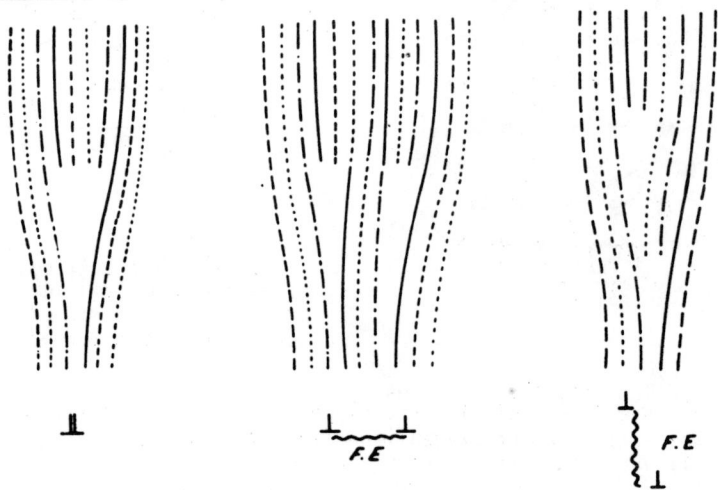

Fig.3 Climb dissociation versus glide dissociation. FE = stacking fault.

TABLE III

Glide systems in oxides. After Ref.[1]

Compound	Oxygen sub-lattice	shortest $\vec{b}$	Easy glide system Low T	Easy glide system High T	simple neutral plane	Secondary system
Al_2O_3-α	HCP	$1/3 <11\bar{2}0>$		$<11\bar{2}0>\{0001\}$		$<10\bar{1}0>\{1\bar{2}10\}$
TiO_2	Pseudo-HCP	$\|001\|$		$<101>\{101\}$		$\|001\|\{110\}$
Y_2O_3	Cubic	$1/2 <111>$	$<110>\{100\}$	$<110>\{100\}$	$\{110\}$	$<111>\{110\}$
MgO	FCC	$1/2 <110>$	$<110>\{110\}$		$\{110\}$	$<110>\{001\}$
NiO	FCC	$1/2 <110>$	$<110>\{110\}$		$\{110\}$	
UO_2	Cubic	$1/2 <110>$	$<110>\{001\}$		$\{110\}$	$<110>\{110\}$
Cu_2O	BCC	$<100>$	$<110>\{110\}$	$<100>\{001\}$	no	$<100>\{011\}$
$MgAl_2O_4$	FCC	$1/2 <110>$	$<110>\{111\}$	$<110>\{110\}$	no	
$MgO(Al_2O_3)_{1.1}$	FCC	$1/2 <110>$	$<110>\{110\}$	$<110>\{110\}$	no	
$Ni_{2/3}Fe_{7/3}O_4$	CFC	$1/2 <110>$	$<110>\{111\}$	$<110>\{111\}$	no	
$Y_3Fe_5O_{15}$	Distorted	$1/2 <111>$		$<111>\{110\}$	no	

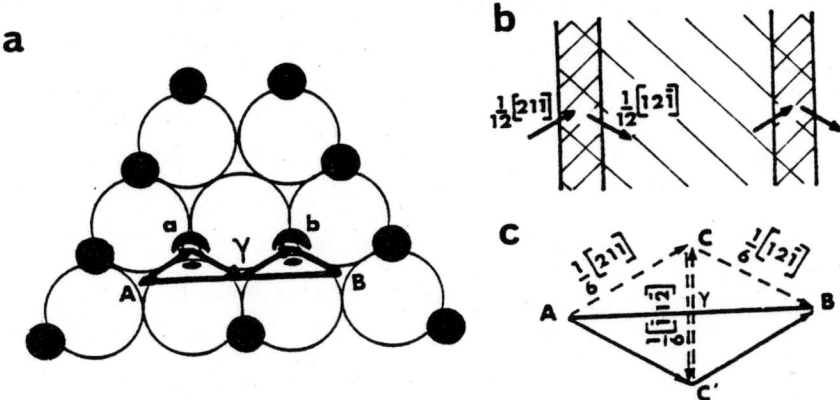

Fig.4 a) Spinel structure, viewed along a $<111>$ direction and showing one anion layer (large open circles) and one trivalent cation layer (small circles).
b) Possible dissociation of the Burgers vector $\vec{AB}$ of perfect dislocation.

Fig.5 Glide (I) and climb (II,III), dissociation of prism plane dislocations in sapphire Al_2O_3-α with stacking faults on prism planes $\{11\bar{2}0\}$(II) or $\{10\bar{1}0\}$(III) c-axis is perpendicular to the plane of the figure.

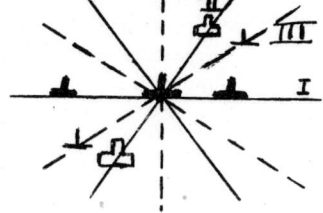

SESSILE DISSOCIATION AND PLASTIC DEFORMATION IN MgO.n Al$_2$O$_3$ SPINELS

R. DUCLOS

Laboratoire de Structure et Propriétés de l'Etat Solide - LA CNRS
Université de Lille I   59655 Villeneuve d'Ascq Cedex - France

ABSTRACT

In this paper the origin of the composition influence on the high temperature plasticity of spinels MgO.n Al$_2$O$_3$ is studied by taking into account the existence of the sessile dissociation mode of dislocations and the presence of composition vacancies. The propounded model is built up from results of mechanical tests performed on samples of composition ratio n = 1.1, 1.8 and 3.

INTRODUCTION

High temperature plasticity of MgO.n Al$_2$O$_3$ spinels is strongly dependent on the composition ratio n = Al$_2$O$_3$/MgO [1-6] (figure 1). Several possible origins which did not take into account the dislocation dissociation mode have been put forward to explain that mechanical behaviour. Contrary to those models the purpose of this paper is to explain the increase in plasticity with n in such spinels by considering the real dislocation core structure. The study of this one by electron microscopy in strained samples has revealed that dislocations are generally dissociated off their slip plane [6,7], whatever be the composition ratio, in two colinear partials as :

(1) $1/2 <110> \rightarrow 1/4 <110> + 1/4 <110>$

The fault which is thus created in between the partials only affects the cationic sublattice. It has been also observed that the dissociation width increases with the composition ratio.

This paper is based on our results of constant stress or strain rate deformation tests performed on $<100>$ specimen of composition ratio n = 1.1 and 1.8, in the temperature ranges 1530 - 1730°C (n = 1.1) and 1350 - 1650°C (n = 1.8) and on the data published by Mac Brayer [1] for the same orientation in the case of samples of composition n = 3 deformed between 1550 and 1850°C. For a $<100>$ compression axis dislocation glide occurs on the {110} planes at 45° of the C.A.

RESULTS AND DISCUSSION

In order to produce a credible model one calculates in the first part of this section the deformation laws for the plateau conditions of σ-ε curves or the steady state of creep curves. This allows us to define the influence of the composition on the different terms of the strain rate law.

Generally high temperature deformation of single crystals is controlled by dislocation climb ; the measured activation energy is only slightly stress dependent. In this way the temperature and stress dependence of strain rate has been analysed following the relation currently observed at high temperature :

(2) $$\dot{\varepsilon} = \dot{\varepsilon}_o (\sigma/\mu)^s \exp(-Q/kT)$$

(In the absence of precise data at high temperatures, the shear modulus μ has been assumed to be independent on the composition as it is the case at room temperature).

Firstly except slight difference in the term $\dot{\varepsilon}_0$, the two kinds of deformation tests, creep or constant strain rate, lead to the same results. One obtains respectively for the three compositions n = 1.1, 1.8 and 3 activation energy values equal to 5.4, 5.5 and 5.7 ev and stress exponent values of 4, 3.7 and 3.4. The measured activation energies are near the self diffusion energy of oxygen anion. The values of the stress exponent are moreover consistent with a number of high temperature deformation models where dislocation climb is the recovery process. The different results are gathered in the figure 2 as a plot of strain rate logarithm versus reciprocal temperature for some stresses.

A second remark concerns the values of stress exponent and activation energy which are relatively insensitive to spinel composition ratio by taking into consideration the experimental errors (± .5 ev and ± .3). This means that the mechanical effect of composition can only stem from the preexponential term $\dot{\varepsilon}_0$, the values of which are :

$\dot{\varepsilon}_0 \simeq 10^{19}$ s^{-1} n = 1.1
$\dot{\varepsilon}_0 \simeq 10^{21}$ s^{-1} n = 1.8
$\dot{\varepsilon}_0 \simeq 10^{23}$ s^{-1} n = 3

or $\dot{\varepsilon}_0(n) \simeq 10^{(2n+17)}$ s^{-1}

These values correspond to ratios

$\dot{\varepsilon}_0(3)/\dot{\varepsilon}_0(1.1) \simeq 10^4$ and $\dot{\varepsilon}_0(1.8)/\dot{\varepsilon}_0(1.1) \simeq 10^2$

The variation of these ratios with n cannot be completly ascribed to the corresponding variation of the oxygen self diffusion coefficient, the maximum ratios measured by Reddy [8] being :

$Do_x(3.5)/Do_x(1) \simeq 10^2$ and $Do_x(1.8)/Do_x(1) \simeq 7$

The cause of the plasticity evolution must be sought elsewhere.

In fact very useful informations can be deduced from the macroscopic study of deformation substructure, the first of which simply resides in the sample shape after deformation.

For the composition $n = 1.8$ dislocation glide on two $\{110\}$ orthogonal planes, or four, produces barreled specimens on the faces of which slip lines can be easily observed. On the contrary samples of composition $n = 1.1$ have an unusual inverted barrel shape (figure 3c) inconsistent with a deformation produced by dislocation glide ; more over no slip line is observed.

The second interesting information is obtained from the study of dislocation substructure by Berg Barret topography [4,6]. For the composition $n = 1.8$ one observe a well defined cellular substructure with subgrain boundaries in the $\{110\}$ planes perpendicular to the slip planes when glide only occurs in two planes (figure 3a) or in the $\{110\}$ planes parallel to the C.A. when four glide systems are active (figure 3b). Inversely only some random subgrain boundaries are present in the $n = 1.1$ samples after deformation (figure 3c).

These two observations concerning the sample shape and the macroscopic dislocation substructure suggest us that deformation largely results from dislocation climb for the composition ratio $n = 1.1$

This point of view agrees very well with the strain rate which can be calculated from the Orowan equation :

(3) $\quad \dot{\varepsilon} = \rho\, v\, b$

which can be written when the controlling mechanism is dislocation climb :

(4) $\quad \dot{\varepsilon} = \rho (L/h)\, v_c\, b$

where L is the mean distance covered by dislocations, h the climb distance in order to free a dislocation and v_c the climb velocity, ρ and b having their usual meaning.

A usual expression for climb velocity [9] give here :

(5) $\quad v_c = \dfrac{4\Pi\, D_{o_x}}{-b\, \ln(b\sqrt{\rho})}\, \dfrac{\sigma_m\, \Omega}{kT}$

by assuming that oxygen anion is the controlling species (σ_m is the climb stress on the supplementary half plane and Ω is presently the volume of oxygen anion).

This gives in the case of a sample of composition $n = 1.1$ strained at 1920 K with a climb stress corresponding to $\sigma_m = 45$ MPa ($\sigma = 90$ MPa) ; $D_{o_x}(1920\ K) = 10^{-16} m^2/S$ [10], the measured dislocation density is $\rho \sim 10^{11} m^{-2}$ and taking $L/h \simeq 1$ for a pure climb deformation : $\dot{\varepsilon} = 3.10^{-7} s^{-1}$ while the experimental creep rate is $\sim 7.10^{-7} s^{-1}$ (figure 2).

The order of magnitude agreement shows that a pure climb strain can account quantitatively for the measured experimental rates.

For $n = 1.8$ the strain rate can be also evaluated by the above relation (4) ; L is then approximated to the cell size (the slip distance) and h to $\rho^{-1/2}$. The agreement is equally good in this case.

We see that the variation of the term $\dot{\varepsilon}_0$ can be explained by a greater slip distance as n increases and the solution of the problem must then explain why dislocation glide is relatively easy for $n = 1.8$ and not for $n = 1.1$ or in other words the higher glide mobility of dislocations when n increases. With this object it is necessary to examine the different possibilities how the observed sessile dislocations can move.

The first possibility consists in recombining the partials before glide. Not only this solution needs the activation of high energy constrictions along the fault ribbon but the recombination of partials seems to be easier when n increases in so far as the dissociation width increases with n ; the invert mechanical behaviour would be more likely in this case.

In the second possibility the dislocation displacement occurs by glide without partial recombination as figure 4 shows. In this process the climb fault is immobile and so partial glide creates two faults of energy γ_g in the $\{110\}$ planes perpendicular to the climb fault plane ; this needs high stresses of the order of :

$$\sigma \sim \frac{2\sigma_g}{b} \geqslant \frac{2\gamma_c}{b}$$

in so far as the glissile fault has a higher energy that the climb one [11]. In our case for $n = 1.1$ with $\gamma_m = 200$ mJ/m^2 this corresponds to stress higher than 700 MPa, about five times the ones we have currently used. For $n = 1.8$ the needed stresses are equally much more higher than the ones used. Moreover the faults necessary created here have never been observed in our deformed spinels. This glide mechanism is therefore unlikely.

In the third possibility dislocations still glide without any recombination of partials, but this time the fault is drawn by the partials. In this case the fault movement corresponds to a climb of this one. The dislocation mobility is then controlled by the fault climb.

The last glide possibility seems to be the most likely and for this reason we now examine, in the case of an edge dislocation dissociated by climb and gliding on the (110) plane, how the composition ratio can influence the fault mobility.

Figure 5 represents, in the vicinity of the dislocation, the idealized projection of the $(1\bar{1}0)$ planes onto the (001) plane perpendicular to the dislocation line ; the fault ribbon is limited by partials P_1 and P_2. For an equimolar spinel the γ planes have the $\left(Al\ O_2\right)^-$ composition and A or B planes the $\left(Mg\ Al\ O_2\right)^+$ one. These two last kinds of plane are deduced from each other by the translation $\pm a/4\ [1\bar{1}2]$.

The sequence of $(1\bar{1}0)$ planes is written in the perfect crystal :
... B γ A γ B γ A γ ... and becomes ... B γ A γ ↓ A γ B γ ... in between the partials. Further glide of such a dislocation on a distance $a/4\ [1\bar{1}0]$ needs only the transformation of the part of the A plane adjacent to the fault into a B one for the γ planes are not affected by the fault. In this transformation all the Al^{3+} and Mg^{2+} cations have to be rearranged : diffusional cationic movements are then necessary; these ones must arise in a cooperative manner in order to keep locally the electroneutrality of the crystal.

In figure 6a the transformation is presented in the case of an equimolar spinels where cations are assumed to occupy the octahedral sites for Al^{3+} and the tetrahedral ones for Mg^{2+}. The ions belonging to the two neighbouring γ planes are also figured : they appear in full circles. The arrows represent the needed movements in the A plane to transform this one in a B plane ; in some places as J or K for example one sees that such movements bring the cations nearer involving thereby high energy barriers.

Such high energy barriers still arise if instead of restricting the site exchange to the cations of A plane only, this transformation is produced with cations of A and γ planes (figure 6b) ; the first jump from I to J produces locally an high deviation from electroneutrality if we consider the magnesium cations in sites K and L unless the cationic movements are synchronized which seems to be problematic. It becomes evident that such a transformation is a very difficult process in an equimolar spinel.

As the composition ratio n increases one replaces three magnesium cations by two aluminium ones ; this produces empty sites called constitution vacancies. It is obvious that these vacancies can help to relieve the hard passing points as the study of the transformation in the case of the MgO 1.8 Al_2O_3 spinel shows. For this particular composition the unit cell - comprising 32 oxygen anions whatever be the composition ratio - contains one constitution vacancy. In the figure 7 we have represented, inside the dotted lines, the equivalent of a unit cell ; the constitution vacancy have been put on an octahedral site in the γ plane and surrounded by three tetrahedral aluminium [12]. Some cationic movements changing the A plane into a B one are represented by the arrows 1 to 13. Cations of both A and γ planes are used for the transformation. We see that the vacancy facilitates in its vicinity the outset of the transformation by avoiding too high energy configurations during the cation displacement.

One then understands how the fault ribbon mobility can increase with the composition ratio ; each constitution vacancy can be compared to a nucleus from which the transformation starts. Therefore the transformation rate and consequently the dislocation glide mobility will increase with the number of such nuclei i.e. with the composition ratio n.

This model is supported by T.E.M. observations which show that for the compositions $n = 1.8$ [13] and 3.5 [7] curved and partly twisted faults are frequently observed contrary to the composition $n = 1.1$ [6] where the fault is well confined in the climb plane. These observations suggest in agreement with our model that the transformation being relatively easy for high composition ratio spinels, it can go faster in some places, due to local divergences to the composition for example, and then partials can move more independently.

CONCLUSION

We have presented a model, taking into account the climb dissociation of dislocations and the presence of the constitution vacancies as $n \neq 1$ which accounts for the higher glide mobility of dislocations, and thus the increase in plasticity, in $MgO \cdot n\ Al_2O_3$ spinels when the composition ratio n increases.

REFERENCES

[1] Mc Brayer : Doctoral dissertation. North Car. state Univ. Raleigh (U.S.A.) (1965)

[2] Radford K.C., Newey C.W.A. : Proc. Brit. Ceram. Soc. 9 (1967) 131.

[3] Lewis M.H. : Phil. Mag. 17 (1968) 481

[4] Doukhan N., Duclos R., Escaig B. : J. Phys. 34 (1973) C9-379

[5] Mitchell T.E., Hwang L., Heuer A.H. : J. Mater. Sci. 11 (1976) 264

[6] Duclos R., Doukhan N., Escaig B. : J. Mater. Sci. 13 (1978) 1740

[7] Donlon W.T., Mitchell T.E., Heuer A.H. : Phil. Mag. A 40 (1979) 351

[8] Reddy K.P.R., Cooper A.R. : J. Amer. Ceram. Soc. 64 (1981) 368

[9] Escaig B. : R. Phys. Appl. 14 (1979) 469

[10] Ando K., Oishi Y. : J. Chem. Phys. 37 (1974) 625

[11] Veyssière P., Rabier J., Grilhé J. : Phys. Stat. Sol.a 24 (1975) 605

[12] Jagodzinski H., Saafeld H. : Z. Kristallogr. 125 (1958) 197

[13] Duclos R., Doukhan N., Escaig B. : Acta Met. 30 (1982) 1381.

FIGURE CAPTIONS

Figure 1 : $<100>$ specimen stress-strain curves obtained at $T \sim 1630°C$ and $\dot{\varepsilon} \sim 1.5 \; 10^{-5} s^{-1}$ (curve n = 3 from [1])

Figure 2 : Plot of the logarithm of the strain rate versus the reciprocal temperature for $<100>$ samples of composition n = 1.1 (dotted lines) 1.8 (mixed lines) and 3 (full lines). The number above each curve refers to the stress (in MPa) and the letter (C) means that the curve is deduced from creep tests.

Figure 3 : Dislocation substructure (B.B.T.) of deformed $<100>$ specimens ((100) face parallel to the C.A.) Scale bar=1 mm
    a) T = 1400°C $\varepsilon = 0.07$ n = 1.8
    b) T = 1650°C $\varepsilon = 0.10$ n = 1.8
    c) T = 1610°C $\varepsilon = 0.05$ n = 1.1, note the concave shape of the left side (the right side has been polished for observations and therefore does not show this shape).

Figure 4 : Partial glide creating pure glide faults.

Figure 5 : Projection of the $(1\bar{1}0)$ planes onto the (001) plane in the vicinity of a climb split edge dislocation.

Figure 6 : Cationic movements changing the A plane in a B one in an ordered equimolar spinel
    a) only cations of A plane are involved in the transformation
    b) transformation occurs with cations of A and γ planes

Figure 7 : Cationic movements changing the A plane in a B one in an ordered spinel of composition ratio n = 1.8. Al_o stands for octahedral aluminium, Al_t for tetrahedral aluminium and V_o for octahedral vacancy. The initial position of the vacancy is A and the final one B for the jump sequence $1 \to 13$.

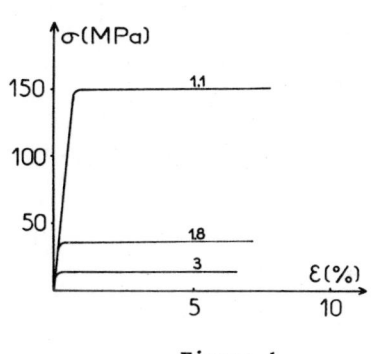

Figure 1

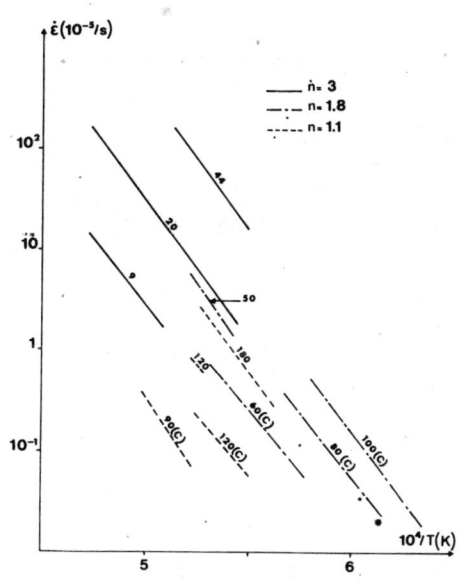

Figure 2

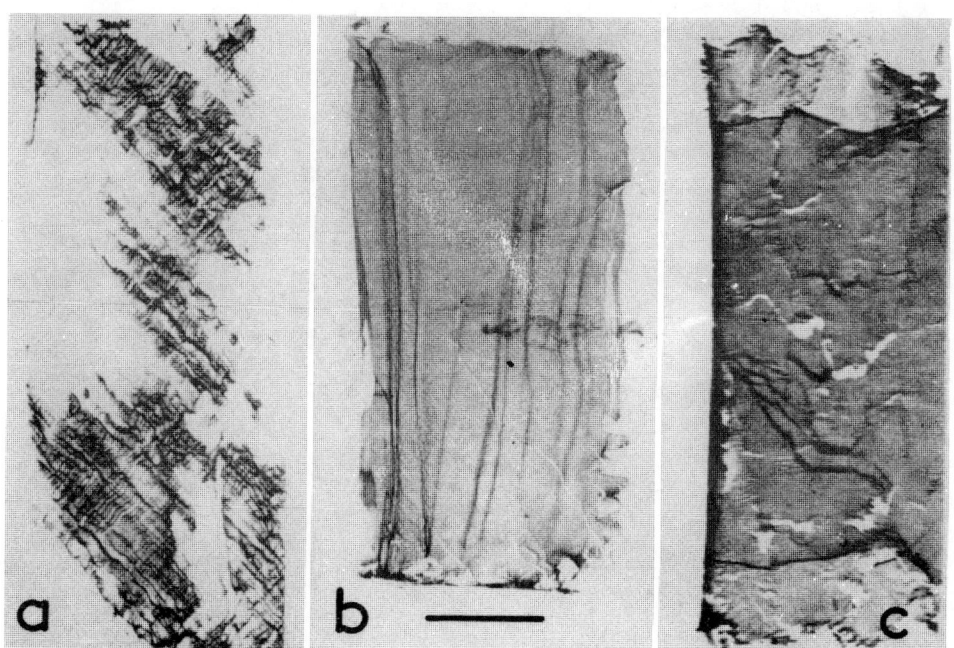

Figure 3

- 273 -

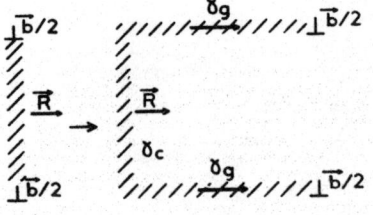

Figure 4

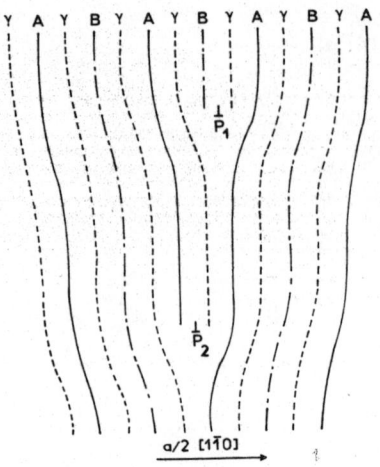

Figure 5

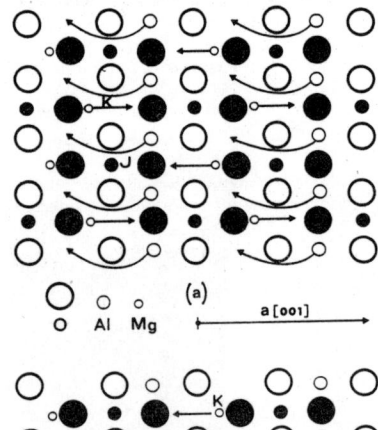

Figure 6

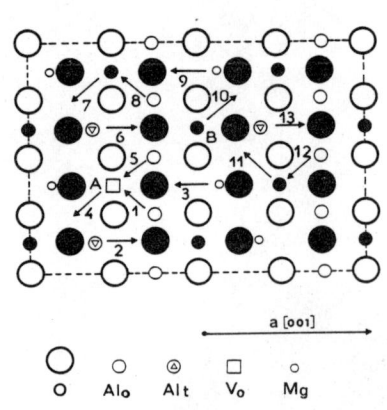

Figure 7

THE EFFECT OF OH⁻ IONS ON DISLOCATION MOBILITY AND THE PLASTIC DEFORMATION PARAMETERS OF LiF CRYSTALS AT LOW TEMPERATURES

S.V. Lubenets, E.I. Ostapchuk, F. Appel[+], H.-J. Kaufmann[++]

Institute for Low Temperature Physics and Engineering, Acad. of Sci. of the Ukr. SSR, Kharkov 310164, USSR, [+] Institute of Solid State Physics and Electron Microscopy, Acad. of Sci. of GDR, Halle/S., [++] Acad. of Sci. of GDR, Berlin 1080

The influence of the growing atmosphere (vacuum for LiF, air for LiF and NaCl, argon for NaCl) on the mechanical properties of LiF and NaCl crystals and on the dislocation mobility in LiF crystals were investigated in a temperature range of 1.6 to 300 K. At the same impurity concentration, the density of obstacles controlling the dislocation velocity is larger if the crystals are grown in the air. In some temperature interval, the reorientation of elastic dipoles in the dislocation core may affect the plastic deformation kinetics and dislocation motion in LiF crystals grown in the air. At the lowest temperature the Peierls mechanism probably controls the dislocation mobility.

1. Introduction

Coulomb binding forces in the NaCl-type crystal lattice as well as covalent binding forces in diamond and in bcc metal lattices predetermine the high energy Peierls barrier for the dislocation motion /1-3/. However, the experimental results on the mobility of individual dislocations and plastic flow kinetics for NaCl and LiF crystals /4-6/ at the lowest temperatures agree to some extent with the double kink model /7, 8/.

The flow stress of alkali halide crystals is mainly determined by divalent impurities. Besides, in air grown material OH⁻ ions are present.

In the present paper, single screw dislocation mobility and the initial stage of the plastic flow were studied in a temperature range of 1.6 to 300 K in pure LiF crystals grown in the air (LiF-1) and in vacuum (LiF-2). Some experiments on the effect of the growth environment on the mechanical properties of NaCl crystals were also carried out.

2. Experimental

The Table given the data on the content of impurity defects obtained by methods of the spectral chemical analysis, ion conductivity and dielectric absorption for LiF crystals. Analogous data are also available for NaCl crystals grown in the air and Ar atmosphere.

Table. Impurity defect concentration in LiF crystals (ppm)

Method	LiF-1	LiF-2
Spectral chemical analysis	2 ± 0.4 Mg 0.1 Al, Ag, Fe, Ti	5.5 ± 1.1 Mg 0.1 Al, Ag, Fe, Ti
Ionic conductivity	10.4 ± 1.4	11.3 ± 1.1
Dielectric losses[+] T = 298 K T = 373 K	4-6 (f_{max} = 50 c) 12 (f_{max} = 7 ks)	8 (f_{max} = 60 c) 15 (f_{max} = 7 kc)

[+]The authors wish to thank Prof. F. Froehlich (Martin Luter Univ., Halle/s, GDR) for help with the d.l. measurements.

The IR absorption spectrum shows that there are ion complexes (Me^{2+} - OH^-) and OH^- "free" ions in LiF-1. In LiF-2 crystal only one peak was found in the absorption band peculiar to (Me^{2+} - OH^-) complexes.

The technique of the sample preparation for the tests is described in /6, 9/. The dislocation density in annealed crystals was of about $10^4 cm^{-2}$. The investigation of the mechanical properties of crystals and of the dislocation velocities were carried out in a temperature range of 1.6 to 300 K.

3. Experimental results

1. Temperature dependences of crss for LiF crystals of two types shown in Fig. 1 differ by the following three peculliarities, i.e. a) for LiF-1 crystal τ_o is larger in the whole tem-

perature range as compared with τ_o of LiF-2 crystal; b) $\tau_o(T)$ of LiF-2 crystal increases monotonically when decreasing temperature whereas a plateau in the dependence $\tau_o(T)$ of LiF-1 crystal in the region of 100 to 200 K; c) the dependence $\tau_o(T)$ is weaker (almost linear) in the lowest temperature region (T < 20 K) for LiF-2 crystals as it is seen in Fig. 1 (insert). The measurements made with one sample when decreasing temperature successively show that this tendency either is kept at T<4.2 K or the dependence $\tau_o(T)$ becomes weaker.

The effect of the growing atmosphere on the mechanical properties was also found in the case of NaCl: Ca^{2+} crystals. Crss of crystals grown in the air increases strongly with increasing calcium concentration ($\tau_o \sim c^{++1/2}$). Crystals grown in Ar atmosphere are essentially softer.

2. There are sharp distinctions in temperature dependences of α_r^{-1} for LiF-1 and LiF-2 crystals. The presence of two minima in the case of LiF-1 may be explained in the framework of the thermally activated process of the plastic deformation assuming a change of dislocation dragging mechanism when decreasing temperature /6/.

In the case of LiF-2 crystals the constancy of α_r^{-1} in a rather wide temperature range of 4.2 to 100 K and its increase at T < 4.2 K and T > 100 K are observed.

The temperature dependence of the activation volume for LiF-1 crystals is nonmonotonic and this peculiarity coincides with the temperature range of the plateau in $\tau_o(T)$ /10/. The activation volume for LiF-2 crystals decreases with decreasing temperature converting to the linear dependence in the range 4.2 K < T < 100 K (Fig. 2).

The growing environment affects also the activation volume in the case of NaCl crystals (Fig. 3). So, in air grown NaCl containing 48 ppm Ca^{++}, it is two times less than in the crystal with the same calcium concentration but grown in Ar atmosphere /11/.

3. Fig. 2 gives the comparison of the temperature dependence $V(T) = kT (\partial \ln v / \partial \tau)$ belonging to the stresses close to crss with the results of macroscopic measurements. The analysis of the data obtained allows one to conclude, i.e. a) individual dislocation velocity at the stresses equal to τ_o at all temperatures $v(\tau_o, T)$ < 10^{-3} cm/s, i.e. it is in the thermal fluctuation region; b) the

values $\partial \ln v / \partial \tau$ and V for both crystals in the whole temperature range are sometimes smaller than these of corresponding quantities obtained by the SR method (it is connected to some degree with the use of the deformation device with a low hardness /6/; c) the similarity of temperature dependences of the analyzed quantities obtained by the SR method and the data on dislocation mobility measurements show that the initial stage of plastic flow of the crystals studied is mainly determined by dynamical properties of individual dislocations in undeformed crystal; d) the dependences $\partial \ln v / \partial \tau (T)$ and V(T) demonstrate the difference of dislocation dragging mechanisms in LiF-1 and LiF-2 crystals in the temperature range studied.

Fig. 4 shows the stress dependences of individual screw dislocation velocities at room temperature and in the low temperature range. Here one more peculiarity is seen. In LiF-2 crystals the dislocation velocity increases monotonically when increasing stress at T = 300 K whereas in LiF-1 crystals the marked decrease of the velocity sensitivity to the stress in the range $v = 10^{-2}$ cm/s and then the sharp dependence $v(\tau)$ in narrow stress interval 5.5 MPa $< \tau <$ 6.5 MPa are observed. At shock loading a gradual transition into the viscous drag region follows. It is important to note that the stress range where v strongly increases falls in the plateau region (Fig. 1).

At low temperatures the dependences $v(\tau)$ in LiF-2 crystals shift to higher stresses in accord with the increasing crss being practically parallel. In the case of LiF-1 crystals an increase of $\partial \ln v / \partial \tau$ is observed at T $<$ 40 K. The comparison of these data with the results of macroscopic measurements given above shows that in a range T $<$ 4.2 K further investigations of single dislocation motion are necessary.

4. Discussion

On the basis of the results given it is possible to see that LiF-1 and LiF-2 crystals differ considerably not only by the magnitude of crss but also by the other parameters characterizing the plastic flow kinetics and single dislocation mobility. This is evidently connected with crystal lattice distortions due to impurity defects.

The greater variety of impurity defects inherent to LiF-1

crystal must change the character of potential barriers overcome by dislocations as compared with LiF-2 crystal grown in vacuum. In LiF-1 crystals large impurity complexes may be present which are overcome by dislocations in an athermal way. This may be one of the reason for the differences of the crss and the relative shift of the dependences $v(\tau)$ at the same temperature (Figs. 1, 4) in LiF and NaCl crystals of two types.

In both LiF and NaCl crystals at the same cation impurity concentration, the density of obstacles controlling the dislocation velocity seems to be less in a crystal grown in vacuum or in the inert atmosphere.

However, such marked peculiarities as the presence of the plateau in the dependence $\tau_o(T)$, nonmonotonic dependence $\lg v(\tau)$ at T = 300 K in the case of LiF-1 crystals and temperature independence of the quantitties α_r^{-1} and $\partial \ln v/\partial \tau$ in the low temperature range in the case of LiF-2 crystals are evidently due to the properties of elementary impurity defects of Me^{2+}-vacancy and Me^{2+} - OH^- types or the properties of a dislocation line itself (for example, the presence of the jogs on it).

The plateau in the dependence $\tau_o(T)$ and nonmonotonic dependence $\lg v(\tau)$ (LiF-1) may be qualitatively explained by the manifestation of some relaxation process that follows dislocation motion. The reorientation of elastic dipoles in the stress field of a dislocation (induced Snoek effect) may be just such a process.

Under this assumption, too low temperature of the plateau in the dependence $\tau_o(T)$ (T $\approx$ 1/8 T_{melt}. in comparison with T $\approx$ 1/4 T_{melt}. where Snoek effect is usually observed) is unclear. This circumstance probably results from the defect properties in the crystals studied.

It can not be excluded, however, that the nature of the effects observed does not consist in the indicated dislocation motion peculiarities in the field of mobile impurity defects. But beyond doubt, it is related to dynamic properties of single dislocations in an undeformed crystal. This follows from the analogy in the behaviour of V(T) measured by means of the SR method and determined from the character of the dependence $v(\tau)$ at room temperature (Figs. 2, 4).

The temperature independences of α_r^{-1} and $\partial \ln v/\partial \tau$ at low temperatures (LiF-2) are a surprising fact but not quite unexpected one. The measurements of dislocation mobility made in a wide temperature range show that in KCl /12/ the quantity decreases with decreasing temperature, this decrease is not connected with an increase of the stress. This peculiarity is not still explained satisfactorily.

In the temperature range below 4.2 K data on LiF-2 crystal may be described on the basis of the theory of dislocation motion in the Peierls relief /7/ with τ_p = 21.8 MPa and H_o = 0.1 eV that agrees with /4/.

In conclusion it is necessary to note that the results of macroscopic experiments and the dislocation mobility measurements in impurity crystals of the NaCl-type agree rather well with dislocation motion theories available /13/. The peculiarities observed in pure LiF crystals show that up to now the nature of dislocation dragging is not quite clear.

References

/1/ Kurosawa T.: J. Phys. Soc. Japan 19 (1964) 2096.
/2/ Granzer F., Wagner G., Eisenblätter: Phys. stat. sol. 30 (1968) 587.
/3/ Hoagland R.G., Hirth J.P., Gehlen P.C.: Phil. Mag. 34 (1976) 413.
/4/ Suzuki T., Kim H.: J. Phys. Soc. Japan 39 (1975) 1566.
/5/ Suzuki T., Kim H.: J. Phys. Soc. Japan 40 (1975) 1703.
/6/ Kaufmann H.-J., Lubenets S.V., Ostapchuk E.I.: phys. stat. sol. (a) 66 (1981) 229.
/7/ Petukhov B.V., Pokrovsky V.L.: Zh. Exper. Teor. Phys. 63 (1972 634.
/8/ Seeger A.Z. Metallkunde 72 (1981) 369.
/9/ Boiko Yu.F., Lubenets S.V., Fomenko L.S., Fedorenko N.M.: Izv. Vuzov, Fizika 7 (1978) 129.
/10/ Kaufmann H.-J., Lubenets S.V., Abraimov V.V.: Fiz. tverd. Tela 25 (1983) 321.
/11/ Appel F.: phys.stat. sol. (a) 61 (1980) 477.
/12/ Lubenets S.V., Ostapchuk E.I., Landau A.I.: Fiz. tverd. Tela 22 (1980) 9.
/13/ Lubenets S.V.: Fizicheskie protsessi plasticheskoy deformatsii pri nizkikh temperaturakh, Naukova Dumka, Kiev 1974, 220

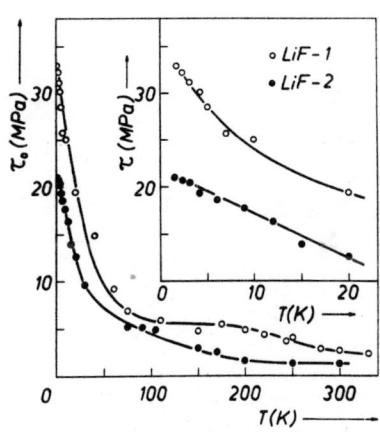

Fig.1 Temperature dependence of c.r.s.s. of LiF crystals.

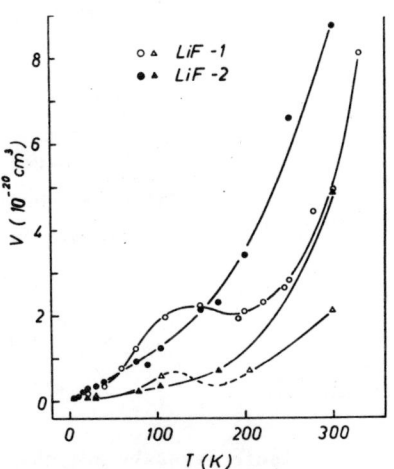

Fig.2 Temperature dependence of the activation volume of LiF crystals obtained by the stress relaxation (o ●) and dislocation mobility (△ ▲) methods.

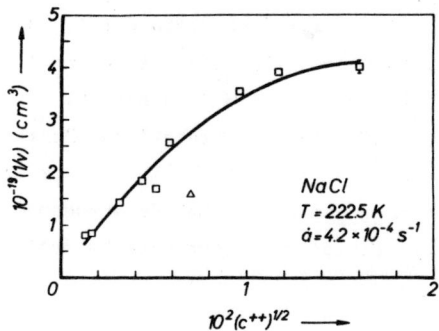

Fig.3 Dependence of $1/v$ on calcium concentration for NaCl crystals. Crystals are grown in the air □ and in Ar atmosphere △. Activation volume was measured by the strain rate cycling method. T = 222.5 K.

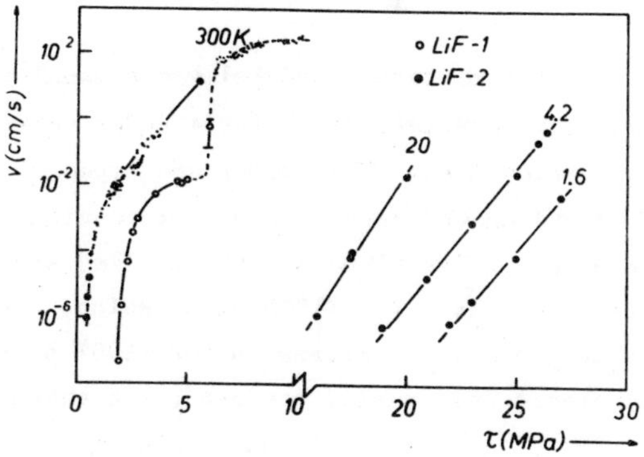

Fig.4 Stress and temperature dependences of dislocation velocities in LiF crystals.

DISLOCATIONS IN IONIC CRYSTALS

M.P. Puls

Materials Science Branch
Whiteshell Nuclear Research Establishment
Atomic Energy of Canada Limited
Pinawa, Manitoba, Canada ROE 1L0

Introduction

Ionic crystals are characterized by the presence of two oppositely charged species. The bonding in the lattice is dominated by the Coulomb interaction, which strongly influences the interaction of dislocations with the lattice, with other dislocations, and with point defects. Because of the presence of two oppositely charged species, significant electrical, as well as mechanical, effects can result from the presence and motion of dislocations. This is discussed in a number of books [1,2] and a review article [3]. Our main focus here will be on the glide behaviour of dislocations in controlling the plasticity of ionic crystals. This topic was covered in a book by Sprackling [4] and in recent reviews by Castaing [5,6], Skrotzki and Haasen [7] and, for binary and ternary oxides, Bretheau et al. [8]. This paper is restricted to effects in ionic crystals having the alkali halide structure. Space limitations also do not permit consideration of either work-hardening or dislocation-velocity measurements.

Glide Planes

Deformation experiments at room temperature and below are usually performed in compression, since most ionic crystals are brittle under tension and fracture after only small plastic extensions. The number and types of slip systems that can be activated depend on the direction of compression. The relation between the shear strain on a given plane and the applied stress is given by the Schmid factor. This gives that, for <100>-compression, four {110} planes are equally stressed, but there is no stress on the {100} planes. For <111>-compression, three {100} planes are equally stressed, but there is no stress on the {110} planes. Slip on single {100} planes, yielding a simpler stress-strain curve, can be achieved using shear strain [9,10] or by compressing the crystal a few degrees away from the <111> orientation [11].

The distribution of gliding dislocations varies with temperature, impurity content, glide system, and sample ionicity. All investigations show that primary slip is in the {110} plane. In the alkali halides, above a temperature T_w, screw dislocations on {110} (<100>-oriented crystals) form wavy slip lines, even at the beginning of deformation. Screw dislocations on {100} (<111>-oriented crystals) always form wavy slip lines [12,13]. Although most investigations of <111>-oriented crystals have determined that secondary slip occurs on {100} [14,15,9], some evidence exists that slip may occur on {111} [9,16,17]. However, Skrotzki [12], referring particularly to the most recent work by Bhagavan Raju and Strung [17], provides persuasive arguments that the latter's interpretation of their results may have been faulty. Recently, Lewis et al. [18] have attempted to obtain evidence for {111} slip by using the intrinsic charge on {111} edge dislocations (not present on {110} or {100} edge dislocations), and have concluded that the electrical effect observed was sufficient to provide some evidence for {111} glide. Appel et al. [19] have examined the fine details of the cross-slip process from 293 K to 4 K in NaCl single crystals, using the gold decoration technique. The cross-slip process was found to be similar throughout this temperature range (primary glide on {110} with cross-slip via {100}, and possibly {111}), and independent of whether the <100>- or <110>-compression axis was used. Since there is no component of applied stress on {100} for <100>-compression, this suggests that the cross-slip process is initiated by long-range internal stresses.

In face-centred-cubic (fcc) metals, primary slip occurs on the most densely packed planes and in the most closely packed direction ({111} <1$\bar{1}$0>}), but this is not the case in fcc ionic crystals, for which the primary slip system is {110}, with secondary slip occurring on {100}, and perhaps {111}. The difference in ease of slip between {110} and the other two slip systems (particularly {100}) is referred to as plastic anisotropy. The characterization and explanation for this anisotropy, which has been the subject of numerous investigations, form the focal point of this review. Qualitatively, it seems easiest to appreciate why glide on {111} would be difficult. These planes contain ions all having the same sign. During glide, there is a strong change in electrostatic interaction between planes, resulting in a high Peierls stress. In addition, the total dislocation energy is expected to be high since the extra half-planes end in rows of like-charged ions. This latter point is also an argument favouring {110} over {100}. As can be seen from Figure 1, although the glide planes in both cases are neutral, the dislocation on {100} has extra planes terminating in ion rows all of one kind. This argument is supported by atomistic calculations of the dislocation's core

energy, E_{core} [20,21]. However, Bücher [22] recently recalculated
$E_{core}\{100\}/E_{core}\{110\}$ for NaCl, obtaining a value of 1.08. When E_{core} was
included in the total dislocation energy, he found that the latter was smaller
on {100} than on {110}. Although these results should be used with caution in
view of the convergence difficulties in calculating the Coulomb sums in the
case of the dislocation on {100}, it appears from this that dislocation energy
is not a viable argument favouring dislocation slip on {110} over {100}.
Other explanations offered for the slip anisotropy involve a high Peierls
stress [14,23], and the differing electrostatic interactions of {110} and
{100} edge dislocations with divalent impurity ions [24]. These explanations
will be considered after we discuss the experimental results on the critical
resolved shear stress (CRSS).

Measurements of the CRSS

The CRSS marks the onset of macroscopic plastic deformation [4].
There are different criteria for determining its value from stress-strain
curves, depending on the shape of these curves [4,12]. In fcc ionic crystals,
the CRSS usually exhibits a decrease with temperature that, for crystals
containing small amounts of aliovalent impurities, falls roughly into four
regimes, described below. (With increasing purity, the four regimes are
expected to reduce to two.) Castaing [5,6] has summarized the data. Much of
the recent work in this area has been carried out by the Göttingen group and
reviewed by Skrotzki and Haasen [7,25,26].

Regime I exhibits both a strong temperature dependence and plastic
anisotropy below a certain temperature, as shown in Figure 2. The CRSS does
not scale with either shear modulus or melting temperature. Doping shifts the
curve to higher stress without altering the temperature dependence. This
effect is greater for {110} than for {100} slip. Determination of the activation volume V* shows that $V^{*\{100\}} \ll V^{*\{110\}}$ and that, in regime I, $V^* < 100$
b^3 [7]. An example of regime II is shown in Figures 3(a) and 3(b), illustrating the smaller temperature dependence of this regime. Decreasing the
impurity concentration decreases the temperature dependence. A plot of CRSS
against concentration of aliovalent impurities (divalent in alkali halides)
yields a roughly parabolic dependence. In regime III, the CRSS depends
linearly on dopant concentration and is approximately independent of temperature. The drop-off temperature in regime IV depends on the material, being
lower for AgCl ($\sim$ 250 K) than for the alkali halides ($\sim$ 500 K). This
correlates with the difference in melting temperatures.

Mechanisms

The strong temperature dependence of the CRSS in regime I and the decrease in activation volume below 100 b^3 indicate the operation of the Peierls mechanism. Skrotzki and Suzuki [27] have recently examined the evidence for the Peierls mechanism in ionic crystals. An analysis based on kink-pair formation using the string model can be used to deduce the stress-temperature relationship (and from that the Peierls stress), the Gibbs free energy for dislocation motion, and the temperature and stress dependencies of the activation volume. In particular, for a quasi-parabolic Peierls potential, the stress dependence is given by [28,29]:

$$(1) \quad \frac{\tau}{\tau_p} = 1 - \left(\frac{T}{T_o}\right)^{1/2}$$

(τ, applied stress; τ_p, Peierls stress; T, temperature; T_o, a constant depending on strain rate). Comparison with experiment shows that relation (1) is fairly well obeyed at low temperature for all crystals investigated. Extrapolation to T = 0 K yields the Peierls stress. This extrapolation procedure was used [27] to determine τ_p using data for slip on both {110} and {100}. For slip on {110}, Suzuki and Kim [30,31] have shown that this method of estimating τ_p is fairly insensitive to the assumed shape of the Peierls barrier. Thus, little change in the estimate of τ_p resulted on choosing a sinusoidal barrier shape (the shape determined from atomistic calculations [32-35]).

For slip on {100}, the rise in the CRSS occurs at a much higher temperature than for slip on {110}, and the extrapolation procedure based on relation (1) may not be as accurate. Confirmation that the estimated $\tau_p^{\{100\}}$ values have, nevertheless, at least the right order of magnitude, can be inferred from the reasonable values obtained for E_L, the dislocation line energy, and for V^*. Comparison of the results shows that (a) $\tau_p^{\{100\}} > \tau_p^{\{110\}}$ and that (b) $\tau_p^{\{100\}}$ (but not $\tau_p^{\{110\}}$) decreases in the sequence MgO to AgCl (roughly correlating with increasing ionicity). Thus, there is an intrinsic plastic anisotropy. Skrotzki and Suzuki [27] have attempted to correlate these results with various properties of the crystal. They have concluded that the correlation between τ_p/Z^2 (Z charge on ion) and $\Sigma\alpha$ (sum of the polarizabilities) originally proposed by Buerger [36] is only roughly obeyed. The decrease of τ_p/Z^2 with increasing $\Sigma\alpha$ is much stronger for {100} than for {110} slip, indicating a change in the primary slip plane at $\Sigma\alpha = 9$. Theoretical values of $\tau_p^{\{110\}}$, based on the most sophisticated methods and potentials [34,35] show good agreement with experimental values. It should be noted that these methods deduce a Peierls barrier having a width of b (the Burgers vector), i.e. one of the two symmetry positions is an energy maximum. Only rough theoretical estimates of $\tau_p^{\{100\}}$ exist [20,23]. Of these, the simple model of Gilman [23] works surprisingly well. Recently, Bücher [22] attempted to calculate τ_p atomistically for both {110} and {100} slip, obtaining almost identical values of about 80 MPa on both slip planes. His Peierls barriers have a width of b/2, are unsymmetrical in shape, and do not go to zero at the endpoints. This latter point, and the fact that the more sophisticated methods of Puls and So [35], using the same potential, yield a symmetrical Peierls barrier of width b for the dislocation on {110}, make Bücher's result seem doubtful. Attempts [25-27] at predicting the plastic anisotropy on the basis of the partially discrete Peierls-Nabarro model proved unsuccessful and point out the need, as expected, for fully atomistic calculations. Precise theoretical estimates of $\tau_p^{\{100\}}$ to compare with the experimental results are currently lacking. Calculations of dislocation properties for other than edges on {110} are problematic because of the difficulties in obtaining convergent Coulomb sums [37,38]. It is worth noting that the postulated dissociation of edge dislocations on {110} [39-41] has not been observed in more elaborate atomistic calculations [35,37]. Although simple estimates based on atomistic calculations of stacking fault energies [42] give separations from 7 to 15 b, the detailed atomistic models yield dislocation cores only slightly more extended than the initial Volterra (linear elastic) configuration.

Still in the early stages of investigation is the combined effect of impurity obstacles and the Peierls barrier in regime I. Preliminary observations indicate that the increase in CRSS is simply additive to that of the 'pure' crystals [12], in contrast to body-centred-cubic (bcc) metals, where impurities are thought to induce softening effects. A theoretical model predicting this effect, which considers the influence of the two barriers, has been derived by Ono and Sommer [43].

In regime II, both the temperature and the impurity concentration dependence (parabolic) of τ_c suggest that the start of deformation is governed by the short-range interaction with impurity-vacancy (IV) dipoles. For low impurity concentrations, the increase in CRSS with impurity concentration at 0 K is given by the Friedel relation [44]:

(2) $$\Delta\tau_{co} = \frac{f^{3/2}}{(2E_L)^{1/2} b} c_p^{1/2}$$

(C_p, areal concentration of dipoles; f, maximum dislocation/solute interaction force). Various authors have determined expressions for the temperature dependence of τ_c. The result depends on the assumed obstacle/dislocation interaction profiles, as discussed by Ono [45]. For many profiles, $\tau_c(T)$ can be given by:

$$(3) \quad \tau_c^{1/2}(T) = \tau_{co}^{1/2}\left(1 - \left(\frac{T}{T_o}\right)^{2/3}\right)$$

A plot of $\Delta\tau_c^{1/2}$ against $T^{2/3}$ should therefore give a straight line. This is indeed the case, as shown in Figure 3, which also clearly illustrates the different temperature dependencies of the CRSS below a certain temperature. Extrapolation of such a plot to 0 K gives $\Delta\tau_{co}$. Note, however, that the smallness of regime II and the limited number of data points introduce a large uncertainty in these estimates. Skrotzki and Haasen [7] have summarized the data for LiF, NaCl, KCl, KBr, KI and AgCl and concluded that the specific hardening, $\Delta\tau_o/C^{1/2}\mu$ (C, solute concentration; μ, shear modulus), is about one order of magnitude greater on {100} than on {110}. Explanation of this effect involves a detailed knowledge of the dislocation/solute interaction. Continuum models of elastic, or shearing, interactions of the dipole with the dislocation as it passes, respectively, very close to, or right through, the dipole have been developed [44]. These have not been able to explain either the anisotropy or the required magnitude of the interaction force, although evaluation of a separate "electrostatic" contribution to the interaction energy showed that this was greater for {100} than for {110} dislocations [24], in agreement with experimental findings. Any agreement with experiment must, however, be considered fortuitous, since linear continuum models are not valid for interactions occurring in the highly distorted region of the dislocation's core and only atomistic models can provide the basis for a realistic assessment. In recent years, results have been published for interaction energy profiles of point defects with {110} dislocations in MgO [46], and are in progress for NaCl [47], but application of this approach to {100} dislocations is hampered by the difficulty of finding a suitable method of Coulomb summation.

The linear dependence of the CRSS on impurity concentration and the temperature independence in regime III are indicative of the operation of the induced Snoek effect [48]. Frank [49,50] has developed a model for ionic crystals based on the elastic field of the dislocation causing a reorientation of the IV-dipole. This model is in substantial agreement with experimental results. In particular, plots of $\Delta\tau_c/\mu C$ for different materials show, as

predicted, no difference between slip on {110} and {100}. The model contains
the tetragonal misfit as a parameter. Comparison between theory and experiment yield misfit values in the reasonable range, 0.50 - 0.15. Until now, it
has not been possible to corroborate these estimates by theoretical calculation, but atomistic methods capable of accurately determining this misfit have
recently been developed [51]. It should be noted that in NaCl the misfit
tensor of the lowest energy Ca^{2+}- vacancy dipole has, in fact, orthorhombic
rather than tetragonal symmetry.

Finally, the high-temperature drop-off of τ_c in regime IV to a
temperature-independent background determined by the long-rang interactions
has been suggested by Skrotzki and Haasen [7], following Frank [50], to be due
to the dragging of Snoek atmospheres. A second suggestion that this is due to
the break-up of the IV complexes appears less likely.

Cross-Slip and Plasticity

According to von Mises' criterion, plastic deformation of a polycrystal requires the operation of five independent slip systems[1]. In fcc
ionic crystals, primary slip on {110}<110> yields only two independent
systems. Hence, slip on the three secondary {100}<110> systems is also
required. The ductility of a polycrystal, therefore, appears to be closely
related to the disappearance of the plastic anisotropy. This seems, however,
to be merely a sufficient condition. Keeping in mind that there are several
ways to define the onset of ductility, a comparison by Skrotzki et al. [13] of
the ductility temperature with the temperature for (a) the onset of wavy slip
lines on {110} and (b) the onset of slip anisotropy suggests that the former
governs ductility; i.e. the cross-slip of screw dislocations on {110}. Note
that the cross-slip process is thought to proceed via slip on the {100} and
perhaps {111} planes. On the other hand, for glide on {100}, the preferred
cross-slip planes are on {110}. As the foregoing discussion has shown, the
latter is always the easier glide system and, hence, this could explain why
slip lines for screws primarily on {100} are wavy at all temperatures.
Skrotzki and Liu [52] have recently used a model developed by Haasen [53] for
fcc metals to analyze the cross-slip process on {110} and found that it also
works fairly well for fcc ionic crystals. This agreement may be fortuitous,
however, since the model assumes that the screw dislocations are dissociated
prior to cross-slip, which does not agree with atomistic model predictions for
edge dislocations [35]. Moreover, the cross-slip process seems to be governed
by unknown internal, rather than external, stresses [52,19]. The latter point

may also be the reason why the disappearance of plastic anisotropy does not seem to be the process governing the ductility of the polycrystal.

Conclusions

The plastic anisotropy of fcc ionic crystals is governed by the anisotropy of both intrinsic (Peierls stress) and extrinsic (dislocation/point-defect interaction) mechanisms. At lower temperatures and for very pure samples, the Peierls mechanism dominates, followed at higher temperatures, or for very impure samples, by the dislocation/solute interaction mechanism. In both cases, resistance to slip on the {100} plane is substantially higher than on the {110} plane. Rationalization of these results involves dislocation core properties and must be based on atomistic models. These have only been developed for {110}<110> slip. Justification for the higher resistance to slip on {100}<110> has been based on plausible, but approximate, models. Ductility of a polycrystal begins at a temperature at which wavy slip lines (cross-slip) are first observed. This is above the temperature at which plastic anisotropy disappears in single crystals. Cross-slip is linked to unknown internal stresses.

References

[1] J.P. Hirth and L. Lothe, "Theory of Dislocations" Second Edition, John Wiley and Sons, New York, 1982.
[2] S. Amelinckx, in "Dislocations in Solids", F.R.N. Nabarro (editor). Vol. 2, p. 67, North-Holland, Amsterdam, The Netherlands 1979.
[3] R.W. Whitworth, Adv. Phys. $\underline{24}$, 203 (1975).
[4] M.T. Sprackling, "The Plastic Deformation of Simple Ionic Crystals", Academic, New York, 1976.
[5] J. Castaing, J. Phys., (Paris), $\underline{41}$, C6, 127 (1980).
[6] J. Castaing, Ann. Phys. Fr. $\underline{6}$, 195 (1981).
[7] W. Skrotzki and P. Haasen, J. Phys., (Paris), $\underline{42}$, C3, 119 (1981).
[8] T. Bretheau, J. Castaing, J. Rabier and P. Veyssière Adv. Phys. $\underline{28}$, 835 (1979).
[9] W. Franzbecker, Phys. Stat. Sol. (b) $\underline{57}$, 545 (1973).
[10] W. Skrotzki, R. Steinbrech and P. Haasen, Mater. Sci. Eng. $\underline{32}$, 55 (1978).
[11] W.H.M. Alsem, Ph.D. Thesis, Groningen University, the Netherlands, 1981.
[12] W. Skrotzki, Ph.D. Thesis, Göttingen University, Fed. Repl. of Germany, 1981.

[13] W. Skrotzki, G. Frommeyer and P. Haasen, Phys. Stat. Sol. (a) **66**, 219 (1981).
[14] E.Yu. Gutmanas and E.M. Nadgornyi, Phys. Stat. Sol. **38**, 777 (1970).
[15] W.H.M. Alsem and J.Th.M. DeHosson, Phil. Mag. A, **46**, 327 (1982).
[16] K.-H. Matucha, Phys. Stat. Sol. **26**, 291 (1968).
[17] I.V.K. Bhagavan Raju and H. Strunk, Phys. Stat. Sol. (a) **53**, 211 (1979).
[18] J.C. Lewis, J. McCardle and R.W. Whitworth, Phys. Stat. Sol. (a) **64**, K67 (1981).
[19] F. Appel, U. Messerschmidt and V. Schmidt, Mater. Sci. Eng. **56**, 211 (1982).
[20] H.B. Huntington, J.E. Dickey and R. Thomson, Phys. Rev. **100**, 1117 (1955).
[21] F. Granzer, V. Belzner, M. Bücher, P. Petrasch and G. Teodosiu, J. Phys. Paris, **34**, C9-359 (1973).
[22] M. Bücher, Phys. Stat. Sol. (b) **114**, 383 (1982).
[23] J.J. Gilman, J. Appl. Phys. **44**, 982 (1973).
[24] P. Haasen, J. Phys., (Paris), **34**, C9 - 205 (1973).
[25] T. Suzuki, W. Skrotzki and P. Haasen, Phys. Stat. Sol. (b) **103**, 763 (1981).
[26] Z.G. Liu and W. Skrotzki, Phys. Stat. Sol. (a) **70**, 433 (1982).
[27] W. Skrotzki and T. Suzuki, Rad. Eff., **72-75**, (1983).
[28] V. Celli, M. Kabler, T. Nonomiya and R. Thomson, Phys. Rev. **131**, 58 (1963).
[29] P. Guyot and J.E. Dorn, Can. J. Phys. **45**, 983 (1967).
[30] T. Suzuki and H. Kim, J. Phys. Soc. Jap. **39**, 1566 (1975).
[31] T. Suzuki and H. Kim, J. Phys. Soc. Jap. **40**, 1703 (1976).
[32] F. Granzer, G. Wagner and J. Eisenblätter, Phys. Stat. Sol. **30**, 587 (1968).
[33] C.H. Woo and M.P. Puls, J. Phys. C: Solid State Phys. **9**, L27 (1976).
[34] C.H. Woo and M.P. Puls, Phil. Mag. **35**, 1641 (1977).
[35] M.P. Puls and C.B. So, Phys. Stat. Sol. (b) **98**, 87 (1980).
[36] M.J. Buerger, Am. Mineralogist **15**, 174 (1930).
[37] M.P. Puls, in "Dislocation Modelling of Physical Systems", M.F. Ashby, R. Bullough, G.S. Hartley and J.P. Hirth, eds., Pergamon, New York, 1981, p. 249.
[38] M.P. Puls, J. Phys., (Paris), **42**, C3, 13 (1981).
[39] G. Fontaine, J. Phys. Chem. Solids **29**, 209 (1968).
[40] G. Fontaine and P. Haasen, Phys. Stat. Sol. **31**, K67 (1969).
[41] P. Haasen, J. Phys., (Paris), **25**, C7, 167 (1974).
[42] P.W. Tasker and T.J. Bullough, Phil. Mag. **43**, 313 (1981).
[43] K. Ono and A.W. Sommer, Met. Trans. **1**, 877 (1970).
[44] T.E. Mitchell and A.E. Heuer, Mater. Sci. Eng. **28**, 81 (1977).
[45] K. Ono, J. Appl. Phys. **39**, 1803 (1968).

[46] M.P. Puls, J. Phys. Paris, 41, C6 - 135 (1980).
[47] M.P. Puls, unpublished.
[48] G. Schöck and A. Seeger, Acta Metall. 7, 468 (1959).
[49] W. Frank, Z. Natuforsch. A22, 377 (1967).
[50] W. Frank, Phys. Stat. Sol. 29, 391 (1968).
[51] M.P. Puls, unpublished.
[52] W. Skrotzki and Z.G. Liu, Phys. Stat. Sol. (a) 73, K225 (1982).
[53] P. Haasen, Phil. Mag. 3, 384 (1958).

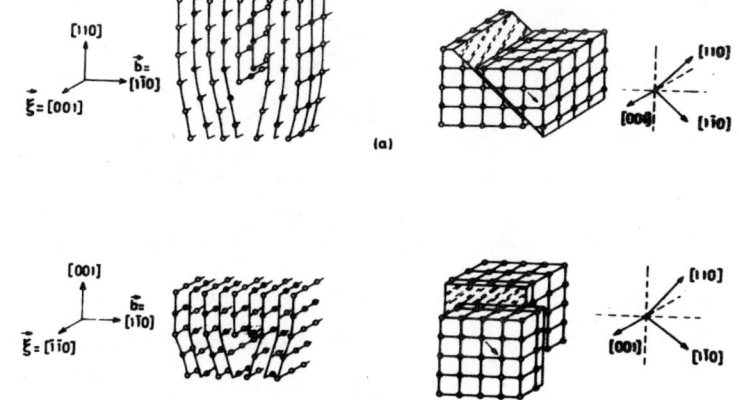

Fig.1 Dislocations and slip in fcc ionic crystals on a) {110} and b) {100} planes ($\vec{\xi}$, dislocation line direction; $\vec{b}$, Burgers vector),(from [11]).

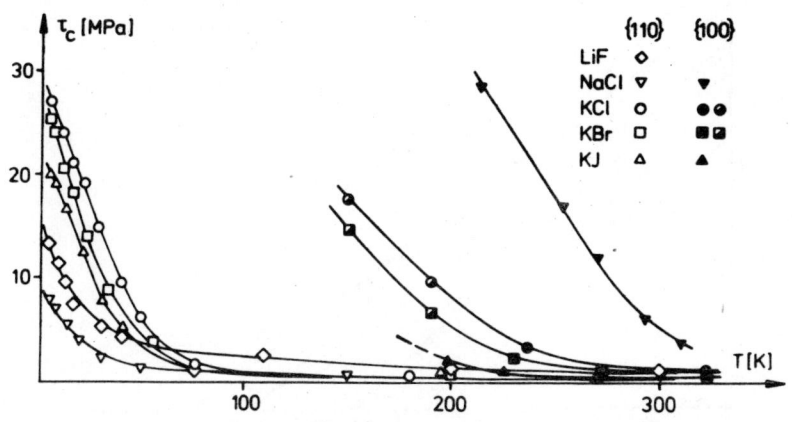

Fig.2 Variation of CRSS with temperature for "pure" crystals (from [12,7]).

Fig. 3(a)

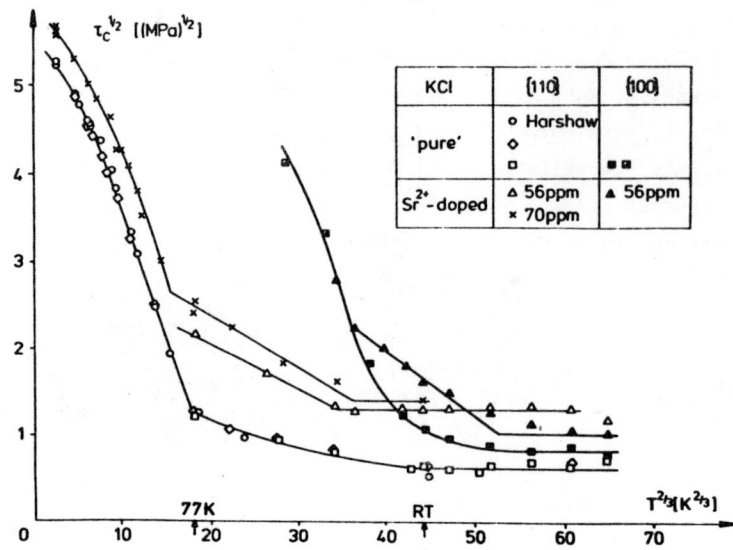

Fig. 3a) Variation of CRSS with temperature for KCl on a $\tau_c^{1/2} - T^{2/3}$ plot. The central portion of the plot constitutes regime II (from /12,7/).

Fig. 3(b)

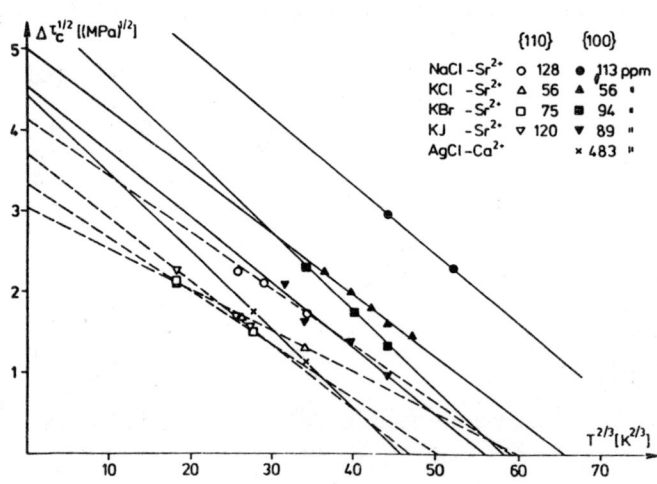

Fig. 3b) Same as for a) but only for the contribution $\Delta\tau_c^{1/2}$ due to the added dopant (i.e. the contribution due to the unknown impurities has been removed); from /12,7/.

DISCLINATIONS IN Sm C* LIQUID CRYSTALS

L. Lejček
Institute of Physics, Czechoslovak Academy of Sciences
Na Slovance 2, 182 00 Prague 8, Czechoslovakia

1. Introduction

Liquid crystals are characterized by the orientational order of long organic molecules whereas their centres of mass show no long range order. With thermotropic liquid crystals the orientational order of molecules depends on the temperature, which leads to the occurrence of different phases. Each phase shows characteristic textures /1/ and their optical contrast can be explained by defects of liquid cristalline order which are present in liquid crystal samples.

The existence of these defects has been well established in many papers and books e.g. /2,3/ where their basic properties were also presented. These defects, dislocations and disclinations, have the same topological properties as the dislocations and disclinations in solids /3/.

In this contribution two examples are chosen to show how the methods of treating the defects in solids can be used for the quantitative description of the disclination behaviour in liquid crystals.

The first example will consider the system of $\pm 2\pi$ twist disclinations in the bulk of chiral smectic liquid crystal using the well-known Peach-Koehler formula adopted to nematic liquid crystal in /3/.

The second example is the use of the Peierls-Nabarro (P.N.) model to the description of the 2π - surface twist disclination core in chiral smectic liquid crystal.

The chiral smectic (Sm C*) liquid crystal is characterized by a layered organization of long chiral molecules tilted by an angle θ with respect to layer normal. The chirality of molecules leads to the helical structure of tilted molecules. The molecules rotate along the layers normal with the helical pitch p_o. The direction of molecular projection into the plane of smectic layers is characterized by $\vec{t}$-vector introduced e.g. in /3,4/.

General expression of the free energy density describing Sm C* liquid crystal was given in /4/. However, in this contribution we utilize an approximation used in /5,6/ supposing that smectic layers perpendicular to the covering glass plates are not deformed. Then the free energy density can be written as

$$f = \frac{B_1}{2}\left(\frac{\partial \phi}{\partial z}\right)^2 + \frac{B_3}{2}\left(-\frac{\partial \phi}{\partial x} + q_0\right)^2. \tag{1}$$

The coordinate system is chosen in such a way that the x-axis is perpendicular to the smectic layers and the z-axis is perpendicular to the glass plates. The angle ϕ is the angle between $\vec{t}$-vector and y-axis, $\vec{t} = (0, \cos\phi, \sin\phi)$. B_1 and B_3 are the elastic constants and q_0 is related to the pitch p_0 as $q_0 = 2\pi/p_0$.

2. The system of $\pm 2\pi$-twist disclinations in Sm C*

In Sm C* liquid crystal with finite thickness 2 h the system of $\pm 2\pi$ - twist disclinations exists as shown in /6/. The $+2\pi$ and -2π disclinations are situated at distances d from upper and lower glass plates limiting the Sm C* sample, respectively, thus separating the parts of Sm C* near the glass covers unwound by surface anchoring from the bulk with perfect helical structure. Suppose further that the boundary conditions are fixed and $\phi(x,z = \pm h) = 0$. By the microscope study /7/ it was found that $\phi(x,z = +h) = \pi$ and $\phi(x,z = -h) = 0$. The assumption $\phi(x,z = \pm h) = 0$ permits to determine the configuration of the disclination system in a simple analytical form. Let us start with the equilibrium conditions.

Introducing the torques C_{xx} and C_{zx} analogously to /3/

$$C_{xx} = \partial f/\partial\left(\frac{\partial \phi}{\partial x}\right) = B_3\left(\frac{\partial \phi}{\partial x} - q_0\right),$$

$$C_{zx} = \partial f/\partial\left(\frac{\partial \phi}{\partial z}\right) = B_1 \frac{\partial \phi}{\partial z}, \tag{2}$$

the equation of equilibrium is

$$0 = C_{xx,x} + C_{zx,z} = B_1 \frac{\partial^2 \phi}{\partial z^2} + B_3 \frac{\partial^2 \phi}{\partial x^2}. \tag{3}$$

The solution of equation (3) can be written in the form

$$\phi = \sum_{m=-\infty}^{+\infty}\sum_{k=-\infty}^{+\infty}(-1)^k\left[\operatorname{arctg}\alpha\frac{z-2hk-h+d}{x-mp_0} - \operatorname{arctg}\alpha\frac{z-2hk+h-d}{x-mp_0}\right], \tag{4}$$

where $\alpha = (B_3/B_1)^{1/2}$. The solution (4) corresponds to the periodic distribution of pairs of $+2\pi$ and -2π twist disclinations parallel to y-axis and situated at $x = np_0$, $z = h-d$ and $x = np_0$, $z = -h+d$, respectively, which satisfied the boundary condition $\phi(x, z = \pm h) = 0$. Its properties are discussed in /6/. Here we will study the equilibrium of this disclination system. The force $\vec{g}$ acting on unit length of disclination at $x = 0$, $z = (h-d)$ by the other disclinations is given by the Peach-Kohler formula proposed for nematic liquid crystal in /3/:

(5) $$g_x = 2\pi C'_{zx}, \quad g_y = 0, \quad g_z = -2\pi C'_{xx}.$$

Torques C'_{zx} and C'_{xx} are given by the equations (2) where disclination at $x = 0$, $z = h-d$ is not included in the summation. The component g_x is zero due to the symmetry of disclination configuration and

(6) $$g_z = \frac{\pi^2 (B_1 B_3)^{1/2}}{h} \sin \frac{\pi d}{h} \sum_{n=-\infty}^{+\infty} \frac{\operatorname{ch} 2\pi Y_n}{\operatorname{ch}^2 2\pi Y_n - \cos^2 \frac{\pi d}{h}} - p_0 q_0^2 B_3$$

with $Y_n = (x-np_0)/4h$. The distance d of the disclinations from the glass plate is determined from the condition $g_z = 0$. Considering the interaction of the nearest $+2\pi$ and -2π disclinations only, i.e. $h\alpha/p_0 < \pi/2$, we take in the sum (6) the term with $n = 0$. Then the condition $g_z = 0$ gives $\sin(\pi d/h) = p_0/4h\alpha$. The distance d for which the system is stable /6/ is $d = h \arcsin(p_0/4h\alpha)/\pi$ at the condition $h \geqslant p_0/4\alpha$. In those samples where $h < p_0/4\alpha$ the system of disclination cannot exist.

3. Peierls-Nabarro model of 2π twist disclination core

In the sample of the thickness $h < p_0/4\alpha$, the system of 2π-twist disclinations does not exist but a single 2π-twist disclination line can appear in the sample bulk /8/. Its existence is a consequence of the molecular rotation throughout the sample in order to connect different molecular orientations on the upper, $\phi(x, z = +h) = \pi$, and lower, $\phi(x, z = -h) = 0$, glass plates. It is possible that this disclination could be also anchored to the cover glass surface. However, in the sample with the boundary conditions $\phi(x, z = \pm h) = 0$ such a 2π-surface disclination is also not excluded and in this case it is stabilized by the surface anchoring only. In this part it will be shown how the core of such a 2π-disclination can be described by P.N. model used first to the description of surface disclinations in nematic liquid crystals in /9/.

Being interested in surface effects only, we will suppose for simplicity that Sm C* liquid crystal fills the half-space, $z > 0$, limited at $z \to 0_+$ by glass plate. In this approximation we neglect the effects of the sample thickness. Let us consider 2π-surface twist disclination to be parallel to y-axis and the core to be spread on glass plate along x-axis.

The analogy between the equation (3) and the equilibrium equation of nematic liquid crystal permits us to write P.N. equation describing the 2π-surface disclination core in the form

$$（7） \quad -\frac{dW_s(\varphi)}{d\varphi} = \frac{(B_1 B_3)^{1/2}}{\pi} \int_{-\infty}^{+\infty} \frac{d\varphi(x')}{dx'} \frac{dx'}{x-x'} ,$$

which is analogous to the P.N. equation in nematic liquid crystal derived and discussed in /9,3/. Integral should be understood as the Cauchy principal value. $W_s(\varphi)$ is the surface anchoring energy and is the function of the angle $\varphi(x) = \phi(x, z \to 0_+)$. Experiments /6,7,8,10/ show that the molecules of Sm C* are anchored to glass plates in the best way when they lay in a direction parallel to the glass plate, i.e. when $\varphi = 0, \pi$ or 2π. For those orientations there are minima of the surface anchoring energy. Suppose that $W_s(\varphi) = 0$ for $\varphi = 0, 2\pi$. In Sm C* the orientation of molecules characterized by $\vec{t}$-vector is not equivalent to the orientation $-\vec{t}$. Thus the minimum $W_s(\varphi = \pi) = W_m > W_s(\varphi = 0, 2\pi)$. The existence of the minimum of $W_s(\varphi)$ with the energy W_m implies a possibility of splitting of 2π-disclination into two $+\pi$-twist disclinations situated at $x = -d$ and $x = d$. So we can propose the solution of (7) in the form

$$(8) \quad \varphi(x) = \operatorname{arctg}\frac{x-d}{\xi} + \operatorname{arctg}\frac{x+d}{\xi} - \pi,$$

where ξ is the half-width of the disclination core. The function $\varphi(x)$ satisfies the conditions $\varphi(x \to -\infty) = 0$ and $\varphi(x \to +\infty) = 2\pi$ which corresponds to the 2π-surface twist disclination. Solution (8) was widely used for the description of dislocation splitting in solids (see e.g. /11,12,13/). Using (8) and (7) the surface anchoring energy $W_s(\varphi(x))$ can be determined in the form

$$(9) \quad W_s(\varphi(x)) = \int_{-\infty}^{x} dx' \frac{dW_s}{d\varphi} \frac{d\varphi}{dx'} = \frac{(B_1 B_3)^{1/2}}{2} \left[\frac{\xi}{\xi^2 + (x-d)^2} + \frac{\xi}{\xi^2 + (x+d)^2} + \frac{1}{d} \left(\text{arctg} \frac{x+d}{\xi} - \text{arctg} \frac{x-d}{\xi} \right) \right]$$

For $\varphi(0) = \pi$ it is

$$(10) \quad W_m = \frac{(B_1 B_3)^{1/2}}{\xi} \left[\frac{1}{1+(d/\xi)^2} + \frac{\xi}{d} \text{arctg} \frac{d}{\xi} \right]$$

If $d \gg \xi$, it is $W_m \approx (B_1 B_3)^{1/2} \text{arctg}(d/\xi)/d$ and maxima W_M of $W_s(\varphi(x))$ are approximately situated at $x = \pm d$. Then $W_M = (B_1 B_3)^{1/2}/2\xi$. Thus the experimental determination of ξ and d can give an estimation of $W_m/(B_1 B_3)^{1/2}$ and $W_M/(B_1 B_3)^{1/2}$. Similar estimation was done for nematic liquid crystal placed on the surface of triglycine sulphate single crystal /14/ where the surface disclinations have the parameter about 0,5 - 2,5 μm what gives the order of W_M about 10^{-6} J/m^2.

The example presented in this contribution shows how the P.N. model of the disclination core was adopted to describe 2π surface twist disclination in Sm C. Previously this model was applied to disclinations in nematics /3,9,14/ and to the edge dislocations in Sm A liquid crystals /15,16/.

References

/1/ Demus D., Richter L.: Textures of Liquid Crystals, Leipzig 1980.
/2/ de Gennes P.G.: The Physics of Liquid Crystals, Clarendon Press, Oxford 1974.
/3/ Kléman M.: Points, Lignes, Parois dans les Fluides Anisotropes et les Solides Cristallins Tome I+II, Édition de Physique, Paris 1977, 1978.
/4/ Rapini A.: J. de Physique 33 (1972) 237.
/5/ Bourdon L., Sommeria J., Kléman M.: J. de Physique 43 (1982) 77.
/6/ Glogarová M., Lejček L., Pavel J., Janovec V., Fousek J.: Mol. Cryst. Liquid Cryst. 91 (1983) 309.
/7/ Glogarová M., Pavel J., Lejček L.: this symposium proceedings Part A, p. 95.
/8/ Glogarová M., Pavel J.: to be published.
/9/ Vítek V., Kléman M.: J. de Physique 36 (1975) 59.
/10/ Brunet M., Williams C.: Ann. de Physique 3 (1978) 237.
/11/ Foreman, A.J.E.: Ph.D. Thesis, Imperial College, London.
/12/ Seeger A., Handbuch der Physik Bd. 7, Berlin 1955, 383.
/13/ Hobart R.: Fundamental Aspects of Dislocation Theory, J.A. Simmons, F. de Wit, R. Bullough Eds., NBS SP 317, 1970, 1157.
/14/ Lejček L.: Czech. J. Phys. B33 (1983) 447.
/15/ Kléman M.: J. de Physique 35 (1974) 595.
/16/ Lejček L.: Czech. J. Phys. B32 (1982) 767.

SECTION 4

THE STRUCTURE AND PROPERTIES OF GRAIN BOUNDARIES

THE STRUCTURE OF GRAIN BOUNDARIES

A.G. Crocker

Department of Physics, University of Surrey
Guildford, England, GU2 5XH

The mechanical properties of polycrystalline materials are in many cases controlled by the structure and mobility of grain boundaries. It is therefore necessary to have an understanding of the shapes of grains, the ways in which they pack together and of the detailed atomic arrangements which occur at their interfaces. This paper reviews the basic ideas of grain boundary structure which have been developed in recent years, presents some new results and discusses their significance.

1. Introduction

Most engineering applications of materials involve their use in polycrystalline form [1]. It is therefore important to have an understanding of the shapes of the grains forming such materials, of the way in which these grains are packed together, of the structure and properties of the interfaces between them, and of the ways in which these boundaries interact with other defects within the grains. In particular the mechanical properties of polycrystals, including yielding, superplasticity, high temperature creep, radiation creep and swelling, and recrystallization, depend strongly on the presence, the structure and hence the mobility of grain boundaries. In recent years powerful experimental, theoretical and computational techniques have been developed to investigate these problems and significant progress has been made [2]. The present paper summarises and discusses some of the principal concepts which have been introduced and reviews some of the important results.

2. The Structure of Polycrystals

An ideal polycrystal is one in which all the grains have the same size and shape and in which all the grain boundaries have the same energy. For such a polycrystal to be in equilibrium, three grain boundaries must meet at equal angles of $2\pi/3$ along each grain edge and four grain edges must meet at equal angles of $\phi = \cos^{-1}(-1/3) = 109.47°$ at each grain corner. No regular array of polyhedral grains with plane faces can satisfy these conditions. However a body centred cubic packing of regular tetrakaidecahedra fills all space and meets the boundary conditions approximately [3]. The tetrakaidecahedron, which is shown in Fig. 1(a), has eight regular hexagonal faces and six square faces. In the b.c.c. packing these faces are shared with the eight first- and six second-nearest neighbours respectively. In this structure the edge angles are ϕ (x1) and $\psi = \cos^{-1}(-1/\sqrt{3}) = 125.27°$ (× 2) and the corner angles are $2\pi/3$ (× 4) and $\pi/2$ (× 2). The exact equilibrium conditions can be met if, as shown schematically in Fig. 1(b), the hexagonal faces become convoluted with 3-fold symmetry and zero net curvature, whilst the square faces remain flat. The detailed shape of such a curved face was first calculated by Kelvin in 1887 [4], as part of a study of the equipartition of space by soap films. A recent more accurate analysis gives the shape shown in Fig. 2(a) [5].

In practice polycrystals do not have grains of uniform size and shape and a more general model which takes into account these variations is therefore required. A very convenient structure to examine is obtained by allowing the tetrakaidecahedra at the corners of the cubic cells of the b.c.c. array of grains to grow at the expense of those occupying body-centred locations [3]. Equal numbers of small and large grains then arise and, assuming that the grain faces are flat, their shapes are as shown in Figs. 1(c) and (d). Each grain corner of the polycrystal is now the junction of two long and two short grain edges but all the angular relations between the faces and edges are unchanged. In practice if the three different grain faces (large squares, small squares and hexagons with 3-fold symmetry) all have the same energy, the square faces will remain flat while the hexagons again become convoluted. An example of the shape of such an hexagonal face is shown in Fig. 2(b). However, if the ratio γ_H/γ_S of the energies γ of the hexagonal (H) and square (S) faces is $\sqrt{3}/2$ rather than unity, the structures with planar grain boundaries are in equilibrium. Furthermore the bimodular structures with large and small grains have exactly the same energy as the original unimodular arrangement [5].

The range of bimodular structures discussed above is clearly limited by the case in which the small grains become octahedra with unstable 8-fold nodes at their corners. These bimodular structures, which may be described as an ordered caesium-chloride arrangement of grains, have formed the basis of a recent analysis of the stability of interconnected pores in nuclear materials of non-uniform grain size. The model is still of course idealized but realistic predictions for materials with a random distribution of grain sizes can be obtained by taking a statistical average of the results for bimodular structures with a range of different ratios of grain volumes [3].

A simple alternative method of generating a non-uniform polycrystal is to allow an individual tetrakaidecahedral grain to change its volume [6]. If this occurs in a uniform manner, the angles at grain edges and grain corners and the total energy will again remain constant. However, as shown in Fig. 1(e), the square faces of the rogue grain will change their size and the regular hexagonal faces become truncated equilateral triangles. Meanwhile seven of the faces of the first nearest neighbours of this grain (Fig. 1(f)) and five of the second (Fig. 1(g)) change their shape. In addition to the original square and regular hexagonal grain faces, the polycrystal now contains four distorted boundaries. The curved forms of these which arise when all of the boundaries have the same energy are currently being calculated [5]. Eventually of course, whether the rogue grain is shrinking or growing, unstable nodes will be generated at its corners. This model is not restricted to a single rogue grain. Indeed, as many as one-quarter of the grains, lying on a face centred cubic superlattice consisting of third nearest neighbours in the original b.c.c. structure, can change size independently. Each of these influences its first and second neighbours so that a pseudo-random distribution of grain sizes and shapes is generated. Remarkably this still has the same energy as the original ideal polycrystal.

The above procedure for generating a model of a polycrystal from an ideal structure is effectively based on introducing point defects in the form of substitutional solute polyhedra into a regular b.c.c. array of tetrakaidecahedra. In practice polycrystalline structures will also contain line and sheet defects. The case of the introduction of an edge dislocation into a two-dimensional array of regular hexagons is well-known [7]. As shown in Fig. 3(a) a pair of 5- and 7-sided grains is then produced at the dislocation core. The corresponding three-dimensional case of introducing edge screw or mixed dislocations into a b.c.c. array of tetrakaidecahedra is far more complex but has been examined in connection with studies of superplasticity [8]. Clearly the grains along the dislocation core become highly distorted and no longer have 14 faces, and indeed it appears that the average number of faces is not 14. Similarly interfaces between regions of grains of differing orientations and size can be examined. A two-dimensional example is shown in Fig. 3(b) [6], but little progress has been made in investigating the three-dimensional analogue.

3. The Geometry of Grain Boundary Structures

In general, as illustrated schematically in Fig. 4, an unrelaxed grain boundary has nine degrees of freedom. Three of these give the relative orientations of the two grains and can be associated with the axis (2) and angle (1) of the rotation between them. A further three are needed to define the orientation (2) and location (1) of the interface plane. Finally the remaining three define the direction (2) and magnitude (1) of the relative displacement between the grains. However, for single lattice structures with only one atom at each lattice point, the location of the boundary may be included in the displacement. This is not true for crystals with a basis such as double lattice structures [9].

As the general description of grain boundaries is so complex, most studies of their structures have concentrated on special cases. In particular twin-, tilt- and twist-boundaries have received detailed attention. Twin boundaries normally obey one of the four conventional orientation relations: (a) reflection in a rational interface, (b) rotation of π about the normal to this interface, (c) rotation of π about a rational direction lying in the interface, (d) reflection in the plane normal to this direction [10]. In general relations (c) and (d) give rise to boundaries with irrational Miller indices. Also in single lattice structures (a) and (b) are equivalent, as are (c) and (d). Non-conventional twins in which the orientation relation is (e) a special rotation of magnitude not equal to π, about a direction lying in the interface and normal to a rational plane may also occur [11]. These five different orientation relations are shown schematically in Fig. 5. In each case six degrees of freedom are in general needed to fully define the structure of the boundaries, if translations between the grains are allowed.

Tilt boundaries are those in which the two grains are related by a rotation about an axis lying in the grain boundary. They may be symmetric, in which case the interface has the same Miller indices when referred to lattice bases in the two grains, or asymmetric when this is not the case. Schematic examples are shown in Figs. 6(a) and (b). Twist boundaries have their axis of rotation perpendicular to the grain boundary. Degenerate cases arise in which for example the interface is a mirror plane and the rotation is about a symmetry axis. However in general both the interface and the rotation axis are irrational. These cases are shown schematically in Figs. 6(c) and (d). Both tilt and twist boundaries have in general eight degrees of freedom. The geometry of any grain boundary can always be resolved into tilt and twist components [1,2].

Two grains meeting at a grain boundary have atoms located at the points of two lattices related by a rotation. If these lattices are considered to interpenetrate and fill all space none of the points will in general coincide (Fig. 7(a)). However a single point from each lattice may be brought into coincidence by translation (Fig. 7(b)), and for special orientation relations an infinite number of points may coincide (Fig. (c)). These points then form a one-, two-, or three-dimensional array which is known as a coincidence site lattice (CSL) [12]. The reciprocal density of coincident sites relative to the original lattice is denoted by Σ, the twin boundary in Fig. 7(c) with one-third of the points coinciding having $\Sigma = 3$. The condition for forming a CSL, especially with a relatively low value of Σ, is very restrictive. In particular the possible rotations between the grains must have specific magnitudes and be about rational crystallographic axes which are perpendicular to rational planes. Hence most analyses of CSLs are restricted to cubic lattices. Also a small rotation or translation of one of the grains immediately destroys the CSL. This is avoided by a generalization of the CSL known as the O-lattice, which is based on coincidences of interior points of the unit cells of the two lattices rather than on the lattice points themselves [12]. Unlike the CSL the size and orientation of the O-lattice change smoothly as the misorientation is varied. If one of the component lattices of a CSL is shifted by one of its own vectors clearly the CSL is fully conserved. This is also true if this lattice is displaced by any vector between the two lattices, except that in general the CSL will then be shifted by a vector of the stationary lattice whilst retaining its structure, size and orientation [13]. An example of this is shown in Fig. 8 for a $\Sigma = 5$ twist boundary on a (001) plane of a simple cubic lattice. Such vector displacements, which are characteristic of the CSL, define a three dimensional array of points known as the DSC lattice [12].

The simplest grain boundaries occur between grains which have a CSL and are parallel to rational planes of this CSL. The structure of the boundary is then periodic having a unit cell based on the CSL. For small values of Σ and boundaries following close packed CSL planes the period is small and the structure correspondingly simple. However for larger values of Σ and boundaries on higher index CSL planes the structures become more complex. Nevertheless the arrangements of atoms at the boundaries tend to lie at the corners of some of the random close packed polyhedra used to discuss the structures of liquids. In particular the seven polyhedra shown in Fig. 9, or distorted forms of these, occur frequently [14]. This is partly because it is always possible to describe a boundary on a high-index plane in terms of one on a low-index plane containing one or two sets of facets or steps [13]. If the original boundary is on a rational plane of the CSL these steps will be uniformly spaced. Departures from such orientations will then be accommodated by irregularites in the step spacings. An interesting example of this effect is provided by the deformation twin boundary in crystalline mercury [15]. This lies on an irrational plane near ($\bar{1}35$) of the face centred rhombohedral crystal structure. The ($\bar{1}35$) plane, as shown in Fig. 10, may be considered to consist of centred ($\bar{1}\bar{1}1$) and primitive ($1\bar{1}3$) facets. The irrational twinning plane which is related to ($\bar{1}35$) by a small rotation about the [$\bar{1}21$] direction is now obtained by reducing the size of approximately one-fifteenth of the ($\bar{1}\bar{1}1$) facets by a factor of two. An example is shown shaded in Fig. 10.

Detailed studies have been carried out of the way in which the structures of tilt boundaries change with the angle of tilt. As a simple example the range of structures for symmetric [$1\bar{1}0$] tilt boundaries in face centred cubic metals lying between $\Sigma = 11$ (113), 130° and $\Sigma = 27$ (115) 149° will be considered. The (113) boundary consists entirely of capped trigonal prims (Fig. 9(d)) which are denoted by the symbol A. The boundary structure may thus be denoted by ..AAA.. Similarly the (115) boundary is composed of units consisting of an irregular pentagon attached to a tetrahedron. These units are denoted by the symbol B so that the boundary may be described by the sequence ..BBB... As the angle of tilt is increased from 130° to 136°, 141°, 145° and finally 149°, the interface changes from (113) to (227), (114), (229) and (115), and Σ changes from 11 to 139, 9, 89 and 27 respectively. Also an increasing number of B type structural units is introduced into the boundaries so that the initial ..AAA.. sequence becomes ..AAB.., ..AB.., ..BBA.. and finally ..BBB.. . Intermediate cases can also be described as mixtures of A and B units so that the boundary structures vary continuously with misorientation. It is particularly interesting to note that a boundary of a CSL structure with Σ as large as 139 can be described as a very simple sequence of structural units [16].

4. Dislocation Description of Grain Boundaries

It is possible to match any two lattices along a boundary by introducing a suitable array of dislocations into the interface. The procedure for determining the total Burgers vector of these dislocations is illustrated in Fig. 11 [13]. The product lattice B is considered to be derived from the parent lattice A by means of a deformation $\underline{S}$. The two lattices are assumed to meet at a surface of unit normal $\underline{v}$ and a vector $OP = \underline{p}$ is chosen in the interface. A Burgers circuit OP_APP_BO, where the parts OP_AP and PP_BO lie in lattices A and B is now drawn as shown in Fig. 11(a). The corresponding circuit in the reference lattice, which is assumed to coincide with A, is given in Fig. 11(b), the total Burgers vector $\underline{b}$ of all dislocations in the interface $\underline{v}$ which cross p being defined by O'O. Unfortunately this procedure is not unique since an infinite number of ways exists for describing each of the two lattices. In practice descriptions corresponding to low dislocation densities are more likely to have physical significance but this is not necessarily the case. For example Fig. 12 shows two possible descriptions of a simple symmetric tilt boundary. The interface in Fig. 12(a) is generated by a large simple shear on the boundary plane and the dislocation content is zero. A more satisfactory description is that the tilt is achieved by a rotation which leads to an array of edge dislocations as shown in Fig. 12(b). The problem of obtaining the most realistic description of a grain boundary is therefore involved. However some intuitive procedures for making the choice are valuable. For example descriptions involving lattice deformations with small principal strains or small rotations may be preferred [13]. These choices may be formalised by making use of the O-lattice theory [12].

In order to describe the dislocation structure of a real interface the net Burgers vector $\underline{b}$ defined in Fig. 11 has to be resolved into components of individual sets of dislocation lines. If the misorientation between the grains is small these will have the same Burgers vectors as lattice dislocations but for high angle boundaries they will have special Burgers vectors associated with the structure of the boundary. In particular they will be vectors of the DSC lattice and both perfect and partial dislocations are possible. As the misorientation of the grains, from either identical orientations or from special CSL orientations, increases the spacing of these grain boundaries dislocations (gbds) decreases. It is anticipated therefore that there will be a corresponding increase in boundary energy. However it is important to note that the strain fields of these intrinsic gbds cancel at long range. They are simply a convenient means of defining the local disorder in a grain boundary. Indeed they are just an alternative way of describing the structural grain boundary units which were introduced in Section 3.

In general, as indicated in Fig. 2, grain boundaries are not planar even at a macroscopic scale and therefore must contain steps [13]. These steps are in addition to any facetting that may occur on irrational or high-index boundaries, such as that shown in Fig. 10. They have the full character of lattice dislocations, including a long range strain field, and indeed often arise at sites where lattice dislocations intersect a boundary. They are therefore known as extrinsic gbds. However they do not in general retain the Burgers vectors of lattice dislocations and often dissociate into dislocations of the DSC lattice becoming indistinguishable from the intrinsic gbds. For example, referring to Fig. 10, if a slip dislocation with a $\frac{1}{2}$ [101] Burgers vector lying on the ($\bar{1}\bar{1}$1) plane intersects the twin boundary an additional double ($\bar{1}\bar{1}$1) facet is created which can dissociate into two facets of the type which is shaded [15].

5. Computer Simulation of Grain Boundary Structures

Grain boundary structures provide a fruitful field of investigation for computer experiments based on inter-atomic potentials. Indeed the geometrical theories of interfaces owe much to the results of these simulations. In particular translations between grains occur frequently in relaxed computer models but were largely ignored in early geometric studies. A good example is provided by the (112) twin boundary in body centred cubic metals which, as shown in Fig. 13, has two distinct possible structures [17]. Traditionally it was assumed that the structure had the reflection orientation relation of Fig. 13(a). However computer simulations revealed that the isosceles structure of Fig. 13(b) is favoured by potentials representing some metals. The case of {112} twins in iron is particularly interesting as the two boundaries are then predicted to have similar energies so that both should occur in practice. Adjacent regions of the two types of boundary will then be separated by a step of height equal to one-half of the {112} interplanar spacing. This step is equivalent to a partial twinning dislocation and perfect twinning dislocations of Burgers vector $\frac{1}{6}$ <11$\bar{1}$> will dissociate into two $\frac{1}{12}$ <11$\bar{1}$> partials. Alternatively this may be described as the dissociation of a DSC perfect dislocation into two partials. Notice that those are extrinsic rather than intrinsic gbds and their motion causes the twin boundary to migrate [18].

The two possible structures of the {112} b.c.c. twin boundary shown in Fig. 13 both exhibit a high degree of symmetry. For the reflection boundary the two grains are clearly mirror images of each other and the isosceles boundary has a 2-fold screw axis in the plane of the interface. Computer simulations also demonstrate that many other grain boundaries have high symmetry. For example {001} twist boundaries in face centred cubic metals are found to have grains in the exact CSL relationship or displaced with respect to each other to one of two alternative symmetric structures [19].

These three structures are illustrated in Fig. 14 for the case of the $\Sigma = 5$ boundary in copper. These diagrams show the way in which atoms adjacent to the boundary relax during the computer modelling and also the symmetry elements of the three resulting structures. These same symmetry elements arise for $\Sigma = 13, 17, 25$ and higher order boundaries and also with some minor changes for b.c.c. crystals. As in the case of the two b.c.c. twin boundaries in iron it is found that these three boundaries in both copper and nickel have similar energies [19]. In practice therefore all three types of structure may arise in different regions of the interface. In addition there are four variants of each of the displaced boundaries. This means that a large variety of partial DSC dislocations may lie between adjacent boundary regions of differing structure.

Computer simulations of other grain boundary structures indicate that symmetry is not always present. For example the $\Sigma = 3$ (110) 71° and $\Sigma = 9$ (110) 39° twist boundaries in a model representing copper have received detailed attention [20]. In each case four distinct highly symmetric structures may arise, three of which involve relative translations of the two grains parallel to the interface. However when long range strains are eliminated by allowing appropriate volume increases, low symmetry structures are found to have marginally lower energies. Indeed the lowest energy relaxed $\Sigma = 9$ boundary exhibits no symmetry. Another example is the (112) twin boundary in copper [21]. The conventional geometrical structure of this interface based on a reflection orientation relation is shown in Fig. 15(a). It involves the close approach of the opposing atoms on either side of the boundary which are marked with asterisks. Large relaxations are therefore anticipated during the computer modelling. In practice the relaxed structure shown in Fig. 15(b) was found. This involves firstly a displacement of the upper grain by $\frac{1}{4}$ [1$\bar{1}$0] which effectively interchanges planes in the two-fold stacking sequence in the [1$\bar{1}$0] direction. Secondly the upper grain is displaced by 0.1623 [11$\bar{1}$] in the orthogonal direction parallel to the interface. Although close to $\frac{1}{6}$ [11$\bar{1}$] the results clearly show that the displacement is distinct from this value. Finally large scale local relaxations occur to give the boundary shown in Fig. 15(b). This is broad, asymmetric and involves planes of atoms parallel to the boundary coalescing and even passing through each other [21]. The result of these three components of the relaxation process which in practice of course occur simultaneously is that none of the atoms are particularly close to any of their neighbours. Clearly complex structures of this kind which depend to some extent on the form of the inter-atomic potential adopted can not be predicted by geometrical theories.

6. Discussion

The structure of grain boundaries is a research field in which there have been very fruitful interactions between theoretical, computational and experimental investigations. The present survey has concentrated largely on geometrical concepts and the results of computer experiments and has attempted to illustrate the elegance of some of the mathematical models and the complexity of some of the computed structures. It is important to realise however that most of this work is only strictly relevant to b.c.c. and f.c.c. crystals. In general no CSL exists for non-cubic crystals so that the formal beauty of the geometrical analyses is irrelevant. Nevertheless grain boundaries in these materials appear to have similar properties to those in cubic crystals. This suggests that basically the same structures and mechanisms arise in all cases and that these can only be elucidated by studying the low symmetry materials. The results will of necessity be independent of the CSL and its generalised forms. Similarly the formal description of the dislocation content of interfaces has serious limitations, as there is no unique solution for the total Burgers vector, no unique way to resolve this into individual dislocations and in any case these intrinsic dislocations have no long range strain field.

Computer simulations of grain boundary structures overcome many of these problems as the relaxation procedures select energetically favourable configurations. Sometimes these have a high degree of symmetry although not the simplest possible geometrical structure based for example on a CSL. However on many occasions the predicted boundaries have little or no symmetry and depend on the detailed form of the inter-atomic potential being used. Indeed one of the problems associated with the simulation technique is that potentials are continually being improved so that it is difficult to compare the results of different research groups. Nevertheless presently available potentials leave much to be desired and most studies are still restricted to cubic crystals. In addition only relatively simple periodic twin, tilt and twist boundaries can be investigated, due to the limitations of the size of the models which can be accommodated in computers. However very stimulating results have been obtained and the structural units which have been found to describe for example the features of tilt boundaries may be used to develop an understanding of more general grain boundaries [16]. The fact that some low index boundaries are broad and asymmetric does suggest however that simple structural models may have little relevance to the general case.

Much of this geometrical and computational work has of course been stimulated by the increasingly sophisticated experimental studies which are proceeding. In particular the observation of primary grain boundary dislocations in low angle tilt and twist boundaries and of secondary gbds in high angle near CSL boundaries using transmission electron microscopy has generated a vast amount of interest [2]. In addition direct images of grain boundary structure have been obtained using both field ion microscopy and TEM. However FIM has many serious limitations and lattice imaging using TEM is again restricted to foils with particular orientations [2]. Electron and X-ray diffraction techniques can also be used to study the structure of grain boundaries and it is interesting that interpretation of the results requires an integrated approach with computer modelling [2]. Again much of this work has concentrated on simple boundaries in metals with cubic structures. Far more effort is needed on lower symmetry materials.

Finally it must be emphasised that structural analyses of grain boundaries are based on flat interfaces. These may contain steps or extrinsic dislocations but little effort is made to consider the convoluted forms which in general grain boundaries adopt. These depend on the geometrical packing of the grains and on the way in which the resulting polycrystal attempts to minimise its energy. The simple model of a polycrystal consisting of a regular array of identical tetrakaidecahedral grains is currently, as described in Section 2, being extended to include a distribution of grain shapes and sizes. Some of the resulting grain faces can become highly distorted. This is particularly true when irregular tetrakaidecahedra based on triclinic rather than cubic symmetry are considered. However these models are based at present on very simple assumptions about the energies of the different grain faces. This is information provided by the computer simulation work and it would be particularly interesting to simulate the structure of a grain edge between three contiguous grains. Also available experimental information on three dimensional grain shapes is very limited.

Thus our existing knowldege of grain boundary structure, although extremely elegant and detailed in certain special cases, is very limited. It may not even provide a useful framework for the development of a general analysis of arbitrary curved boundaries in low symmetry materials. However interactions between those investigating the problem using widely differing approaches is currently leading to rapid advances in our understanding and this will surely continue.

References

[1] Chadwick G.A., Smith D.A. (eds.) : Grain boundary structure and properties, Academic Press, London 1976.

[2] Balluffi R.W. (ed.) : Grain boundary structure and kinetics, American Society for Metals, Metals Park, Ohio 1980.

[3] Rinous P.J., Tucker M.O., Crocker A.G.: Proc. Roy. Soc. Lond. $\underline{A383}$ (1982) 201.

[4] Thompson W. : Phil. Mag. $\underline{24}$ (1887) 503.

[5] Ahmed I., Crocker A.G. : to be published.

[6] Crocker A.G., Rinous P.J., Tucker M.O. : Dislocation modelling of physical systems, Ashby M.F. et al. (eds.) Pergamon, Oxford 1981, p.519.

[7] Hirth J.P., Lothe J. : Theory of dislocations, MacGraw Hill, New York 1970.

[8] Morral J.E., Ashby M.F. : Acta Metall. $\underline{22}$ (1974) 567.

[9] Pond R.C. : Proc. Roy. Soc. Lond. $\underline{A357}$ (1977) 471.

[10] Bilby B.A., Crocker A.G. : Proc. Roy. Soc. Lond. $\underline{A288}$ (1965) 240.

[11] Bevis M., Crocker A.G. : Proc. Roy. Soc. Lond. $\underline{A313}$ (1969) 509.

[12] Bollmann W. : Crystal defects and crystalline interfaces, Springer, Berlin 1970.

[13] Christian J.W., Crocker A.G. : Dislocations and lattice transformations, in Dislocations in solids $\underline{3}$, Nabarro F.R.N. (ed.) North Holland, Amsterdam 1980.

[14] Vitek V., Sutton A.P., Smith D.A., Pond R.C. : In ref. [2], p. 115.

[15] Guyoncourt D.M.M., Crocker A.G. : Acta Metall. $\underline{16}$ (1968) 523.

[16] Sutton A.P., Vitek V. : Phil. Trans. Roy. Soc. $\underline{A309}$ (1983) 1.

[17] Bristowe P.D., Crocker A.G. : Phil. Mag. $\underline{31}$ (1975) 503.

[18] Bristowe P.D., Crocker A.G. : Acta Metall. $\underline{25}$ (1977) 1363.

[19] Bristowe P.D., Crocker A.G. : Phil. Mag. $\underline{38}$ (1978) 487.

[20] Ingle K.W., Crocker A.G. : Phil. Mag. $\underline{41}$ (1980) 713.

[21] Crocker A.G., Faridi B.A. : Acta Metall $\underline{28}$ (1980) 549.

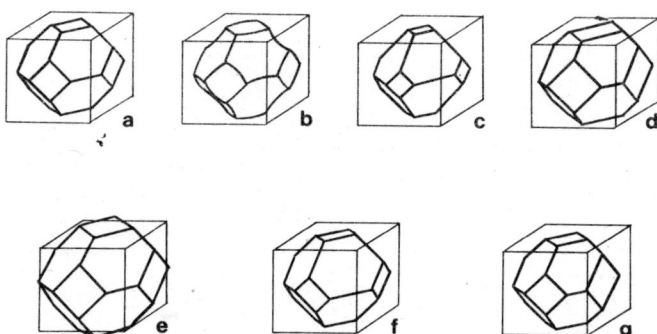

Figure 1. Examples of tetrakaidecahedral grains. The regular 14-hedron with eight hexagonal and six square flat faces is shown at (a) and the relaxed form with convoluted hexagons at (b). The small and large grains of the flat faced bimodular structure are given at (c) and (d) respectively. The effects of the large rogue grain (e) on its first and second nearest neighbours is indicated at (f) and (g).

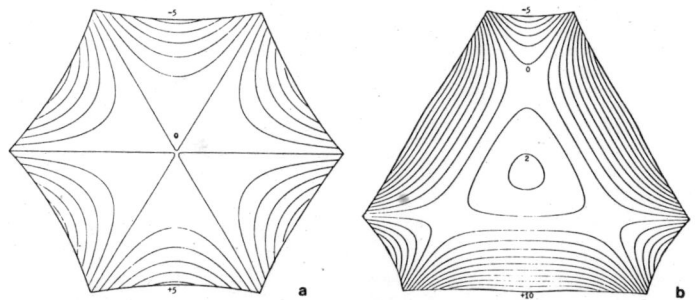

Figure 2. The convoluted forms of the relaxed hexagonal faces of (a) uni-modular and (b) a particular bimodular polycrystal. The contours give heights in units of $10^{-4}a$ where a is the edge of the b.c.c. unit cell.

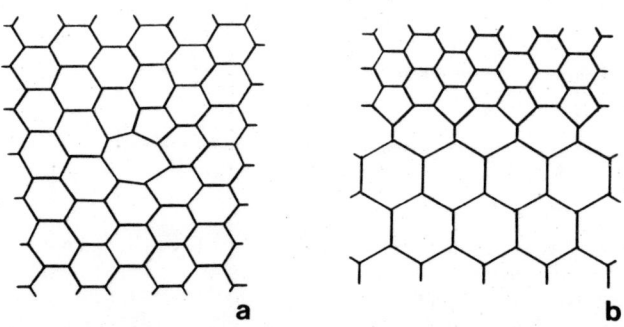

Figure 3. Schematic structures of (a) a dislocation and (b) an interface in two-dimensional polycrystals. Note the pairs of five- and seven-sided grains in both cases.

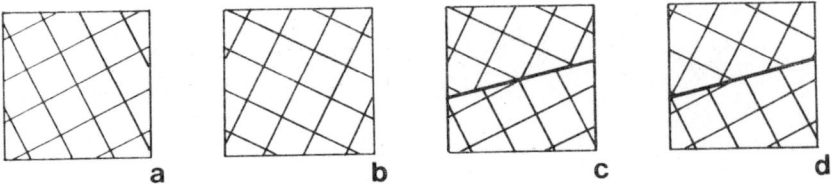

Figure 4. Schematic illustration of the nine degrees of freedom associated with an unrelaxed grain boundary. Three arise from the axis and magnitude of the rotation which relates the two grain orientations shown at (a) and (b), three from the choice of interface between these two grains as shown in (c) and three from the magnitude and direction of the relative displacement of the two grains as shown in (d).

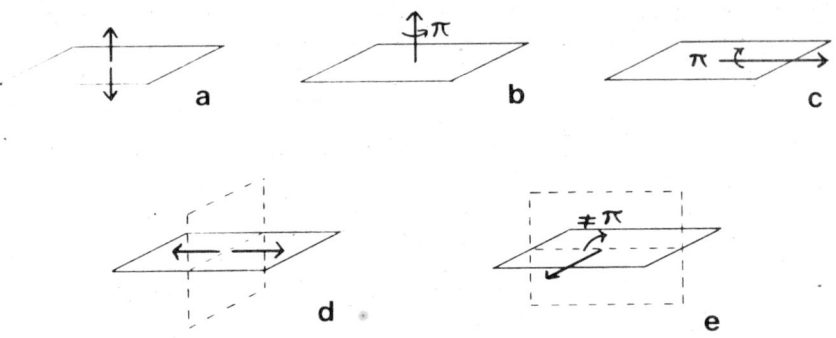

Figure 5. The four conventional, (a)-(d), and one non-conventional, (e), orientation relations for a twinned crystal. The interface in each case is represented by continuous lines, other planes by broken lines, reflections by double headed arrows and rotations, either equal or not equal to π, by single headed arrows.

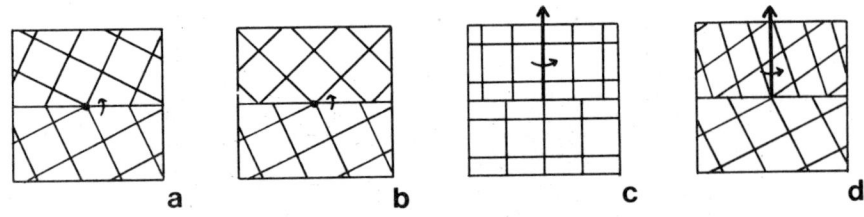

Figure 6. Schematic illustrations of (a) and (b) tilt boundaries, with the axis of rotation relating the two grains in the interface and (c) and (d) twist boundaries with the axis perpendicular to the interface. Boundary (a) is symmetric and (c) is a mirror plane whereas (b) is asymmetric and (d) is a general interface.

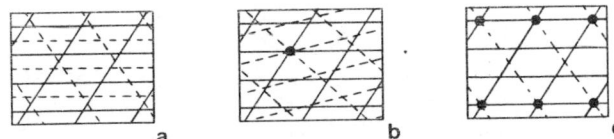

Figure 7. Illustrating the Coincidence Site Lattice (CSL). In (a) no points of the two lattices coincide, whereas in (b) one point does and in (c) one-third of the points ($\Sigma = 3$).

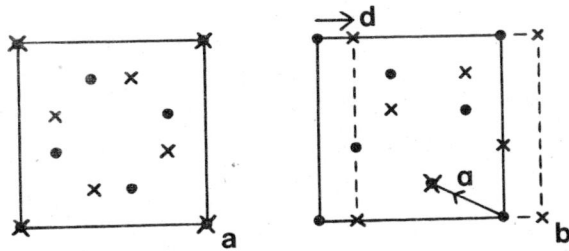

Figure 8. A $\Sigma = 5$, 37° twist boundary on a (001) plane of a simple cubic lattice. In (a) unit cells of the separate grains, represented by dots and crosses, are superimposed to give coincident sites at the corners. In (b) the cell of crosses is shifted by the vector d of the DSC lattice which results in the CSL being displaced by the vector $\underline{a}$ of the lattice of dots.

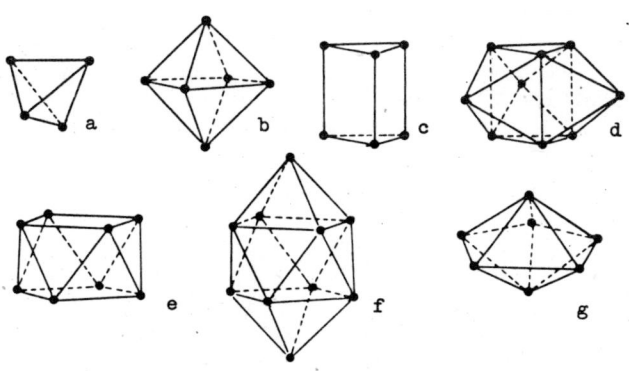

Figure 9. Examples of compact polyhedra of atoms found in grain boundaries: (a) tetrahedron, (b) octahedron, (c) trigonal prism, (d) capped trigonal prism, (e) archimedean square antiprism, (f) capped archimedean square antiprism, (g) pentagonal biprism.

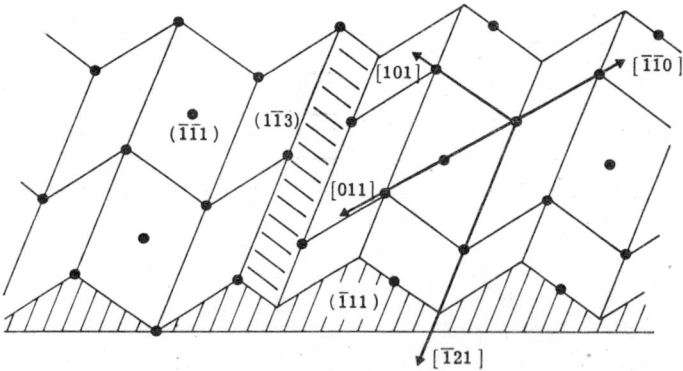

Figure 10. The structure of the irrational twin boundary of crystalline mercury which lies near $(\bar{1}35)$ of the face centred rhombohedral lattice. The boundary consists of facets on $(\bar{1}\bar{1}1)$ and $(1\bar{1}3)$.

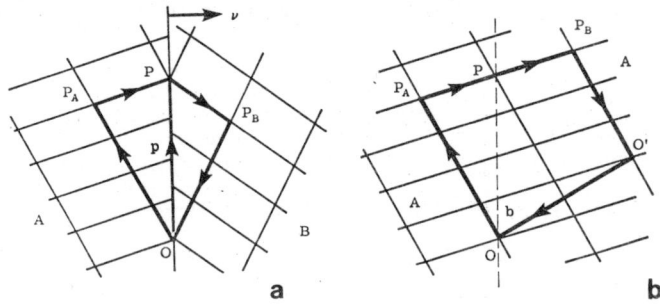

Figure 11. The procedure for defining the total effective Burgers vector of interfacial dislocations. A Burgers circuit OP_APP_BO in (a) is repeated in (b) in the reference lattice. The closure failure $O'O$ in (b) defines the Burgers vector $\underline{b}$.

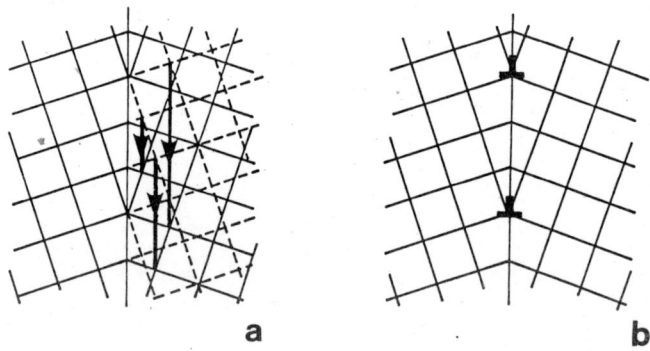

Figure 12. The structure of a rational symmetrical tilt boundary produced by (a) a homogeneous shear and (b) a rotation.

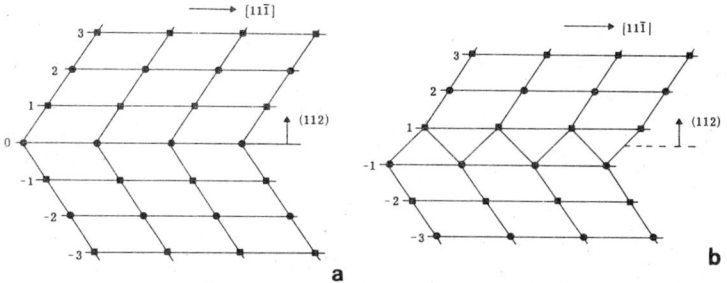

Figure 13. Two possible structures of a (112) twin boundary in body centred cubic crystals projected on to the (1$\bar{1}$0) plane. Atoms represented by circles and squares lie on adjacent (1$\bar{1}$0) planes. The conventional reflection twin is shown at (a) and the alternative isosceles structure at (b).

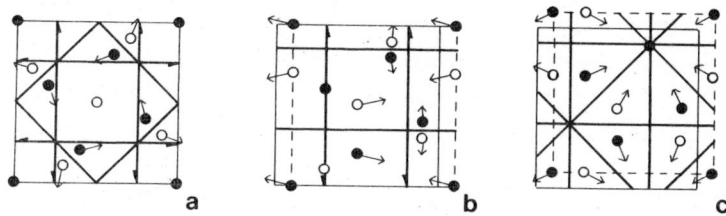

Figure 14. Three possible structures for the $\Sigma = 5$ (001) twist boundary in copper. The CSL structure is shown in (a) and two displaced but symmetrical structures in (b) and (c). Open and closed symbols represent atoms in planes immediately above and below the interface respectively. Displacements ($\times$ 5) are represented by arrows from initial to relaxed positions. Bold lines represent two-fold and two-fold screw axes, the latter being distinguished by half arrow-heads. There are additional two- and four-fold axes perpendicular to the boundaries.

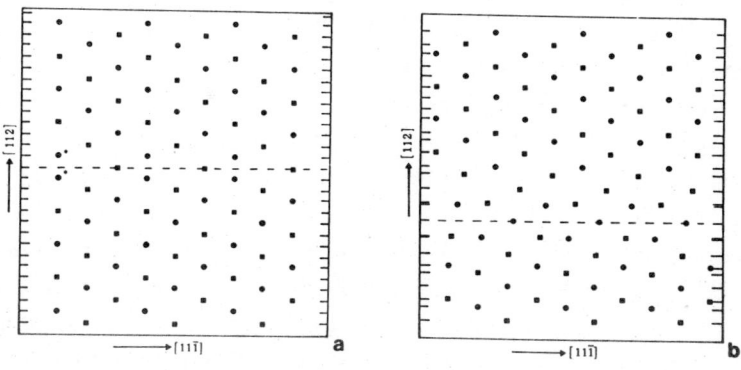

Figure 15. The relaxed (b) structures of the (112) twin boundary in copper projected on to the (1$\bar{1}$0) plane. Atoms in adjacent (1$\bar{1}$0) planes are represented by different symbols. The boundary in (b) is broad and translated both parallel and perpendicular to itself.

- 317 -

IDEAL AND NON-IDEAL COHERENT INTERFACES BETWEEN F.C.C. AND H.C.P. METALLIC CRYSTALS

A.P. Sutton and J.W. Christian

Department of Metallurgy and Science of Materials, University of Oxford, Parks Road, Oxford OX1 3PH, U.K.

Introduction

When the nearest neighbour separation in a f.c.c. structure (f) is equal to the interatomic distance in the basal plane of a h.c.p. (h) crystal, the two structures may be related by an invariant plane strain in which the invariant (habit) plane is $(111)_f$ and $(001)_h$. (We use the non-orthogonal three axis system for the h.c.p. lattice and the lattice correspondence given in /1/; the lattices then have the Wassermann /2/ orientation relation with $[11\bar{2}]_f$ parallel to $[\bar{1}10]_h$. For an ideal axial ratio, $\gamma = (8/3)^{\frac{1}{2}}$ the invariant plane strain reduces to a simple shear of magnitude $8^{-\frac{1}{2}}$ on the system $(111)_f[11\bar{2}]_f$. The migration of the $(111)_f/(001)_h$ interface into the f.c.c. crystal may be effected by the gliding of elementary transformation dislocations, with Burgers vector $\underline{b} = a_f/6<11\bar{2}>_f$ on alternate $(111)_f$ planes /3/, where a_f is the lattice parameter of the f.c.c. crystal. Each elementary transformation dislocation is associated with a step of two $(111)_f$ planes height. This dislocation model has been proposed /3/ as the mechanism for the martensitic transformation in cobalt. For non-ideal γ the Burgers vector of the elementary transformation dislocation has a component normal to the $(111)_f/(001)_h$ interface.

In an earlier paper /4/ we reported the relaxed structures and energies of the $(111)_f/(001)_h$ interface and the conjugate habit plane $(55\bar{7})_f/(\bar{3}3\bar{1})_h$ for ideal γ. Empirical, central force, pair potentials, representing atomic interactions in Co, were constructed specifically for these calculations. In this paper we first report a small error in the construction of those potentials and give the corrected coefficients. The corrections to the relaxed structures and energies of the interfaces are negligible.

Elementary transformation dislocations and perfect steps were introduced into the $(111)_f/(001)_h$ interface with use of the anisotropic elastic solution for an interfacial dislocation derived in ref./5/. In this work we have modelled perfect steps as an array of three transformation dislocations on alternate $(111)_f$ planes, with zero net Burgers vector. More precisely, the effect of these dislocations is to introduce a step of six $(111)_f$ planes height with the long-range elastic field of a dislocation tripole. The atomic structures of these interfacial defects have been relaxed with use of two interatomic potentials.

Interatomic Potentials

The method of constructing the potentials was as described in ref./4/. For completeness we repeat here the analytic form:

(1) $$\phi(r) = \phi_{sr}(r) + \phi_{as}(r)$$

where the short range potential, $\phi_{sr}(r)$ is

(2) $$\phi_{sr}(r) = \frac{A\, e^{-K_1 r}}{r^m}$$

A is a fitted constant, m an integer such that $1 \leq m \leq 20$ and K_1 is a positive constant. The long range asymptotic potential, $\phi_{as}(r)$, is

(3) $$\phi_{as}(r) = \left[\frac{B\cos(2K_F r)}{(2K_F r)^3} + \frac{C\sin(2K_F r)}{(2K_F r)^4} + \frac{D\cos(2K_F r)}{(2K_F r)^5} \right.$$
$$\left. + \frac{E\sin(2K_F r)}{(2K_F r)^6} + \frac{F\cos(2K_F r)}{(2K_F r)^7} + \frac{G\sin(2K_F r)}{(2K_F r)^8} \right] e^{-\alpha^2 r^2}$$

where B-G are fitted constants, $\alpha = 0.3 a_f^{-1}$ or $0.4 a_f^{-1}$ or $0.5 a_f^{-1}$ and K_F is the Fermi vector. K_1 is 0 or k_{TF} or $2k_{TF}$ where k_{TF} is the Thomas-Fermi vector. Assuming Co has a valence of 2, and the free electron approximation, $K_F = 1.746 \text{Å}^{-1}$ and $k_{TF} = 2.050 \text{Å}^{-1}$. The coefficients A-G reported in table 1 of ref. /4/ are incorrect owing to an error in the evaluation of long range forces in the potential construction. The corrected coefficients are given in table 1:

Table 1

Potential	A(eV)	B(eV)	C(eV)	D(eV)
V1	2.54252×10^{-3}	3.20367	2.10864×10^2	-2.38835×10^3
V2	2.85737×10^{-6}	2.18421	1.43883×10^2	-1.26396×10^3
V3	6.72931×10^2	2.52188	8.71763×10^1	-2.07733×10^3

Potential	E(eV)	F(eV)	G(eV)
V1	-9.33951×10^4	1.42686×10^6	5.05541×10^5
V2	-8.23030×10^4	5.81872×10^5	6.02205×10^6
V3	-3.45696×10^4	7.89047×10^5	1.33236×10^6

The other parameters for these potentials are listed in table 2:

Table 2

	$\alpha(a_f^{-1})$	k	m	E_c (eV/atom)
V1	0.3	0	12	-2
V2	0.3	0	16	-1
V3	0.4	$2k_{TF}$	2	-1

Potential V3 is new and has been used in this work because it is much 'softer' than V1 and V2 and because it has a larger damping factor, α. Potentials V1 and V3 were used in this work; they are shown in fig. 1. E_c is the pair potential contribution to the cohesive energy per atom.

As in ref./4/, all of the constructed potentials gave very similar sets of the five elastic constants of the h.c.p. crystal which were all in fair agreement with those for Co. These elastic constants are given in table 3 for potentials V1, V2 and V3 and the last row gives the elastic constants for h.c.p. Co. /7/ for comparison:

Table 3

	c_{11}^h	c_{12}^h	c_{44}^h	c_{13}^h	c_{33}^h (eV/Å^3)
V1	2.209	0.816	0.523	0.642	2.214
V2	2.169	0.803	0.516	0.635	2.236
V3	2.135	0.791	0.508	0.627	2.244
Co	1.916	1.030	0.470	0.643	2.235

With these corrected potentials it is found that the relaxed structure of the $(111)_f/(001)_h$ interface is identical to the unrelaxed structure. Thus the very small expansion found in ref./4/ was an artefact of the incorrect potentials used. For a cut-off radius, r_c, equal to $4.25a_f$, the energies of this interface are -2.7 and 0.1 mJ/m^2 for potentials V1 and V3 respectively.

Calculations of the atomic structures of interfacial steps

The introduction of interfacial dislocations

Barnett and Lothe /5/ derived the anisotropic elastic solution for the displacement field of an interfacial dislocation. The dislocation coordinate system we adopt is as follows: x_1 along $[11\bar{2}]_f$, x_2 along $[111]_f$ and x_3 along $[1\bar{1}0]_f$. The i'th component of the displacement field, $\underline{u}$, is then given by

$$(4) \quad u_i^{(f)} = \frac{1}{\pi} \text{Im} \sum_{\alpha=1}^{3} A_{i\alpha}^{(f)} E_\alpha^{(f)} \ln(x_1 + p_\alpha^{(f)} x_2), \quad x_2 > 0$$

$$(5) \quad u_i^{(h)} = \frac{1}{\pi} \text{Im} \sum_{\alpha=1}^{3} A_{i\alpha}^{(h)} E_\alpha^{(h)} \ln(x_1 + p_\alpha^{(h)} x_2), \quad x_2 < 0$$

where the interface is at $x_2 = 0$ and the f.c.c. and h.c.p. crystals occupy the half-spaces $x_2 > 0$ and $x_2 < 0$ respectively. In each half-space the $A_{i\alpha}$ and p_α are determined from the elastic equilibrium condition. The E_α are determined from the conditions of continuity of displacements on $x_2 = 0$, $x_1 > 0$ and continuity of tractions on $x_2 = 0$, $-\infty < x_1 < \infty$ ($x_1 \neq 0$), together with the 'zero body force' condition and the Burgers condition (equations 43-46 of ref./5/). Thus the Volterra cut is made along $x_2 = 0$, $-\infty < x_1 \leq 0$. The elastic strain field energy of the dislocation is given by:

$$(6) \quad E = E^{f-h} \ln(R/r_o)$$

where E^{f-h} is the interfacial dislocation energy factor and R and r_o are the radii of outer and inner cylinders centred about the dislocation. Formulae for E^{f-h} are given in ref./5/. Following Head /8/ we have calculated the inverse Wulff plot for $E^{f-h}(\theta)$ for all dislocations considered below to establish their elastic stability with respect to changes in orientation. θ is the angle between the dislocation line and an arbitrary reference direction. For both V1 and V3 potentials the inverse Wulff plot deviated very slightly from a circle, with $1/E^{f-h}(\theta)$ being 0.4% less at $<2\bar{1}\bar{1}>_f$ than $<1\bar{1}0>_f$ orientations. We consider this energy anisotropy negligible. All the dislocations and perfect steps considered here are parallel to $[1\bar{1}0]_f$.

Elementary transformation dislocations with Burgers vectors $+^a f/6[11\bar{2}]_f$ and $-^a f/6[11\bar{2}]_f$ were introduced successively into the $(111)_f/(001)_h$ interface by imposing the corresponding elastic displacement fields (equs.4-5) on all atoms in the block. These dislocations are distinguishable because there is no symmetry operation of the holosymmetric $(111)_f/(001)_h$ interfacial structure which relates atoms in the f.c.c. and h.c.p. lattices. Thus $+^a f/6[11\bar{2}]_f$ in $(111)_f/(001)_h$ is equivalent only to $-^a f/6[11\bar{2}]_f$ in $(001)_h/(111)_f$. With respect to a given location of the $(111)_f/(001)_h$ interface $+^a f/6[11\bar{2}]_f$ and $-^a f/6[11\bar{2}]_f$ dislocations change the location by two $(111)_f$ planes in opposite senses. Thus these dislocations are associated with steps of height equal to two $(111)_f$ planes.

Perfect steps were modelled by arrays of three dislocations centred on a line normal to the interface with Burgers vectors $-^a f/6[11\bar{2}]_f$, $-^a f/6[11\bar{2}]_f$ and $+^{2a} f/6[11\bar{2}]_f$. These dislocations were introduced between the first and second, third and fourth, and fifth and sixth $(111)_f$ planes. Again, perfect steps in $(111)_f/(001)_h$ of opposite senses are distinguishable. In this work we have considered only one sense for perfect steps. However, three arrangements of the above set of dislocations are possible, with the $+^{2a} f/6[11\bar{2}]_f$ dislocation either between the first and second or third and fourth or fifth and sixth $(111)_f$ planes. All three possibilities have been considered here.

Each 'block' of atomic coordinates consisted of 201 layers parallel to $(111)_f$ with the interface as close as possible to the central layer. Within each layer there were 201 atoms in the $[11\bar{2}]_f$ direction and periodic boundary conditions were applied to the $(1\bar{1}0)_f$ faces. The dislocations were introduced as close as possible to the centre of the block. Table 4 summarises the atomistic calculations carried out.

Table 4

Burgers vector	potentials used
$+^a f/6[11\bar{2}]_f$	V1 and V3
$-^a f/6[11\bar{2}]_f$	V1 and V3
Perfect Steps $\begin{cases} (+^{2a}f/6[11\bar{2}]_f, -^a f/6[11\bar{2}]_f, -^a f/6[11\bar{2}]_f \\ (-^a f/6[11\bar{2}]_f, +^{2a} f/6[11\bar{2}]_f, -^a f/6[11\bar{2}]_f \\ (-^a f/6[11\bar{2}]_f, -^a f/6[11\bar{2}]_f, +^{2a} f/6[11\bar{2}]_f \end{cases}$	V3 V3 V3

Method of Relaxation

Once the elastic displacements have been introduced the block is divided into two regions I and II. Atomic relaxation is carried out only in region I. Region II surrounds region I and consists of a mantle along the four faces parallel to $[1\bar{1}0]_f$, of thickness equal to twice the cut-off radius of the potential. The only displacements suffered by atoms in region II throughout the calculation are those due to the elastic field (equs.4-5). Periodic boundary conditions are applied to the $(1\bar{1}0)_f$ faces. A modified gradient method is used to minimise the internal energy of the atomic assembly in region I. The relaxation is terminated when the maximum force on any atom is less than 0.03 eV/Å. Tests showed that reducing the maximum admissible atomic force to 0.003 eV/Å resulted in a negligible change to the relaxed structure and energy.

Results

A feature of the elementary transformation dislocations is that for a given Burgers vector the relaxed atomic structures are virtually identical for potentials V1 and V3. This indicates that the detailed nature of the atomic interactions is not governing the relaxed dislocation structures.

To determine how localised the dislocations remain after relaxation we have calculated the atomic level hydrostatic stresses /9/, and displayed them in 'hydrostatic stress field maps'. In the framework of central forces the hydrostatic stress p_i at atomic site i is given by

$$(7) \quad p_i = \frac{1}{6V_a} \sum_{j \neq i} |\underline{r}_{ij}| \frac{d\phi(|\underline{r}_{ij}|)}{d|\underline{r}_{ij}|}$$

where V_a is the local atomic volume (assumed here to be the ideal crystal atomic volume), $\phi(r)$ is the pair potential, $\underline{r}_{ij}$ is the position vector of atom j relative to atom i and the summation is over all atoms interacting with atom i. When p_i is evaluated in the ideal f.c.c. or h.c.p. lattices we obtain the negative of the Cauchy pressure, p_c. Since we are interested only in the field of the dislocation we add p_c to each p_i and display this reduced p_i. In a hydrostatic stress field map each reduced p_i is represented by an arrow, centred on the i'th relaxed atomic site, the length of which is proportional to the magnitude of the reduced p_i and the direction of which indicates the sign of the reduced p_i. Arrows pointing to the right/left indicate hydrostatic compression/tension, respectively. It was found that for both potentials the hydrostatic stresses at the relaxed ideal $(111)_f/(001)_h$ interface were negligible relative to those caused by steps.

Figs. 2 and 3 show the hydrostatic stress field maps of the relaxed $-^a f/6[11\bar{2}]_f$ and $+^a f/6[11\bar{2}]_f$ dislocations respectively, obtained with potential V3. The dislocation centres are indicated and the interface planes are shown by broken lines. The only discernible difference between these fields and those obtained with potential V1 is that the magnitudes of the stresses obtained with the former are approximately half as large as those obtained with the latter. The elastic energy factors, E^{f-h}, obtained for $\pm{}^a f/6[11\bar{2}]_f$ dislocations with elastic constants corresponding to potentials V1 and V3 are 0.173 and 0.170 eV/Å respectively (1 eV/Å = 1.602 × 10^{-9} N).

Figs. 4-6 show the hydrostatic stress field maps of the relaxed structures of three perfect steps obtained with potential V3. Centres of the three dislocations used to construct these perfect steps are indicated, the larger symbol corresponding to the $^{2a}f/6[11\bar{2}]_f$ dislocation. We note that, because of the outer mantle of fixed atoms (region II), the relative displacements of $(111)_f$ planes far from the steps are fixed and therefore relaxation from one perfect step configuration into another is impossible. Owing to the arrangements of the three dislocations in figs. 4-6 the steps have interstitial, neutral or vacancy characters, respectively. By comparing the number of atoms within a large, closed contour around the step with the number within an equivalent contour in the ideal interface, the number of interstitials or vacancies associated with a $^a f/2[1\bar{1}0]_f$ repeat can be deduced. It is found that there are $+4\frac{1}{2}$, $+\frac{1}{2}$ and $-3\frac{1}{2}$ atoms per $^a f/2[1\bar{1}0]_f$ repeat associated with the interstitial, neutral and vacancy character steps, respectively. Simple calculations, based on the Burgers vectors and separations of the dislocations comprising the perfect steps, indicate that +4, 0 and -4 atoms per $^a f/2[1\bar{1}0]_f$ repeat should be associated with the steps. The discrepancy of $+\frac{1}{2}$ atom for each step is not understood. The energies per unit length of the vacancy and neutral character steps are 1.097 and 1.514 eV/Å, respectively. We have not yet calculated the energy of the interstitial character step.

Discussion

The martensitic transformation, observed in Co and its alloys, between f.c.c. and h.c.p. structures may be effected by the gliding of $^a f/6[11\bar{2}]_f$ elementary transformation dislocations on the observed $(111)_f/(001)_h$ habit plane. On the other hand diffusion is involved in the movement of the perfect steps with interstitial or vacancy characters, and perfect steps are not expected to respond to a shear stress. Hence we do not expect perfect steps to be the agents of the martensitic transformation.

The shearing of the f.c.c. lattice into the h.c.p. lattice on close packed planes by elementary transformation dislocations is analogous to deformation twinning on {112} planes in b.c.c. crystals by elementary twinning dislocations /6/. Atomistic studies of the Σ=3(112) boundary /10, 11/ have indicated that two metastable structures exist, and consequently a variety of twinning dislocation configurations and splittings can occur /12, 13/. Moreover, the twinning dislocation structure varies markedly with the interatomic potential /13/. This is in contrast to the results reported here, where only one metastable structure of the $(111)_f/(00\bar{1})_h$ interface was found, and virtually identical transformation dislocation structures were obtained with two dissimilar potentials.

References

/1/ Christian J.W.: Interfaces Conference (1969), ed. by R.C. Gifkins, Butterworths, Sydney, 159.
/2/ Wassermann G.: Arch.Eisenhüttenw. $\underline{11}$ (1932) 61.
/3/ Christian J.W.: Proc. Roy. Soc. A$\underline{206}$ (1951) 51.
/4/ Sutton A.P., Christian J.W.: J. de Physique Colloque C4, $\underline{43}$ (1982), 197.
/5/ Barnett D.M., Lothe J.: J.Phys.F: Metal Phys., $\underline{4}$ (1974) 1618.
/6/ Christian J.W., Knowles K.M.: Intern. Conf. on Solid-Solid Phase Transf., ed. H.I. Aaronson, 1981 to be published, AIME.
/7/ Smithells C.J.: Metals Reference Book, 5th ed. (1976) Butterworths, London.
/8/ Head A.K.: Phys.Stat.Sol. $\underline{19}$ (1967) 185.
/9/ Sutton A.P., Vitek V.: Phil.Trans.Roy.Soc. $\underline{309}$ (1983) 1.
/10/ Vitek V.: Scripta Met. $\underline{4}$ (1970) 720.
/11/ Bristowe P.D., Crocker A.G., Norgett M.J.: J.Phys.F: Metal Physics $\underline{4}$ (1970) 1859.
/12/ Yamaguchi M., Vitek V.: Phil. Mag. $\underline{34}$ (1976) 1.
/13/ Bristowe P.D., Crocker A.G.: Acta Met. $\underline{25}$ (1977) 1363.

Acknowledgement

APS acknowledges the support of the SERC in the form of a research fellowship.

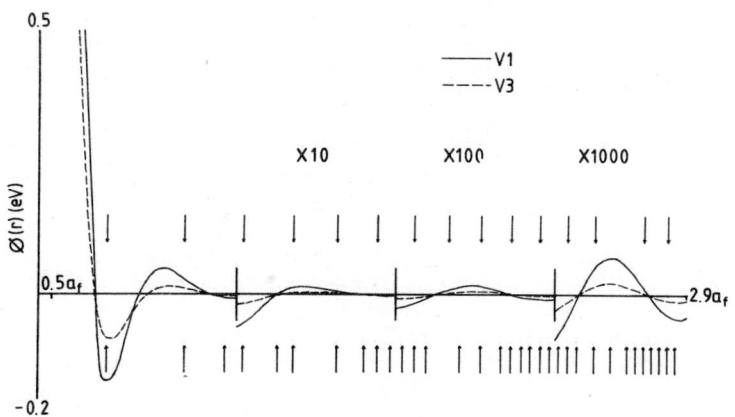

Fig.1: Potentials V1 and V3. Upper/lower arrows indicate nearest neighbours in f.c.c./h.c.p. respectively.

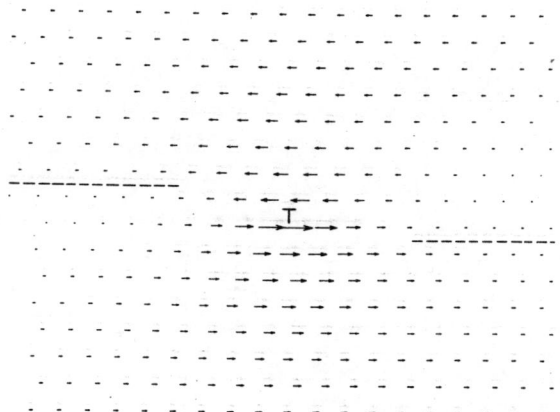

Fig.2: Hydrostatic stress field map of $-a_f/6\ 11\bar{2}_f$ in $(111)_f/(001)_h$. Maximum hydrostatic stress = 0.0666 eV/Å^3, potential V3.

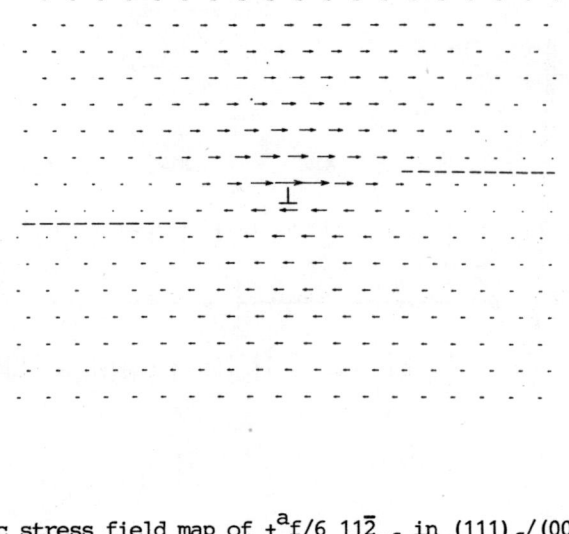

Fig.3: Hydrostatic stress field map of $+\frac{a_f}{6}11\bar{2}_f$ in $(111)_f/(001)_h$. Maximum hydrostatic stress = 0.0688 eV/Å^3, potential V3.

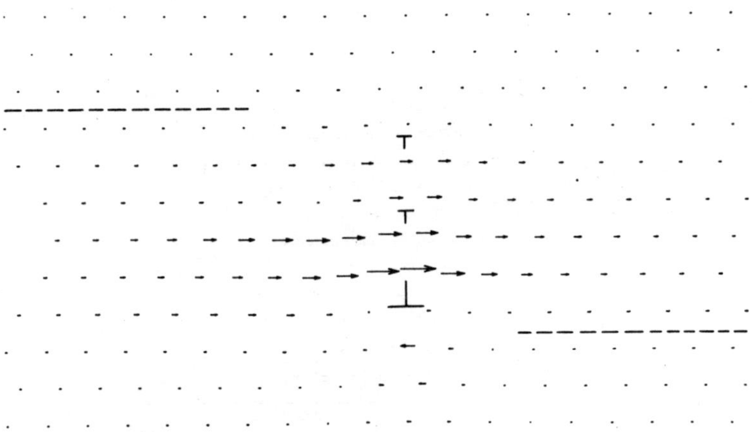

Fig.4: Hydrostatic stress field map of perfect step with interstitial character. Maximum hydrostatic stress = 0.2532 eV/Å^3.

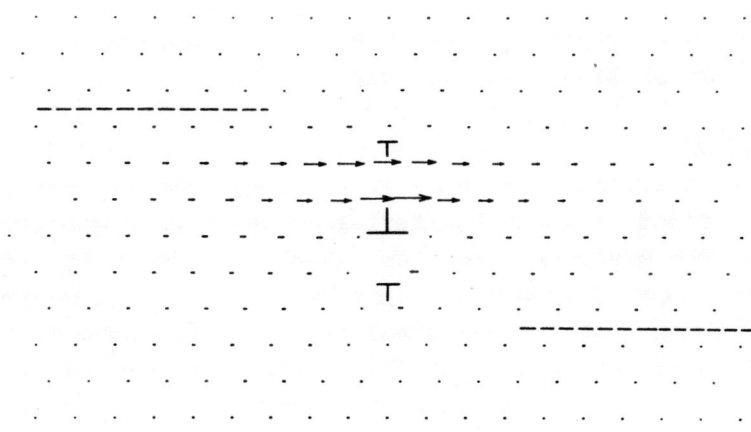

Fig.5: Hydrostatic stress field map of perfect step with neutral character. Maximum hydr static stress = 0.1568 eV/Å^3.

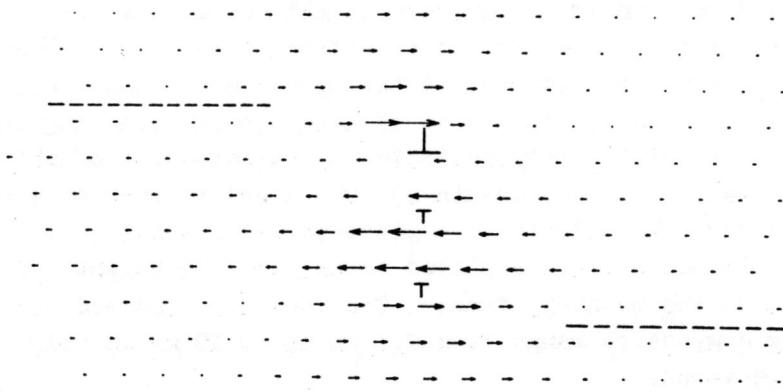

Fig.6: Hydrostatic stress field map of perfect step with vacancy character. Maximum hydrostatic stress = 0.0668 eV/Å^3.

GRAIN BOUNDARY SLIDING IN METALS AND RELATED PHENOMENA

I. Saxl, V. Sklenička, J. Čadek

Institute of Physical Metallurgy, Czechoslovak Academy of Sciences, Žižkova 22, 616 62 Brno, Czechoslovakia

1. INTRODUCTION

Grain boundary sliding (GBS) is the most striking manifestation of the effect of grain boundaries on the high temperature deformation. The mounting attention given to it recently (after the long-time lack of interest caused by usually small contribution of GBS to the total elongation) is the consequence of its close relation to the intercrystalline creep fracture mechanisms.

GBS may be simply observed on the surface of polycrystalline specimens deformed above 0.4 T_m as the offset at the boundaries. Its magnitude and direction determine the total sliding vector $\vec{p}$, that constitutes a vector point function on the idealized grain boundary surface. Its value at given external conditions (stress, temperature and time) is a function of the boundary type and orientation, of the grain size, of the position within the grain facet etc. The vector $\vec{p}$ is usually resolved into three mutually perpendicular components: u - in the direction of the stress axis, v - in the direction of the surface normal and w - perpendicular to the both of them. Clearly, it is difficult to measure $\vec{p}$ and its components in the interior of the specimen and the specimen surface is the predominant source of data (only technologically introduced rows of impurity particles or embedded net of thin wires may serve as interior markings). The u and w components can be deduced from the offsets of surface scratch marks, whereas interferometric methods are employed to measure the height v of surface steps at the boundary traces. The commonly observed values of sliding components range from 0.1 μm up to 10 μm in polycrystalline specimens.

The inhomogeneity and anisotropy of $\vec{p}$ make the characterization of the amount of sliding in the specimen very difficult. Therefore, the isotropy of boundary and sliding vector orientation is assumed and the possible difference between the surface and interior sliding is neglected. Accordingly, the mean values of sliding components are all equivalent and the contribution of GBS to the total deformation may be estimated by /1/

$$\varepsilon_{gb} = \frac{1}{2} S_V \cdot E_s u \, . \tag{1}$$

Here S_V is the grain boundary area per unit volume of the specimen and $E_s u = S^{-1} \int_S u dS$ is the average value (with respect to the area S) of u, that may be estimated by measurement in randomly chosen points of the boundary traces at the specimen surface.

2. MODELS OF GRAIN BOUNDARY SLIDING

The nature of GBS is not yet precisely known, but two types of sliding are commonly distinguished:

i) <u>GBS due to vacancy flow</u> (GBS with diffusional accommodation, Lifshitz sliding) proceeds by diffusion either through the lattice (Nabarro-Herring creep) or along the grain boundaries (Coble creep) /2/. It is equivalent to say that sliding is accommodated by diffusion or that sliding is inevitable consequence of diffusional creep.

ii) <u>GBS due to dislocation movement</u> (Rachinger sliding) is based on a nonconservative dislocation motion either in the grain boundaries (glide and climb of grain boundary dislocations) or in zones adjacent to them (climb of lattice dislocations along the boundaries)/3/.

The theories of GBS have been reviewed recently by Langdon and Vastava /4/ and their results may be summarized as follows:

a) <u>Intrinsic models</u> (applicable for bicrystals) do not take into account the hindrance effect of three grain junctions and neighboring grains. They predict the rate of sliding in the form

$$\dot{p} = KD \sigma^{\alpha}/kT \, , \tag{2}$$

where D is the appropriate diffusion coefficient (D_{gb}, D_V or their combination) and σ is the shear stress acting in the boundary. The constant K includes the effect of grain size and differs according to the type of sliding whereas $\alpha = 1$ for sliding due to vacancy flow /5/ as well as for sliding due to dislocation movement /6/, /7/.

b) <u>Extrinsic models</u> consider at least partly the accommodation of stresses arising at three grain junctions and/or another grain boundary irregularities (see bellow) and give the rate of sliding also in the form of Eq. (2), but $\alpha = 1 \div 2$ for models based on the climb of lattice dislocations in the boundary zone /8/, /9/, $\alpha = 1$ for the accommodation by nonuniform plastic flow within the grains /10/ and $\alpha = 3.5$ for the accommodation by the formation of folds /11/.

The results of experiments performed on different metals and alloys (Al, Pb, Sn, Zn, Cu, Ni, W, Fe, α-brasses, CuAl, CuFe, austenitic stainless and low-carbon steels etc.) and consisting in the determination of stress and temperature dependences of mean sliding rates have shown that the activation energy of sliding lies within the range $(0.6 \div 1)Q_{SD}$. The lower bound corresponds to GBS controlled by boundary diffusion, the upper bound indicates that the lattice diffusion is controlling. This result does not contradict the rate Eq. (2) at least. On the other hand, the comparison of theoretical and experimental stress dependences of sliding rates is less encouraging, as the experimentally determined stress exponent α varies between 2 and 6, being usually only slightly lower than the stress exponent of dislocation creep inside the grains - Tab.I. The data for Al and its alloys, Pb, Sn, Zn relate to bicrystals, for which the value $\alpha = 1$ is predicted by the theoretical models.

Tab.I Stress exponent of sliding rate (for detailed references see /4/).

α	material
2	W
2.2 - 6.1	Al, Al-alloys
2.3	Ni
2.8	Sn, Pb
3.3	α-brass
4.5	Zn
4.7	low C steel

3. GRAIN BOUNDARY SLIDING IN COPPER AND COPPER ALLOYS

As a part of the investigation of creep fracture process, a study of GBS in copper and its alloys CuZn, CuAl, CuFe has been performed over a considerable range of total creep rates (e.g. for copper was $\dot{\varepsilon}$ varied between 10^{-10} s^{-1} and 10^{-2} s^{-1} by the change of stress and temperature) /12 - 15/. The main attention has been focused to the local values of sliding component u. A representative sample of facet traces has been chosen and the mean value u appropriate to any individual facet has been determined. As it was found that an appreciable number of facets does not slide (at least at the early stages of loading) the parameter describing the homogeneity of sliding was introduced, namely $\mathcal{H} = N_S/N$, where N_S is the number of facets with $u \neq 0$ and N is the number of all investigated facets. Simultaneously the mean value (with respect to the number of sliding facets) $\tilde{u} = E_{N_s}\bar{u}$ was calculated. Under the assumption that all facets are of the same area the relation $E_s u = \mathcal{H}\tilde{u}$ holds.

a) Homogeneity of sliding

The parameter $\mathcal{H}$ is a function of stress, temperature, time and composition and its maximum value ranges between 0.5 and 1 — Fig.1. The occurrence of simultaneous sliding at all facets is slightly surprising, the effect of composition is pronounced.

b) Time dependence of sliding

The time dependence of sliding has been studied by means of the graphical method proposed by DeHoff /17/ on a set of copper specimens. The method enabled us to determine the time dependences $\bar{u}_\tau(t-\tau)$ of longitudinal sliding pertaining to facets that started to slide at the time $t = \tau$. The rate of sliding is the highest just at the time τ for each facet and then decreases parabolically thus revealing an appreciable deformation hardening — Fig.2.

c) Stress dependence of sliding

Two ranges of different stress dependence $\dot{\bar{u}}$ have been observed in copper at 773 K; namely $\alpha = 4.6$ for higher stresses ($\sigma_a > 15$ MPa) and $\alpha \approx 1$ for low stresses ($\sigma_a < 10$ MPa) — Fig.3. The values of 4.3 and 3.3 describe the stress dependences of $\dot{\bar{u}}$ in Cu-20Zn and Cu-30Zn, respectively (only the range of higher stresses was examined).

The mean rate of sliding was in all cases higher (at least by 10^2) than that predicted by Eq. (1) for sliding with diffusional accommodation.

d) Temperature dependence of sliding

The activation enthalpy of sliding as determined from the temperature dependence of $E_{N_s}\dot{\bar{u}}$ (thus excluding the temperature dependence of $\mathcal{H}$, which is necessarily included in $E_s\dot{u}$) was in all examined cases $(0.6 - 0.7)Q_{SD}$ and confirmed that GBS is controlled by the grain boundary diffusion in copper and its alloys.

e) Contribution of GBS to the total elongation

The problem of mutual relation between the deformation inside the grains and on their boundaries has been frequently tackled by considering the ratios of ε_{gb} to the total (ε) or intragranular (ε_g) deformations. At the common "laboratory" creep rates 10^{-6} s^{-1}, the ratio $\varepsilon_{gb}/\varepsilon$ only rarely exceeds the value of 20% — Fig.4, which led to the conclusion that the effect of GBS on deformation process is unimportant. But the results obtained by examination of coarse-grained copper and its alloys have shown that just the opposite may be true. Bellow the mean creep rate of 10^{-7} s^{-1}, the component ε_{gb} starts to prevail and at even lower creep rates nearly all fracture elongation is due to it - Fig.5. But what is even more surprising, the fracture value ($\varepsilon_{gb})_f$ remains practically constant over the range of several orders of magnitude of the creep rate $\dot{\varepsilon}$, whereas the fracture value of intracrystalline deformation varies considerably - Fig.6. This result allows to formulate the hypothesis that GBS controls the fracture process and is responsible for the loss of plasticity.

4. PHENOMENA ACCOMPANYING GRAIN BOUNDARY SLIDING

To understand the role of GBS in fracture process we must turn our attention to the fact that grain boundaries are not smooth but rugged. Therefore several accompanying processes must be invoked to accommodate the high local stresses created at boundary undulations and irregularities. At least three main sources of such quasiperiodical undulations with considerably different wave lengths Λ must be mentioned: the grains and subgrains - Λ is proportional to the grain and subgrain size, the line defects (ledges, intersections of slip bands with grain boundary surface etc.) - Λ of the order of microns and smaller, structural units of the grain boundary structure - Λ of the order of several lattice spacings. Beside these line irregularities also the grain boundary particles must be included in the consideration. The most important accommodating processes are:

a) diffusion - especially significant to maintain the compatibility at the intercrystalline particle interfaces,
b) elastic accommodation - effective only in the case of very small sliding vector $p \leqslant 5$ nm,
c) plastic accommodation - local slip manifested by the formation of grain boundary serrations, by the formation of folds at three grain junction etc.,
d) grain boundary migration - accommodates especially the "atomic" ruggedness of grain boundaries; the migration distance must be comparable with the sliding vector $\vec{p}$ - Fig.7.

If the accommodation by the above listed processes is not sufficiently effective, another process enter into the play, namely the nucleation and growth of intercrystalline voids - cavities - Fig.8. Their formation in the interior of the specimen is frequently accompanied also by the occurrence of shallow intercrystalline surface cracks.

Whereas the importance of GBS in the process of void nucleation seems to be indisputable, the processes competing in the promotion of cavity growth are beside GBS also lattice, grain boundary and surface diffusion and plastic flow inside the grains. Nevertheless, it may be shown by direct comparison of cavity size and growth rate that the cavity growth is controlled nearly exclusively by GBS in copper and its alloys /12 - 16/.

5. CONCLUDING REMARKS

i) The inability of contemporary theories to explain the experimentally evaluated stress exponents α reflects our poor understanding of the nature and complexity of GBS. The ommission of dislocation interactions could be the probable source of this disagreement.

ii) The attention has been paid exclusively to the role of GBS in high temperature creep in tension. It should be stressed that similar effect of GBS may be expected also in the high temperature fatigue and especially in the case of complex multiaxial cyclic loading. The outstanding role of GBS in superplasticity is also well known /19/.

iii) The importance of GBS in metals is far from being purely scientific. On the contrary, its technical aspects are the main stimulus of recent increased efforts for better description and understanding of this phenomenon that lies in the background of limitations posed on the effective high temperature exploitation of engineering materials.

REFERENCES

/1/ Bruner H., Grant N.J.: Trans. AIME 215 (1959) 48.
/2/ Burton B.: Diffusional Creep of Polycrystalline Materials, Trans.Tech.Publications, Aedermannsdorf 1977.
/3/ Harris E., Roberts G.: Metals Forum 4 (1981) 29.
/4/ Langdon T.G., Vastava R.B.: ASTM Spec.Tech.Publ. 765, Philadelphia 1982, p.435.
/5/ Raj R., Ashby M.F.: Met. Trans. 2 (1971) 1113.
/6/ Gates R.S.: Acta Met. 21 (1973) 855.

/7/ Pond R.C., Smith D.A., Southerden P.W.J.: in Proceedings of 4th International Conference on the Strength of Metals and Alloys, Laboratoire de Physique du Solide, E.N.S.M.I.M., Nancy, France 1976, Vol.1, p.378.
/8/ Langdon T.G.: Phil. Mag. 22 (1970) 689.
/9/ Veršok B.A., Rojburd A.L.: Fiz. Tverd. Tela 13 (1971) 1693.
/10/ Crossman F.W., Ashby M.F.: Acta Met. 23 (1975) 425.
/11/ Gifkins R.C.: J. Austr. Inst. Met. 18 (1973) 137.
/12/ Sklenička V., Saxl I., Čadek J.: Mezikrystalový lom při vysokoteplotním creepu kovů a slitin, Studie ČSAV č.8, Academia, Praha 1977.
/13/ Sklenička V., Saxl I., Čadek J., Ryš P.: Res Mechanica 1 (1980) 301.
/14/ Saxl I., Sklenička V., Čadek J.: Z. Metallkde 72 (1981) 499.
/15/ Sklenička V., Saxl I., Čadek J.: in B. Ilschner (Ed.): Festigkeit und Verformung bei hoher Temperatur, Symposium der Deutschen Gesellschaft für Metallkunde, Erlangen, October 1982 (in press).
/16/ Sklenička V., Saxl I., Čadek J.: in D. Francois (Ed.): Advances in Fracture Research, Proc. 5th Int. Conf. on Fracture, Vol.4, Pergamon Press, Oxford 1981, p.1643.
/17/ DeHoff R.T.: Treatise on Materials Science and Technology, ed. H. Herman, Vol.1, Academic Press, New York 1972, p.248.
/18/ Procházka K., Saxl I., Sklenička V., Čadek J.: Scripta Met. 17 (1983) No.6.
/19/ Langdon T.G.: Metals Forum 4 (1981) 14.

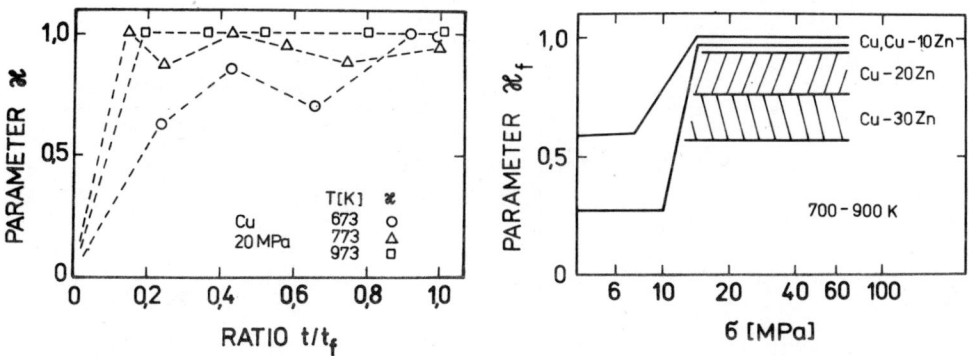

Fig.1 The effect of time, stress, temperature and composition on the homogeneity parameter $\mathcal{H}$; $\mathcal{H}_f$ is the fracture value of $\mathcal{H}$.

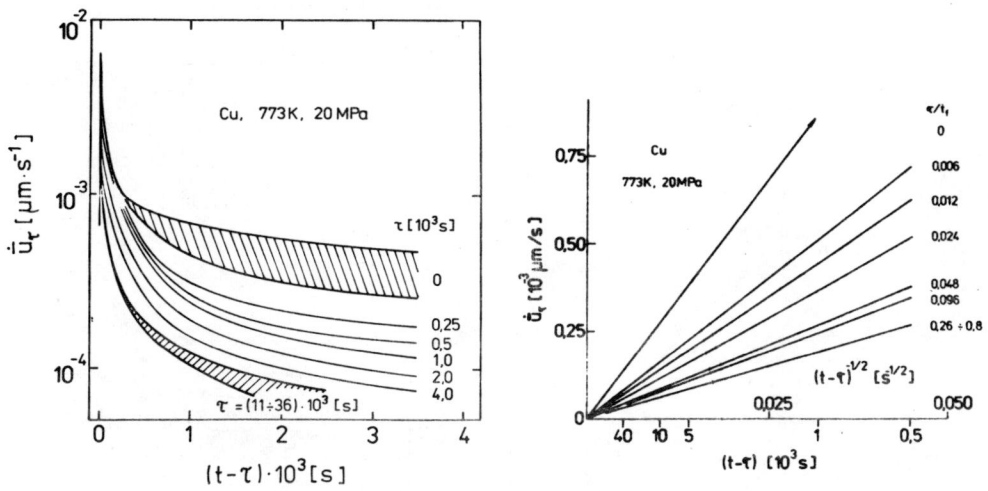

Fig.2 The time dependence of sliding rate $\dot{\bar{u}}_\tau$ along individual facets distinguished by the time τ at which the longitudinal sliding component $\bar{u}$ becomes perceptible (time of the initiation of sliding along the given facet). The dependence $\dot{\bar{u}}_\tau$ vs $(t-\tau)^{-1/2}$ has been obtained by linear regression analysis.

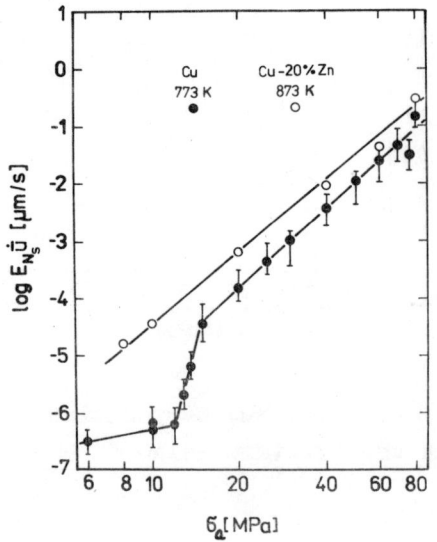

Fig.3 The stress dependence of the mean sliding rate $\tilde{\bar{u}} = E_{N_s}\bar{u}$ (σ_a is the applied stress).

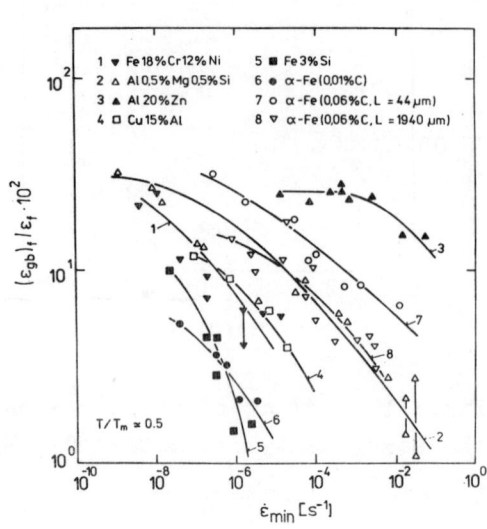

Fig.4 The dependence of the ratio $(\varepsilon_{gb})_f / \varepsilon_f$ on the minimum creep rate $\dot{\varepsilon}_{min}$ for different metals and alloys.

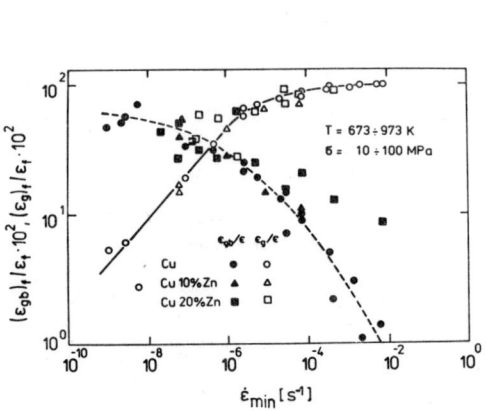

Fig.5 The relative contributions of GBS and of the intragranular creep to the fracture elongation for copper and its alloys.

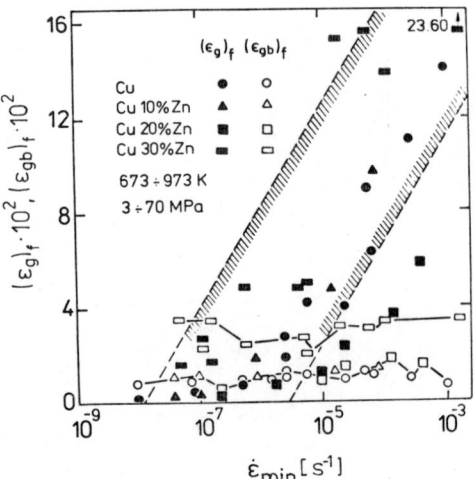

Fig.6 The magnitude of the fracture elongation due to GBS and due to intragranular creep.

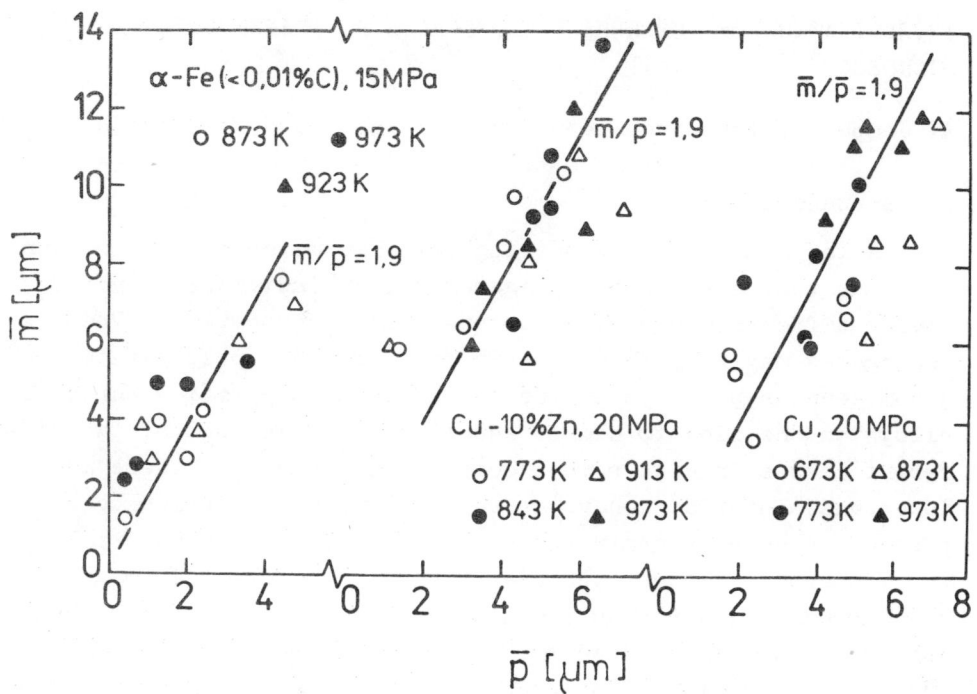

Fig.7 The mutual relation between the mean values of total sliding vector p and the mean migration distance.

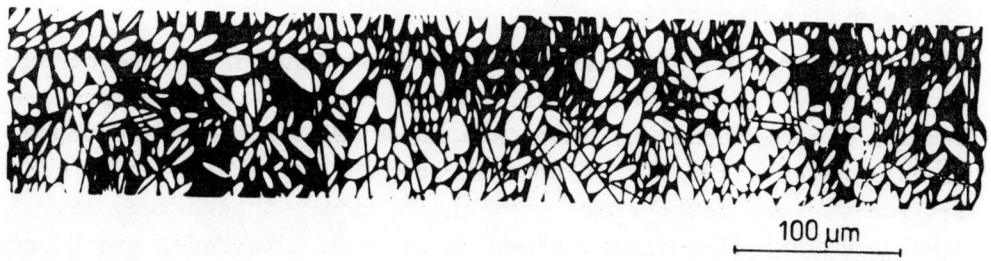

Fig.8 Intercrystalline voids in the grain boundaries of copper deformed at 625 K, 15 MPa (reconstruction of cracked area performed by the method of serial sections /18/).

INVESTIGATION OF INTERPHASE INTERFACES BY TRANSMISSION ELECTRON MICROSCOPY

A. Gemperle, Iron and Steel Research Institute, Karlštejn

1. Introduction

A large part of engineering metallic materials are non-uniform and they are formed by aggregates of individual crystals having different crystal structure and/or composition. These aggregates may vary from distribution of small precipitates in a homogeneous polycrystalline matrix in precipitation hardened alloys on one side to almost equal volume fractions of two different phases in e.g. some steels on the other. In these materials interphase interfaces have an equally important influence on their properties as have grain boundaries in homogeneous materials.

Interphase interfaces are primarily different from grain boundaries by separating two crystals of different structures and/or compositions. However, it is clear that their proper structure must be in many instances similar to the structure of grain boundaries. In interphase interfaces special orientations having a very simple structure are rather frequently observed due to the fact that they are formed by phase transformations where the two phases are joined along preferential habit planes. Grain boudaries are oriented far more randomly. From the similarity of the basic structure of interphase and grain boundaries it follows that analogous methods may be used for its investigation.

2. Classification of interphase boundaries

According to Christian /1/ interphase boundaries are classified by their structure as fully coherent, semi-coherent and incoherent. Fully coherent interface is an analogue of the composition plane of a twin. Corresponding crystallographic planes and lattice vectors match exactly at the boundary though they may have different directions. Examples of such interfaces are boundaries between f.c.c. and a h.c.p. phases and boundaries separating regions having different ordered structures or ordered and disordered regions in ordered alloys. Small crystals may form fully coherent boundaries even in cases that the two lattices are slightly different. The two crystals are brought into coherency by elastic strains. The opposite type is a fully incoherent boundary. At such boundary there are no continuity conditions for lattice planes and vectors. Its basic structure is fully disordered. They are analogous to high angle grain boundaries. A transition type between these two ones is the semi-coherent boundary. It separates two phases whose crystal lattices do not match exactly. In certain regions coherency is forced by elastic strains. These coherent regions are separated by regions of disorder, the misfit dislocations, which accomodate the misfit between the two lattices. If the boundary is curved it contains further regions of disorder e.g. steps and defects analogous to twinning dislocations.

Semi-coherent boundaries are of two types. The martensitic type, where the Burgers vectors of the interfacial dislocations do not lie in its plane and the dislocations are not of pure edge type. The epitaxial type in which two or more crossing systems of parallel pure edge dislocations have Burgers vectors lying in its plane.

3. Analysis of TEM images of interphase boundaries

The characteristics of a boundary image depend on the type of the boundary and on its orientation in respect to the foil surface and electron beam direction. A fully coherent boundary parallel to the foil surface exhibits some contrast only in regions where it terminates in the foil. A fully coherent boundary inclined to the foil surface which separates two crystals having different structure factors of the operating reflection exhibits a fringe contrast similar to stacking fault fringes. These fringes are characterised by the parameter $\delta = s_1 \xi_{g_1} - s_2 \xi_{g_2}$ /2/, where ξ_{g_1}, ξ_{g_2} are the extinction distances of the operating reflections in the two crystals and s_1, s_2 are their excitation errors. This type of contrast was observed e.g. by Fourdeux et al. /3/ on a cubic-hexagonal interface for c/a ratio deviating from the ideal value. Generally the only information which can be gained from this type of contrast is the morphology of the boundary.

A special type of stacking fault-like fringe contrast is observed in the cases where the regularity of continuous diffracting planes is disturbed in the boundary by a small displacement of one of the crystals. From the comparison of experimental images with calculated contrast profiles the magnitude and direction of the displacement may be deduced. This was used e.g. by Gemperlová et al. /4/ for antiphase boundaries and by Pond /5/ for coincidence grain boundaries, but no examples are known as yet for interphase interfaces.

The most common type of contrast of inclined incoherent boundaries is the orientation contrast. Here, one of the crystals is diffracting strongly and the other only weekly. Fringes similar to those observed on a perfect wedge appear /6/.

The contrast of semi-coherent boundaries is more different. Besides the fringe contrast on inclined boundaries it is mainly moiré contrast and contrast of arrays of interfacial dislocations on interfaces inclined and parallel to the foil surface. Moiré contrast was analysed in details by Gevers /7/. For a boundary parallel to the foil surface it consists of fringes whose spacing D is given in a kinematical approximation by the relation

$$D = \frac{\frac{1}{g_1 g_2}}{\left(\frac{1}{g_1^2} + \frac{1}{g_2^2} + \frac{2}{g_1 g_2} \cos \phi \right)^{1/2}}$$

where g_1, g_2 are the diffracting vectors in both crystals and $\emptyset$ is the angle between them. In common cases $\emptyset = 0$ and the above relation is simplified to $D = 1/|g_1 - g_2|$. In this case the fringes are always straight and perpendicular to $\vec{g}$. Dynamical moiré fringe patterns and fringe patterns on inclined interfaces are rather comlicated. The fringes are not necessarily straight and their spacing is non-uniform.

Hirsch at al. /8/ derived the relation $1/g_1 < b$, where b is the Burgers vector of structural dislocations, for observation of moiré fringes on a semi-coherent interface. The relation is derived under the assumption that the spacing of the dislocations is in accordance with Brooks' criterion of the coherency loss. The probability of the presence of moiré fringes in the image increases with increasing the diffracting vector. In many instances it is difficult to distinguish moiré fringes from images of dislocations. One criterion may be useful as follows: moiré fringes are always nearly perpendicular to $\vec{g}$.

The contrast of dislocations in interfaces has some special features in comparison with dislocations in the interior. It was shown by Marukawa et al. /9, 10/ that in common cases of one crystal diffracting strongly and the other weakly, only the part of the strain field of the dislocation lying in the diffracting crystal contributes to the image. This facilitates the determination of the sign of the Burgers vector of the dislocations.

Dense arrays of structural dislocations may be resolved using the weak-beam technique. However, similarly to grain boundaries, also the periodicity of structural dislocations is best studied by electron diffraction. Even for interphase boudaries the relations of the diffraction pattern to the arrangement of dislocations found in the papers /11, 12/ hold. Every system of parallel straight dislocations having spacing d_D which lies in a plane nearly perpendicular to the electron beam creates in the neighbourhood of the main reflections a row of diffraction spots. These spots lie on a line perpendicular to the direction of dislocations and their spacing is $1/d_D$. If there are several crossing systems of dislocations the additional diffraction spots are arranged in regular planar patterns. Careful interpretation of these patterns is needed as they are often complicated by double and multiple diffraction.

The resolution of the smallest details of atomic dimensions of the interphase boundary structure as also of the grain boundary structure is made possible by the lattice imaging technique. As early as 1960 Cowley and Moodie /13/ have shown that lattice images taken with axial illumination using several beams and under suitable conditions of the foil thickness and defocus may be interpreted in terms of the space charge distribution i.e. as images of the atomic structure. Columns of atoms are imaged as spots, atomic planes as rows of spots. By comparison of theoretical image calculations with experimental images taken with the best present microscopes structural resolution of 0.25 nm is attained (See e.g. /14/).

Optimum conditions for revealing fine details of the interphase boundary structure are obtained with the boudary plane and a low-index zone axis in both crystals oriented parallel to the electron beam. Therefore, it is rather difficult to take high quality images of incoherent interfaces. Only by chance would it be possible to image the atomic structure of both crystals.

Hirsch et al. /15/ postulated that the lattice image of a dislocation viewed end-on i.e. parallel to the electron beam, formed by the diffraction on planes having $\vec{g}$ diffraction vector, contains $\vec{g}\vec{b}$ = N terminating fringes ($\vec{b}$ is the Burgers vector of the dislocation). From this relation the same condititon $\vec{g}\vec{b}$ = 0 follows for invisibility of the dislocation as in conventional diffraction contrast imaging. Later it was shown by Cockayne et al. /16/ that the existence of terminating fringes in a lattice image does not indicate necessarily the presence of dislocations. A detailed analysis for dislocations in interfaces was accomplished by Smith and Goodhew /17/. They have shown that the relation of terminating fringes in a boundary and the presence of dislocations is more complicated. The number of fringes cutting a certain length of the boundary in each crystal depends on the expression $\vec{g}(\vec{S} + \vec{h} + \vec{b})$, where $\vec{S}$ is a lattice vector parallel to the boundary and perpendicular to the beam and $\vec{h}$ is the height of the step associated with the dislocation, measured perpendicularly to the boundary. The expression is evaluated for both crystals separately. The influence of interfacial steps on the image i.e. $\vec{g}_1\vec{h}_1 - \vec{g}_2\vec{h}_2$ is in many instances more significant than the Burgers vector of the dislocation, as h can be substantially larger than b. The absence of terminating fringes in the image does not indicate necessarily that $\vec{g}\vec{b}$ = 0. The height of the step and the Burgers vector of an interfacial dislocation can be deduced with some care from the position and number of terminating fringes but it is not always possible.

Further details of the interface boundary structure revealed by lattice imaging are larger facets and eventually some amorphous layer. If there is no amorphous layer, it is possible to compare theoretically calculated images of suitable models with experimental lattice images and to find the exact crystallographic relationship of the two crystals in the boundary plane.

4. Some recent investigations of the structure of interphase boundaries

The results of microscopical investigations of phase boundary structures using classical imaging techniques have been carefully reviewed by Aaronson /18/ and Laird and Sankaran /19/.

Therefore in this article only the results obtained by using the lattice imaging technique will be treated.

Earlier works on metallic systems e.g. /20, 21/ made the use of a more simple imaging technique with only one reflection contributing to the image in each crystal. In this case the corresponding lattice planes are represented by fringes. An example of a more recent work of this type is the observation of a martensite-austenite interface in an equiatomic NiTi alloy /22/. A growing martensite plate in austenite matrix was imaged by (110) planes of austenite (d = 0.213 nm) and (020) planes of martensite (d = 0.231 nm). The boundary was fully coherent until a distance of 26 nm from the tip where the first interface dislocation was recorded. The change of the phase was manifested only by a change of the direction of fringes. Careful measurements of the fringes in martensite revealed occasional irregularities in their spacing which are likely to be due to transformation dislocations. Wu /23/ studied the interface between the f.c.c. Al matrix and the semi-coherent Θ' precipitate in an Al-4%Cu alloy. The interface was oriented parallel to the electron beam. Fringe spacings in Al, Θ' and the boundary region have been measured directly and by laser optical diffraction. Irregularities in the spacings found in the boundary region were attributed to a compositional gradient or to a strain field.

However, much more detailed investigations of interphase interfaces using lattice imaging have been accomplished recently on metal silicide-silicon epitaxial systems important for the semiconductor technology. They show in full the potentialities and limitations of the technique in revealing the structure of interfaces on an atomic scale and therefore they will be shortly reviewed here.

The specimens are prepared by the vacuum deposition of several tenth of nm thick metallic layer on an oriented silicon crystal substrate. The following annealing in an inert atmosphere transforms the metal to silicide, which grows epitaxially on Si. A thin foil perpendicular to the silicide-silicon interface is finally prepared by embedding the crystal in epoxy resin, cutting it in platelets, metallographic grinding and ion beam thinning to perforation /24/.

Föll et al. /25, 26/ investigated Ni-Si and Pd-Si systems. Ni film on Si forms upon annealing at increasing temperatures successively Ni_2Si, $NiSi$ and $NiSi_2$. The epitaxially growing NiSi layer on (111) Si is hexagonal and the misfit between $\{11\bar{2}0\}$ NiSi and $\{1\bar{2}0\}$ Si planes is rather large (15%). A misfit dislocation array with 1.5 nm spacing is needed to accomodate it. This spacing is smaller than the resolution of conventional TEM techniques including the weak beam. The lattice image of the interface oriented with $\langle 110 \rangle$ Si parallel to the electron beam is presented in fig. 1. The fringes correspond to (111) planes in Si and ($1\bar{1}00$) planes in NiSi. The presence of misfit dislocations manifests itself by termination of nearly every sixth NiSi fringe at the boundary. The Burgers vector of the dislocations is supposed to be $a/2 \langle 110 \rangle$ in Si and $a/3 \langle 11\bar{2}0 \rangle$ in NiSi.

$NiSi_2$ is cubic and its lattice parameter is only by 0.3 % smaller than the lattice parameter of Si. Lattice images of the boundary revealed that it is atomically sharp and lying on a single plane in parts up to 100 nm long. Occasionally dislocations connected with steps and larger facets were observed. In some regions $NiSi_2$ was twinned with respect to Si.

Pd film on Si is formed upon annealing hexagonal Pd_2Si oriented with $(11\bar{2})$ Si$\|(2\bar{1}\bar{1}0)$ Pd_2Si. The misfit of the two lattices is 1.8 %. In lattice images the interface had no facets but it was wavy with a period of about 2 nm and atomically sharp. By counting (111) Si and ($22\bar{4}0$) Pd_2 Si fringes cutting a certain length of the interface differences in their number were detected and they were attributed to misfit dislocations and steps. Their exact character could not be assessed.

Further work on the Pd-Si system is the paper by Cherns et al. /27/. They analysed the possible transformation dislocations which transform the Si structure on (111) plane into the Pd_2Si structure. They found that the transformation may be accomplished by the motion of $1/6 \langle 11\bar{2} \rangle$ dislocations which form a step in the boundary and simultaneously relieve the natural misfit. Besides them dislocations $1/2\langle 110 \rangle$ without steps are possible Fig. 2 presents a lattice image of the interface by using the axial illumination in seven silicon and nine silicide beams. In both crystals cross-grating spot patterns are visible. The interface is sharp and atomically smooth in 3-5 nm parts limited by steps. By counting the number of fringes along circuits similar to the one marked by AA'B'B in fig. 2 surplus fringes were recorded in some cases in Si and in others in Pd_2Si. These differences were explained by the presence of steps with various heights and dislocations with either mixed or edge character. However, an unambiguous determination of the type of dislocations in singular cases was not possible.

In order to determine the exact crystallographic relationship of the two crystals in the boundary theoretical images of two model structures were calculated. In both silicon was terminated by identical (111) layers but Pd_2Si was terminated by two alternate layers. One interesting feature common to all computed and experimental images was the existence of broader fringes parallel to the interface with brighter and darker spots which bear no relation to the structure of the boundary. They are the result of interference of beams from the two crystals. Though the computed images were significantly different for the two models, it was not possible to decide by comparison with experimental micrographs which one of the two is correct. This was attributed to the relatively high density of interfacial dislocations and to the existence of an unknown surface layer.

In a further paper Cherns at al. /28/ demonstrated that the establishment of the exact crystallographic relationship by means of the comparison of computed and experimental images is possible in the case of an $NiSi_2$/Si interface. They calculated images of both basic orientations, I (untwinned) and II (twinned), with $NiSi_2$ terminated either by Ni or by Si layers (figs. 3, 4). The comparison of computed and experimental structural images is presented in figs. 5, 6. In fig. 5 it may be seen that in the top computed image the silicon and silicide spot rows viewed along C are exactly in line, in the bottom computed image they are just a little out of line. The experimental image in the center corresponds more nearly to the top image. A similar reasoning applies also to fig. 6.

5. Conclusion

The lattice imaging seems to be the most promising technique for the study of the detailed structure of interphase boundaries which can supply the maximum amount of useful information. There are two reasons for which it is not used for the study of interphase boundaries in metals to a larger extent. One of them is general and is connected with the very complicated specimen preparation. The other applies specially to common metals and is connected with the fact that present microscopes cannot as yet resolve the core structure of defects in them.

References

/1/ Christian J.W., The theory of transformations in metals and alloys, Pergamon, Oxford 1965, p. 331.
/2/ Gevers R., Van Landuyt J. and Amelinckx S.: Phys.Stat.Sol. 11 (1965), 689.
/3/ Fourdeux A., Gevers R. and Amelinckx S.: Phys. Stat. Sol. 24 (1967), 195.
/4/ Gemperlová J., Gemperle A. and Paidar V., Symposium on the Structure and Properties of Crystal Defects, Liblice 1983, Part A, p. 114.
/5/ Pond R.C.: J. Microsc. 116 (1979), 105.
/6/ Gevers R.: Phys. Stat. Sol. 3 (1963), 1672.
/7/ Gevers R.: Philos. Mag. 7 (1962), 1681.
/8/ Hirsch P.B., Howie A., Nicholson R.B., Pashley D.W. and Whelan M.J., Electron microscopy of thin crystals, Butterworth, London 1965, p. 343.
/9/ Marukawa K. and Matsubara Y.: Trans. Japan Inst. Metals 20 (1979), 560, 724.
/10/ Marukawa K., Electron microscopy 1982, The congress organizing committee, Hamburg 1982, p. 355.
/11/ Baluffi R. W., Woolhouse G. and Komen Y., AIME symposium on nature and behaviour of grain boundaries, Plenum Press, New York 1972, p. 41.
/12/ Baluffi R.W., Sass S.L. and Schober T.: Philos. Mag. 26 (1972), 585.
/13/ Cowley J.M. and Moodie A.F.: Proc. Phys. Soc. 76 (1960), 378.
/14/ Bourret A., Desseaux J. and Renault A.: Philos. Mag. 45 (1982), 1.
/15/ Ref. sub. /8/, p. 371.
/16/ Cockayne D.J.H., Parsons J.R. and Hoelke C.W.: Philos. Mag. 24 (1971), 139.
/17/ Smith D.A. and Goodhew P.J.: Philos. Mag. A 46 (1982), 161.

/18/ Aaronson H.I.: J. Microsc. 102 (1974), 275.
/19/ Laird C. and Sankaran R.: J. Microsc. 116 (1979), 123.
/20/ Phillips V.A. and Tanner L.E.: Acta Metall. 21 (1973), 44.
/21/ Sinclair R., Schneider K. and Thomas G.: Acta Metall. 23 (1975), 873.
/22/ Sinclair R. and Mohamed H.A.: Acta Metall. 26 (1978), 623.
/23/ Wu C.K., Electron microscopy 1982, The congress organizing committee, Hamburg 1982, p. 357.
/24/ Föll H., Ho P.S. and Tu K.N. J. Appl. Phys. 52 (1981), 250.
/25/ Föll H.: Phys. Stat. Sol. (a) 69 (1982), 779.
/26/ Föll H., Ho P.S. and Tu K.N.: Philos. Mag. A 45 (1982), 31.
/27/ Cherns D., Smith D.A., Krakow W. and Batson P.E.: Philos. Mag. A 45 (1982), 107.
/28/ Cherns D., Anstis G.R., Hutchison J.L. and Spence J.C.H.: Philos. Mag. A 46 (1982), 849.

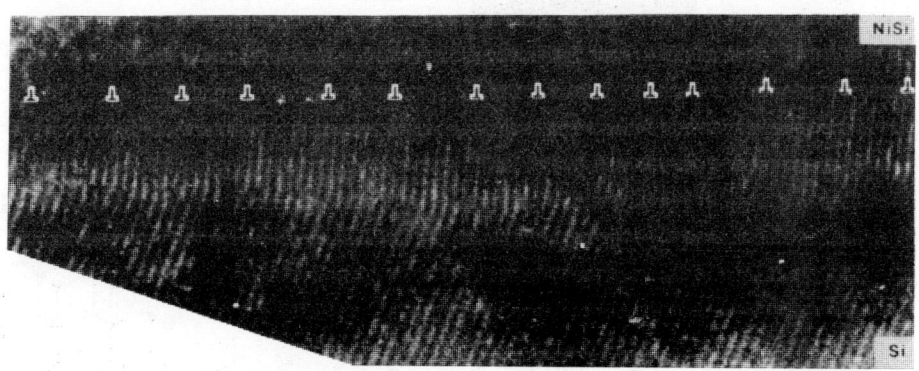

Fig. 1 NiSi-Si interface with marked NiSi terminating fringes (/26/ with permission).

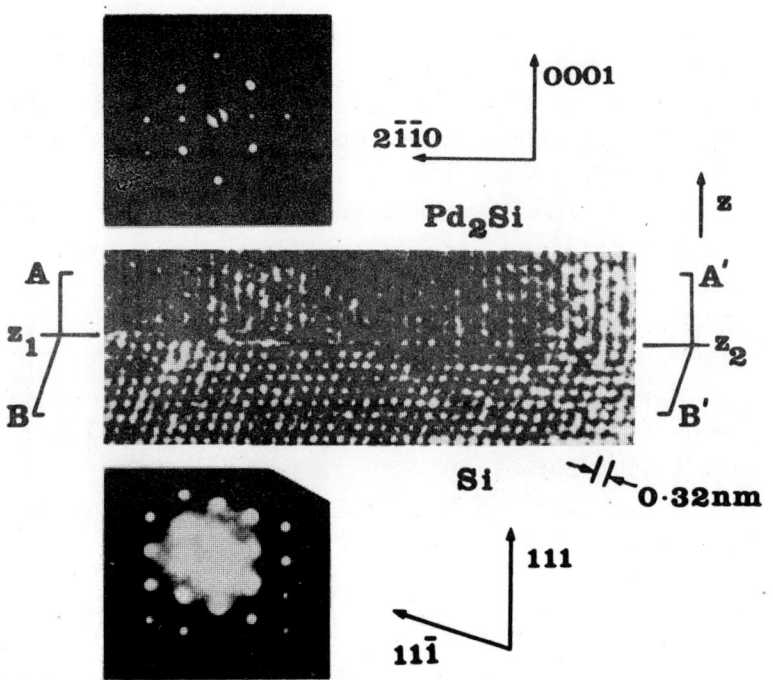

Fig. 2 Lattice image of Pd_2Si-(111)Si interface using 7 Si and 9 Pd_2Si beams. Diffraction patterns show the orientations of both crystals. (/27/ with permission)

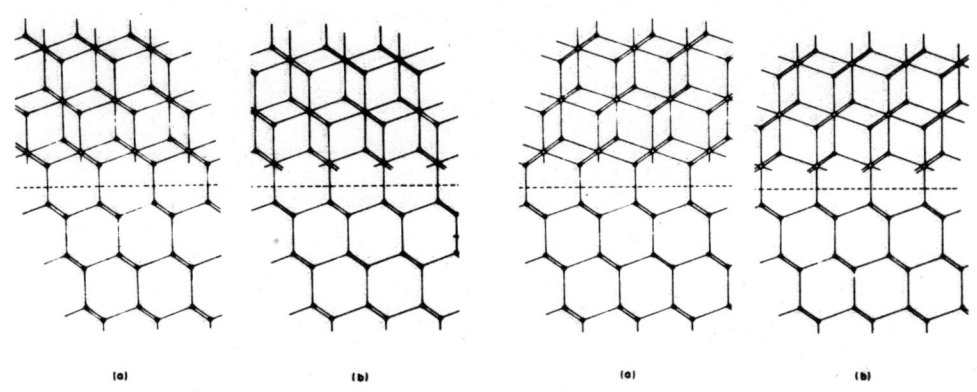

Fig. 3   Fig. 4

Fig. 3 Orientation I of $NiSi_2$-(111)Si interface having seven- (a) and five-coordinated (b) nickel atoms. Filled circles Ni, open circles Si. (/28/ with permission)

Fig. 4 Orientation II of $NiSi_2$-(111)Si interface. (a) and (b) cf. fig. 3 (/28/ with permission)

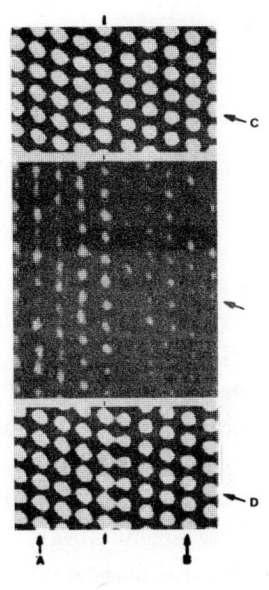 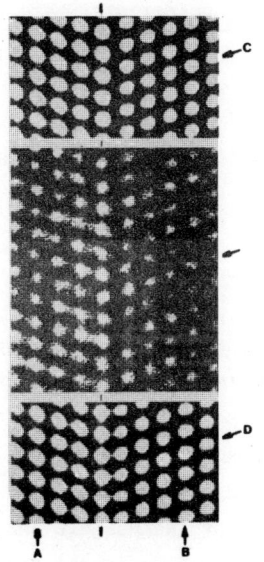

Fig. 5   Fig. 6

Fig. 5 Comparison of theoretical calculations with experimental images of type I $NiSi_2$-(111)Si interface. From top to bottom computed image of model fig. 3(a), experimental image, computed image of model fig. 3(b). A silicon, B silicide. The position of interface is marked. (/28/ with permission)

Fig. 6 Comparison of theoretical calculations with experimental images of type II $NiSi_2$-(111)Si interface. Top to bottom: computed image of model fig. 4(a), experimental image, computed image of model fig. 4(b). A silicon, B silicide. The position of interface is marked. (/28/ with permission)

TEM AND DIFFRACTION STUDIES OF THE Mo-Mo$_2$C PHASE BOUNDARY

M. Florjancic and M. Rühle

Max-Planck-Institut für Metallforschung, Institut für Werkstoffwissenschaften, Seestraße 92, 7000 Stuttgart 1, West-Germany

1. Introduction

The solubility of carbon at room temperature in molybdenum is very low. Precipitates of Mo$_2$C form easily intergranularly and intragranularly in molybdenum-carbon alloys. The Mo$_2$C precipitates influence strongly the mechanical properties of the polycrystalline molybdenum. Therefore, it is necessary to understand not only the structure of the Mo grain boundaries, but also the structure of the Mo-Mo$_2$C phase boundary down to the atomic level, if possible.

Grain boundaries belong to the group of homophase boundaries which are regions in space where two crystals of the same structure and composition meet. In contrast, phase boundaries belong to the group of heterophase boundaries which are regions in space where two crystals, possessing different structures and/or chemical composition, are in contact. For the analysis of a phase boundary it is important to analyse not only the structural aspects of the interface (i.e. the arrangement of atoms and Burgers vectors of possible dislocations) but also the chemical variation across and along the phase boundary.

Cahn and Hilliard /1/ have shown that, for thermodynamical reasons, a phase boundary should be "diffuse" at high temperatures (that means the concentration of the different atoms does not change abruptly across the boundary but within a certain region). For the low temperature regime "sharp" phase boundaries are expected (Becker /2/). In the present paper results of the study of the Mo-Mo$_2$C phase boundary by means of high resolution electron diffraction and transmission electron microscopy will be presented.

2. Experimental Procedure

For the high resolution electron diffraction /3/ it is assumed that an interface can be regarded as a separate crystal (interface crystal) of thickness t with a structure different from the structures of the adjacent crystals. Therefore, additional reflections are expected in the diffraction pattern. The additional reflections are elongated normal to the interface plane (streaks); the length of the streaks is 1/t. The position of the maximum intensity of the streak with respect to the origin of the reciprocal space, L, is correlated to the mean strain field $<\varepsilon>$ normal to the interface /4/.

One type of phase boundary between the bcc molybdenum (M) and the hexagonal Mo_2C precipitates (P) was studied where $(0001)_P$ and $(110)_M$ are approximately parallel to the phase boundary planes.

3. Experimental Observations

Fig. 1 shows a TEM micrograph of a typical Mo_2C precipitate embedded in the molybdenum matrix. The largest dimension of the precipitate is about 2 μm. The long interface (planes parallel to $(0001)_P$ and $(110)_M$, respectively) were analysed. Fig. 2 shows a TEM of the same phase boundary inclined with respect to the incoming electron beam. Periodic dislocations (spacing 13.5 nm) are visible. The dislocation lines are parallel to the $|\bar{1}13|_M$ and $|1\bar{1}00|_P$ directions, respectively. The Burgers vector b of the interface dislocation is parallel to the $|1\bar{1}1|_M$ direction, the magnitude of b could not be determined. If the phase boundary is oriented parallel to the beam (Fig. 3a), black dots are visible on the TEM image. These contrast features are caused by residual strain contrast of dislocations (the direction of the dislocation line is parallel to the beam). In addition to the reflections of molybdenum and Mo_2C, streaks are visible on the diffraction pattern, see Fig. 3b. From the (maximal) length of the streaks (0.5 nm^{-1}) the thickness t of the interface crystal is determined to t = 2 nm which corresponds to 9 plane spacings of the $(110)_M$ planes. The site of the maximum of the streaks possesses the distance L from the origin of reciprocal lattice; L = 4.4 nm^{-1} ± 0.01. This results in a mean strain field normal to the interface of $<\varepsilon>$ = + 2.15 %.

4. Discussion of the Experimental Results

4.1 Structural Analysis

It is well established that low energy grain boundaries possess a high density of coincidence lattice points /5/. The Burgers vectors of dislocations in relaxed grain boundaries can be determined from the DSC lattice. It is expected that the structure of phase boundaries can also be deduced by a similar model (Balluffi and Brokman /6/). Therefore, we calculated the CSL and DSC lattice of the $Mo-Mo_2C$ phase boundary. The results of the calculations demonstrate the observed average direction of the interface planes which is not connected with the highest density of coincidence plane (Fig. 4). The lowest energy configuration should follow the $(0001)_P$ and $(110)_M$ planes, respectively, which would result in a facetting of the interface. Experimental high resolution TEM studies should explore those details in the future.

On the other hand, the calculated DSC lattice shows a good agreement with the experimentally determined Burgers vector of the interface dislocation. From the two possible DSC Burgers vectors $\underline{b}_1 = 1/20\ |\bar{1}11|$ and $\underline{b}_2 = 1/2\ |1\bar{1}1|$, $\underline{b}_2$ was experimentally observed. The magnitude of $\underline{b}_1$ is probably too small to be determined. It is reasonable that the Burgers vector of the phase boundary dislocation is equivalent to a bcc crystal dislocation.

3.2 Discussion of the Diffraction Results

The mean strain field was calculated to be $<\varepsilon> = +\ 2.15\ \%$ from the diffraction pattern (Fig. 3b). This can be represented by expansion of the plane spacing in the interface crystal with respect to the molybdenum matrix. Since the precipitates form during cooling from 2600 K, the resulting strain field due to the difference in thermal expansion coefficients /7, 8/ has to be considered. The Mo_2C precipitate shrinks with respect to Mo in the c-direction by 0.35 % and expands in the a-direction by 0.32 %. The strain fields due to thermal mismatch between Mo and Mo_2C are, therefore, too small to explain the large experimentally determined strain field of about 2 %. A reasonable explanation of those large dilatation fields can be made by the assumption of a concentration gradient of carbon in the phase boundary (Cahn and Hilliard /1/). Fig. 5 shows schematically the concentration profile (identical with the variation in plane spacing) calculated from the experimental results, compared to those calculated from Cahn and Hilliard's theory. Both profiles fit quite well. Therefore, one can conclude, that the Mo-Mo_2C phase boundary is diffuse and the carbon concentration decreases continuously from the concentration of Mo_2C over 9 Mo-planes to the very low carbon concentration in molybdenum.

References

/1/ J.W. Cahn, J.E. Hilliard, J. Chem. Phys. 28, 258 (1958).
/2/ R. Becker, Ann. Phys. 32, 128 (1938).
/3/ M. Florjancic, M. Rühle, S.L. Sass, Proc. of the 10th Int. Congress on Electron Microscopy, Hamburg, FRG, Vol. 2, 359 (1982).
/4/ M. Florjancic, M. Rühle, S.L. Sass, to be published.
/5/ R.W. Balluffi, Grain Boundary Structure and Kinetics, ASM, Metals Park, Ohio, 1980.
/6/ R.W. Balluffi, A. Brokman, A.H. King, Acta Met. 30, 1453 (1982).
/7/ L.E. Toth, Transition Metal Carbides and Nitrides, Acad. Press, N.Y., London 6 (1971).
/8/ Molybdän-Drenst 28, 6 (1964).

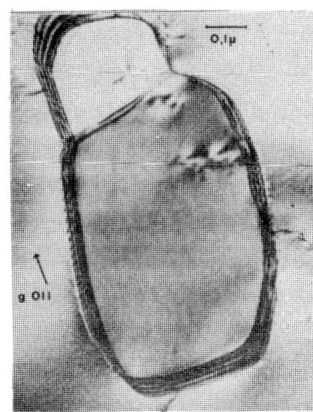

Fig. 1: A typical Mo_2C precipitate embedded in the molybdenum matrix.

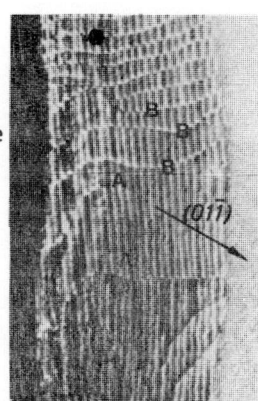

Fig. 2: TEM of the inclined Mo-Mo_2C phase boundary with dislocations A-A $\underline{b} = \frac{1}{2} |1\bar{1}1|$.

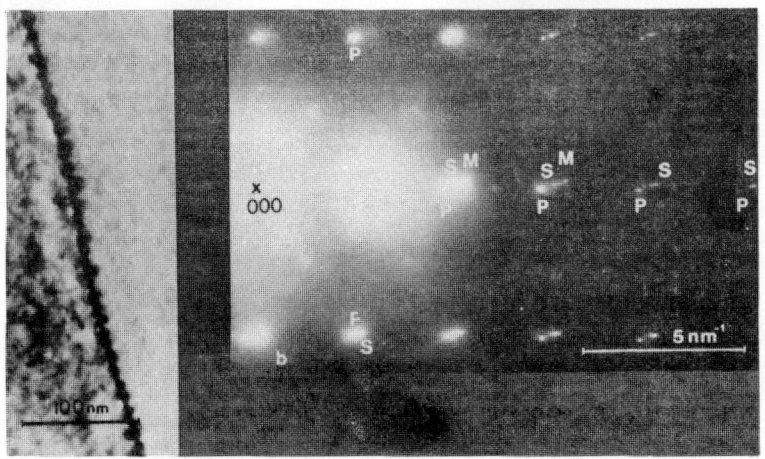

Fig. 3: (a) TEM of the phase boundary parallel to the beam. Black dots are caused by the residual strain of the dislocations.
(b) Diffraction pattern with the Mo reflections M and Mo_2C reflections P; in addition streaks S are present.

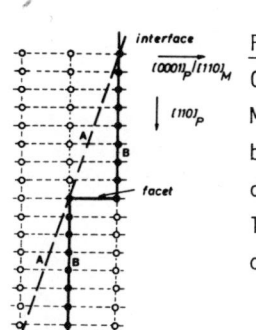

Fig. 4: CSL of the Mo-Mo_2C phase boundary. Average direction A-A, lowest energy configuration B-B.

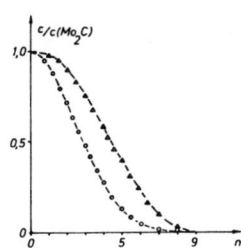

Fig. 5: Concentration profile across the boundary (n = 9, number of planes) results O-O and the profile calculated from the Cahn-Hilliard's theory Δ-Δ.

SECTION 5

COLLECTIVE BEHAVIOUR AND INTERACTION
OF DEFECTS

FIELD THEORY OF DEFECTS IN BRAVAIS CRYSTALS

E. Kröner

Institut für Theoretische und Angewandte Physik, Universität Stuttgart, Stuttgart, F. R. Germany

The present state of the field theory of defects in Bravais crystals is reviewed. The elementary defects are treated in analogy to elementary particles in the otherwise empty universe (vacuum). A continuized crystal is defined by a limiting process which leaves the crystallographic directions at each point intact. Every distribution of intrinsic defects - dislocations, vacancies and self-interstitials - defines a configuration of the crystal and is described by a linear connexion of the (crystals) space. External defects, e.g. atoms of another species, do not belong to the physical system "Bravais crystal". They are not internal to the system and therefore appear as external source terms in the field equations for the connexion.

Beside the <u>strain space</u> discussed so far a <u>stress space</u> is considered that has the same structure as the strain space. The identities of the curvature tensor of this space form the equilibrium equations in the absence of external (generalized) forces. Stress and strain space are mutually dual. They are connected by constitutive laws not discussed here.

1. Introduction

In 1964 a summer school on the Theory of Crystal Defects was held in Hrazany, CSSR under the direction of F. Kroupa. This summer school certainly belonged to the outstanding events of this kind in our field. Almost 20 years later another congregation takes place with the theme of Crystal Defects. It might be appropriate also at this occasion to recall that there exists the possibility of a broad theoretical basis for the phenomenon "defect in crystal". The theory developed on this basis is sometimes called "field theory of crystal defects". In this theory, the perfect crystal plays the role of the empty universe (vacuum), whereas the defects are compared with the elementary particles moving around in the real universe. It is a fascinating feature that, unlike to what is usually considered in the field theories of the universe, the elementary defects can also possess line shape (dislocations, disclinations etc.). Only topological defects shall be discussed in this lecture.

The field theory of crystal defects does not yet exist in a form that is similarly complete as for instance Maxwell's theory. The dynamical theory is even less complete whereas major parts of the static theory are developed satisfactorily. Above all this is true for the (statical) "Dislocation Field Theory" and the (static) theory of "Dia- and Para-Elasticity" (field theory of point defects) where within quotation marks the titles of my contributions to the Hrazany school are reproduced /1/. The two theories, there given in linearized description, are completely separate, due to the approximation involved in the linearization. In reality, there is a strong nonlinear coupling between dislocations and point defects of all sorts which manifests itself, among others in the creation and annihilation of point defects during nonconservative motion and intersection of dislocations. The interaction responsible for such processes will be called "topological interaction" in order to distinguish it from the "energetical interaction" that acts via the elastic stresses and is present also in a linearized theory.

The topological interaction implies that a theory which speaks only of dislocations, is rather restrictive in its applications. In fact, many applications of dislocation theory to materials behaviour do involve nonconservative motion, intersection etc., and in these problems the linearized theory is certainly not good enough.

In this lecture I shall attempt to report on the present state of the (statical) field theory of defects in Bravais lattices. In section 2 we discuss the compatible deformation of the perfect crystal (i.e. a crystal without defects) and introduce crystallographic coordinates. An essential point is here the limiting process in which the atomic distance goes to zero under conservation of the crystallogrphic directions. In section 3 we show that the crystallographic coordinates of a dislocated crystal are anholonomic. Distances between atoms retain a quantitative meaning only if they are infinitesimal (in a macroscopic sense).

We also demonstrate the equivalence of Frank's Burgers circuit and Cartans's circuit. This comparison leads to the identification of dislocations and Cartan's torsion. The curvature tensor is introduced as a measure of incompatibility, a notion also explained in section 4. The definition, given by eq.(3) is more general than that usually found in text books (eq.(5)). It permits us a more intuitive understanding of curvature. The essential results of the geometrical theory are listed in section 5, where in particular the field equations are introduced.

The concept of strain space and stress space, discussed in section 6 reveals a fundamental symmetry which gives the theory a particularly compact form. In section 7 we discuss future extensions of the theory, in particular extensions to dynamics and to structures that are more complex than Bravais crystals, e.g. lattices with basis, liquid crystals and spin structures. In several points, this lecture goes beyond the author's extended review in ref. /2/ where most of the relevant literature is cited.

2. The perfect crystal and its deformed configurations

Perhaps the most distinguished feature of a perfect crystal as compared to an amorphous arrangement of particles is that distances can be measured by counting atomic steps. Here we shall consider only Bravais crystals. Then any particle B, for simplicity called atom, is identified with respect to a given other atom A by the numbers of steps along the three crystallographic directions that have to be taken when hopping from A to B. In this way the so-called crystallographic coordinate system is introduced that is discrete in the sense that only integer values of coordinates have a meaning.

In many applications the atomic distance is very small compared to any other distance of importance. It is then appropriate to consider a limiting process towards a continuum in such a way that it is at the same time a process for the crystallographic coordinate system which in the limit becomes continuous. In other words, we consider the crystal as a continuum in which at each point three crystallographic directions can be identified.

The undeformed state or configuration, of the perfect crystal is also called the crystal's ideal state or ideal configuration. Its crystallographic coordinates are rectilinear. They are cartesian in the case of the simple cubic lattice considered for simplicity in fig. 1a. A deformation of the ideal crystal is called compatible if it does not induce defects (fig. 1b). We say that the crystallographic coordinate system is carried along during the compatible deformation. Obviously, the crystallographic coordinates of the atoms remain unchanged under compatible deformation. Therefore, a fictive internal observer who can orient himself only by counting atomic steps does not feel any difference between compatibly deformed configurations and the ideal state of the crystal. In contrast to the internal observer the external observer can distiguish the various compatibly deformed states of the perfect crystal, for instance by use of an external cartesian coordinate system.

3. The crystal with dislocations

Consider now a crystal containing many dislocations but no other defects. An idealized situation of this kind is shown in fig. 2. Three crystallographic directions can be identifed at each point of the lattice except at the points in the centers of the dislocations. In fig. 2 the crystal is divided into blocks each of which does not contain dislocations. These are rather located in the boundaries between the blocks. It follows that within each block we have an intact crystallographic coordinate system, but, due to the presence of the dislocations, the manifold of these systems does not form an intact global crystallographic coordinate system. By the introduction of dislocations the originally holonomous crystallographic coordinate system has become anholonomous, as one says.

Consequently, the identification of atoms by counting steps as well as the measurement of the distance between two more distant atoms is no longer possible. It can be done only for infinitesimal distances, say ds. The presence of the dislocations induces an uncertainty of the size db in the length measurement, if db is the amount of Burgers vector or dislocations piercing through an area of size ds^2. Thus the relative uncertainty db/ds goes to zero like ds. It is worthwhile to note already here that the uncertainty is independent of ds when the counting of steps is disturbed by vacancies or self-interstitials. In fact, the probability per step to meet one of these defects is independent of the length of the path. Since the counting is not defined at the defects we have the situation that in the presence of vacancies and self-interstitials the metricity breaks down even for infinitesimal distances, for which it is preserved in the presence of dislocations.

It should be clear by now that the mathematical language of our theory should be that of differential geometry. This was first recognized by Kondo /3/ and by Bilby, Bullough and Smith /4/ in 1952/54, who independently noticed that the so-called Cartan circuit considered in differential geometry is just the continuum version of Frank's Burgers circuit commonly used to define the dislocation. This is illustrated by fig. 3. Quantitatively we define our continuized crystal as a linear space L_3 in three dimensions to which the law of parallel displacement of a vector v^l,

$$(1) \quad dv^k = - \Gamma_{ml}{}^k v^l dx^m$$

along the infinitesimal curve dx^m applies. Eq.(1) is valid for instance in the cartesian frame of the external observer. Reference to the anholonomic crystallographic coordinates is also possible, but not convenient for our purpose.

The knowledge of the linear connexion $\Gamma_{ml}{}^k$ permits us to construct the defected crystal by repeated parallel displacements. Eq.(1) can be interpreted either as a classification of those crystals (Bravais!) to which this theory applies or as a fundamental equation of the theory. Applying Cartan's procedure, one finds

$$(2) \quad db^k = - T_{ml}{}^k dS^{ml}$$

where db^k is the closure failure (Burgers vector) of the circuit around the area element dS^{ml}. Fig. 3c shows the discretized version of this. The Cartan's torsion tensor $T_{ml}{}^k$ is defined as the part of the linear connexion $\Gamma_{ml}{}^k$ antisymmetric in m, l. If in eq.(2) db^k is interpreted as the resulting Burgers vector of the dislocations enclosed by the mentioned circuit and $T_{ml}{}^k$ as Cartan's torsion, then eq.(2) expresses first important identification of the differential geometry of defects.

4. The curvature tensor

Going beyond our representation in ref. /2/, let us introduce the concept of incompatible deformation of a (continuized) Bravais crystal as follows: Assume that at the beginning we do not have one big single crystal, but rather an assembly of "infinitesimal", in general, defected crystal elements which do not fit together to give the macrocrystal. Imagine that the elements are deformed in such a way that they can be fitted together without holes between them. We say that the so built-up macrocrystal is in an incompatibly deformed state. The present, somewhat rough description of this state will become more precise later in this section.

Assume that the incompatibility of the deformed state can be specified by a tensor field $\Delta\gamma_l^{\ k}$ which depends continuously on the position $\underline{r}$ in the macrocrystal. Assume furthermore, that $\Delta\gamma_l^{\ k}$ can be related to the infinitesimal area element ΔS^{nm} by

$$(3) \quad \Delta\gamma_l^{\ k} = \frac{1}{2} R_{nml}^{\ \ \ k} \Delta S^{nm}$$

Eq.(3) defines the 4th rank tensor $R_{nml}^{\ \ \ k}$ which we call "curvature tensor" for reasons to become clear shortly. Since $R_{nml}^{\ \ \ k}$ is continuous together with $\Delta\gamma_l^{\ k}$, we obviously describe a continuous incompatibility. In other words, the original nonfitting is supposed to be distributed in such a way that it possesses macroscopic continuity.

In general, a vector v^l at point $\underline{r}$ will be transformed into a vector $v^k + \Delta v^k$, also at $\underline{r}$, by application of $-\Delta\gamma_l^{\ k}$ so that

$$(4) \quad \Delta v^k \equiv -v^l \Delta\gamma_l^{\ k} = -\frac{1}{2} R_{nml}^{\ \ \ k} v^l \Delta S^{nm}$$

(the signs in eqs.(3) and (4) are chosen by convention).
If the special form

$$(5) \quad R_{nml}^{\ \ \ k} = 2[\partial_n \Gamma_{ml}^{\ \ k} - \Gamma_{mp}^{\ \ k} \Gamma_{nl}^{\ \ p}]_{[nm]}$$

is given to the curvature tensor, where [nm] denotes antisymmetrization in n,m, then eq.(4) can be written in terms of line integrals along the oriented edge line C of ΔS:

$$(6) \quad \Delta v^k = \oint_C dv^k = -\oint_C v^l d\gamma_l^{\ k} = -\oint_C \Gamma_{ml}^{\ \ k} v^l dx^m .$$

This is the formula for the parallel transport of the vector v^l along the circuit C (cf. eq.(1)).

The first eq.(6) allows us to give a topological interpretation to the vector v^k at $\underline{r}$. Imagine a very thin infinitesimal ring of crystalline matter which may contain dislocations but no other defects (fig. 4a). Assume that a vector v^l at point $\underline{r}$ in the ring undergoes a parallel transport once around the ring back to $\underline{r}$, and that we find $\Delta v^k \equiv \oint_C dv^k = 0$. If we now cut through the ring at point $\underline{r}$ in order to make it simply connected, then the ring may show a gap (fig. 4b). If we remove this gap by bending back to the closed form (fig. 4c) we expect that the vectors v^k at corresponding points of the two cut-faces are equal, i.e. $\Delta v^k = 0$. Now fill the intact ring (state of fig. 4a) with point defects, here not specified, and cut as before (fig. 4d). Bend back to the closed form (fig. 4e). Then the two vectors v^k are not the same but have a difference Δv^k.

The situation just described arises when we cut out an infinitesimal ring along the circuit C at any point $\underline{r}$ and at any orientation of the circuit C (or the area element ΔS). The totality of the so measured Δv's determines the incompatibility field $\Delta \gamma_1{}^k$ according to eq.(4) and the curvature field $R_{nml}{}^k$ according to eq.(3). A procedure related to that described here, but more in the language of continuum mechanics, has been described by Kunin.

Originally we had defined the curvature tensor by eq.(3) and found the special form (5) that is usually given as the definition of the curvature tensor (see e.g. Schouten /5/). Eq.(5) implies the existence of a linear connexion, therefore of a connected macrobody. In order to have such a situation the curvature tensor must satisfy the well-known identities (/5/, ch. III §5). These equations, e.g. the Bianchi identity, have vanishing source terms. The general definition (3) of the curvature tensor would also permit source terms. In their presence no connexion would exist so that the assembly of crystal elements would not form a compact, i.e. everywhere connected macrocrystal. A realization of such a situation is perhaps a crystal with microcracks distributed continuously over the body. Therefore, the mentioned source terms can be interpreted as crack densities in a general sense. For the rest of this lecture we shall exclude them.

A very special situation arises if $R_{nml}{}^k = 0$. This is the case of teleparallelism, in which a distorsion function $\gamma_1{}^k$ exists. It has been shown by Kondo /3/ and by Bilby, Bullough and Smith /4/ that this case includes dislocations as lines which do not end in the interior of the crystal. In this case the connexion possesses 9 independent components. This means that the curvature identities which are equivalent to eq.(5) imply 9 independent equations for the components of the curvature tensor.

5. Results of the geometrical theory

Space and time do not allow me to continue with the same prolixity. Besides, the theory is not worked out in all details so that it may suffice to list without much explanation some of the relevant results.

a) The components of the linear connexion are straintype quantities when judged from outside. The internal observer prefers to speak of configurations rather than of strains.

b) The $\Gamma_{ml}{}^k$ satisfy the field equations

$$(7) \quad R_{nml}{}^k = M_{mnl}{}^k$$

where $\underline{R}$ is taken from eq.(5) and the 4th rank tensor $\underline{M}$ describes the external sources. These sources are <u>extrinsic</u> defects, e.g. atoms of a different species on interstitial or substitutional sites. $\underline{M}$ must satisfy the same identies as $\underline{R}$, it therefore represents 18 functions of position.

c) The elementary <u>intrinsic</u> defects dislocations, vacancies and self-interstitials are described by the connexion, since they define configurations.

d) Whereas dislocations are described by the in m,l antisymmetric part (the torsion) of the affine connexion $\Gamma_{ml}{}^k$, the vacancies and self-interstitials determine the nonmetric part of $\Gamma_{ml}{}^k$.

e) The structure of the connexion and the field equations contain the topological interaction.

f) A metric tensor, say g_{lk} exists also in the presence of intrinsic point defects. This is so, although the connexion $\Gamma_{ml}{}^k$ is nonmetric with respect to g_{lk}, which means that $\nabla_m g_{lk} \neq 0$. The metric g_{lk} defines a new prescription for counting atomic steps: vacancies are counted like ordinary atoms whereas self-interstitials are ignored.

g) The linear connexion is completely exhausted by the mentioned intrinsic defects. In particular, there is no more space for a further elementary, i.e. irreducible, intrinsic defect that could be called disclination (see also section 7). Where disclinations in

Bravais lattices are discussed, these are composed of dislocations
and therefore not elementary defects.

6. Strain space and stress space

The geometry considered so-far will from now on be called
the geometry of the (crystals) strain space because the aim was
essentially the study of (generalized) strains in a defected crystal. In order to complete the static part of the theory we have
now to consider (generalized) stresses and shall speak of the
differential geometry of the (crystals) stress space. This space
has formally the same structure as the strain space. We can identify the metric tensor with the stress function tensor, the torsion tensor with the moment stress tensor, the nonmetric part
of the connexion with a generalized stress tensor, sometimes called microstress tensor, and the Einstein tensor with the ordinary
force stress tensor. The curvature identities correspond to the
equilibrium equations in the absence of external influences (forces, moments etc.).

7. Conclusion

The differential geometry of the strain and stress space
of the Bravais crystal has just enough freedom to include all those
crystal defects that we consider as elementary, i.e. irreducible.
In particular, it gives us the field equations of the theory of
defects. So-far, strain and stress space are separate spaces the
theory of which has been developed independently. It is clear
that they are not independent with respect to real processes, but
rather have the status of dual spaces in some sense. The connexion between the two spaces is given by the constitutive law for
statics. Sometimes it may suffice to use some sort of generalized
Hooke's law. The two spaces retain their significance also in
dynamics where the constitutive laws are much more involved. It
may well be that realistic laws cannot be established on the basis of Lagrangian formalism since the topological interaction
leads to high irreversibility of the elementary processes.

So-far, everything was restricted to Bravais crystals. Crystals with basis have more functional degrees of freedom (optical
waves!) and need a more general geometry (e.g. Finsler's or

Kawaguchi's geometry). The same is true for liquid crystals and spin structures where the particles are no longer point-like, but have a preferred orientation. Since the geometry of these structures deviates considerably from that of the Bravais crystal, it is clear that also their defects may be different. In particular, one finds that these structures may have an important elementary line defect, the disclination.

The theory discussed here is the fundamental (statical) field theory of defects in Bravais crystals. It should not be identified with what sometimes is called theory of continuous distributions of dislocations (or defects) or simply continuum theory of defects in crystals. The present theory does not assume that defects occur in the form of continuous distributions. The emphasis is rather on the elementary defects, like the emphasis of the fundamental physical field theories is on the elementary particles.

References

/1/ B. Gruber, ed., Proc. Summer School Theory of Crystal Defects, Hrazany, CSSR, 1964 (Academia, Prague, 1966).

/2/ E. Kröner, Continuum Theory of Defects, in: R. Balian et al., eds., Les Houches, Session 35, 1980 - Physique des Défauts (North-Holland, Amsterdam 1981), p. 215.

/3/ K. Kondo, On the Geometrical and Physical Foundations of the Theory of Yielding, in: Proc. 2nd Japan Nat. Congr. Applied Mechanics (Tokyo, 1952).

/4/ B. A. Bilby, R. Bullough and E. Smith, Proc. Roy. Soc. London A 231 (1955), p. 459.

/5/ J. A. Schouten, Ricci-Calculus, 2nd ed. (Springer, Heidelberg, 1954).

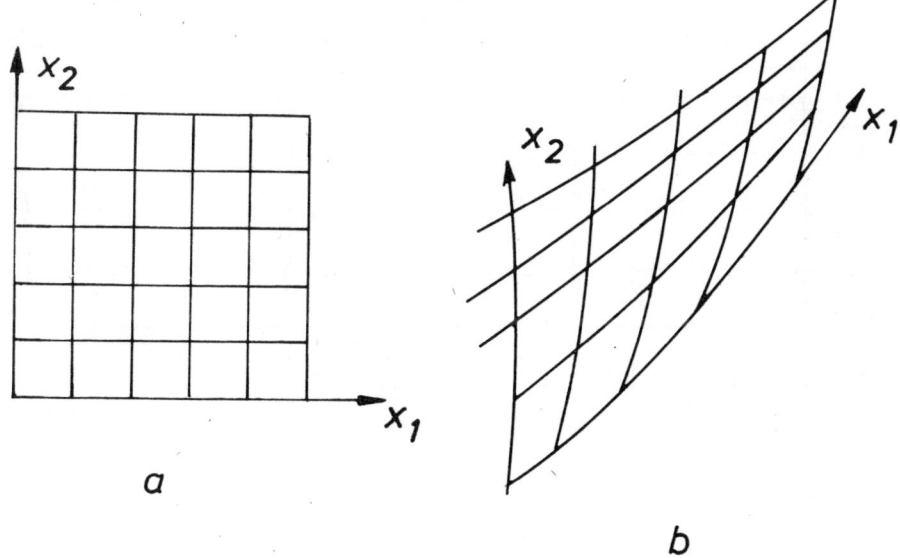

Fig. 1 a: Lattice plane of a simple cubic lattice in the ideal state.
b: Same lattice plane as in fig. a, after compatible deformation.

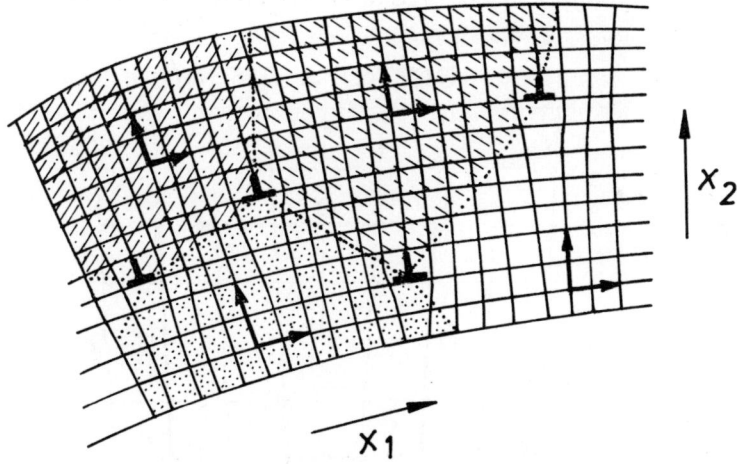

Fig. 2 The crystallographic coordinates system becomes anholonomic in the presence of dislocations.

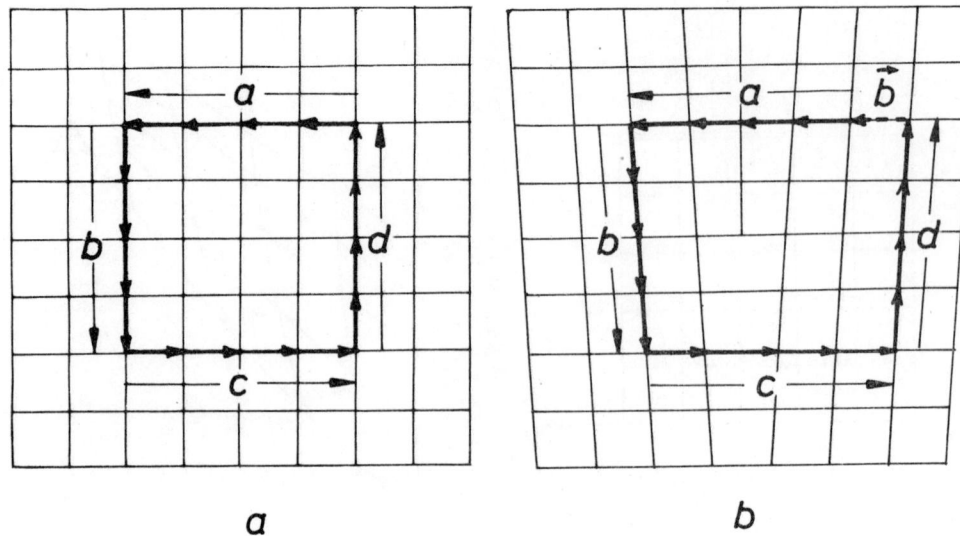

a   b

Frank's Burgers circuit

Fig. 3 a,b: Frank's Burgers circuit defines the dislocation. Fig. a can be replaced by program (a,b,c,d) = (4,4,4,4).

c: Cartan's circuit implies parallel displacement of a along b and c along d. The closure failure defines the torsion.

Cartan's circuit

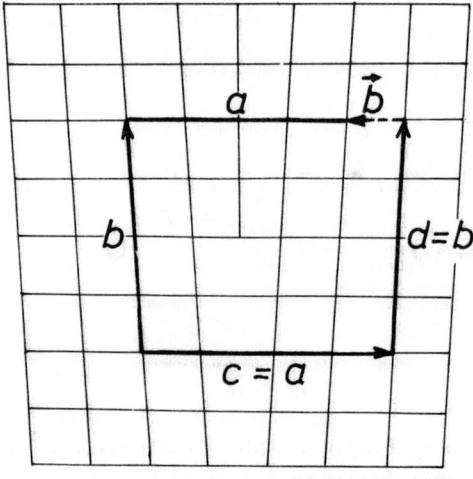

c

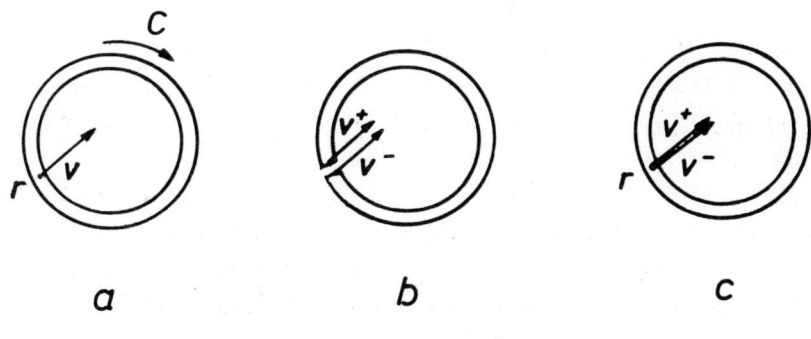

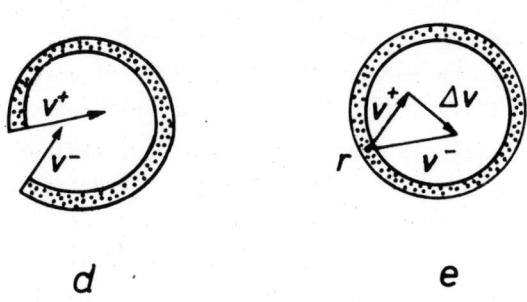

Fig. 4 a: Crystalline ring, may contain dislocations. Observe vector v at point r.
b: Opening of ring after cut at r. Vector v splits in v^+ and v^-.
c: After bending back of ring: $\Delta v = v^- - v^+ = 0$.
d: Ring of fig. a filled with point defects, then cut. Vectors v^+ and v^- are rotated and stretched relative to v.
e: After bending back of ring: $\Delta v = v^- - v^+ \neq 0$

DISLOCATION FIELDS

H.O.K. Kirchner

Institut fuer Festkoerperphysik, Universitaet Wien, A-1090 Boltzmanng.5, and Department of Mechanical Engineering, M.I.T., Cambridge, Mass. 02139 USA

§1. INTRODUCTION

Classical Elasticity starts with the concept of a displacement between two different states. By differentiation a displacement gradient is obtained, and the elastic energy associated with the difference between the two states depends only on this gradient. Unless the history of how one state is obtained from the other is known, there is no way to determine the displacement by a physical experiment. Only the displacement gradient can be observed by, say, a diffraction experiment. The displacement gradient, being a tensor with 9 components, cannot be arbitrary, if it is to be derived as the gradient of a vector with 3 components. It has to obey certain differential relations that are called compatibility conditions. The question arises if elasticity can be carried out if the notion of displacements is disregarded. The answer is yes. In order to test if a given candidate (called distorsion) is the gradient of a vector field, it is not actually necessary to construct the vector field by integration, but it suffices to check if the rotation of the tensor field vanishes. If the rotation of the distorsion vanishes, one has classical elasticity with a displacement function. If not, dislocations are present. Of the numerous treatises on the subject one should mention Kroener's [1] fundamental book, Noll's very rigid exposition [2] and Gairola's review paper [3].

In this sense dislocations are the sources of distorsions just as forces are the sources of stress, or the other way round. Just as one proceeds to find the stresses produced by body forces, the task arises to find the distorsions when the dislocation density is given. Both can be done using Green's functions, either for a finite or the infinite body. The next question to be asked is if these dislocations (and forces) feel forces in the presence of distorsions and stresses. This is equivalent to asking if the energy of the body depends on the position of either. This notion touches upon a concept now quite familiar to physicists: nowadays textbooks derive conservation laws from the invariance of the energy with respect to one or the other transformation. In mechanics the conservation of momentum and angular momentum are consequences of the translational and rotational invariance of space. The fundamental idea that invariance of the energy with respect to something gives rise to a conservation law is due to Emmy Noether [4]. It leads to the concept of the energy-momentum-tensor and other surface-independent integrals. The energy-momentum-tensor was introduced by Eshelby [5] to elasticity as early as 1951. It is a convenient means to compute the forces felt by defects. In the following it will be used to obtain the forces felt by continuous dislocation distributions for the case of nonlinear elasticity.

§2. FUNDAMENTALS OF THE LINEAR THEORY

Consider an energy density $w = \sigma_{ij}(x)\beta_{ij}(x)$ over a finite volume V

(2.1) $$\hat{w} = \frac{1}{2} \int_V \sigma_{ij}(x)\beta_{ij}(x) \, d^3x$$

where $\sigma_{ij} = \sigma_{ji}$ is a symmetric stress tensor and β_{ij} is a nonsymmetric infinitesimal distorsion tensor. Because of the symmetry of σ one might also write $\varepsilon_{ij} = (\beta_{ij} + \beta_{ji})/2$ instead of β in w. The local constitutive relation shall be

(2.2) $$\sigma_{ij}(x) = C_{ijkl}(x)[\beta_{ij}(x) + \beta_{ji}(x)]/2$$

with the usual symmetry of the elastic constants

(2.3) $$C_{ijkl} = C_{jikl} = C_{ijlk} = C_{klij}$$

In view of the fact that the linear differential operators ∂_p and $\varepsilon_{rsp}\partial_s$ are orthogonal in the sense that, applied to anything, they yield identically zero, it is suggestive to decompose the fields according to

(2.4) $\quad\quad\quad\quad \sigma = \text{rot}\emptyset + \text{grad}A$
(2.5) $\quad\quad\quad\quad \beta = \text{grad}u + \text{rot}Z$

Commonly these decompositions are called internal and external stress and distorsion, respectively.

(2.6) $\quad\quad\quad\quad \sigma_i = \text{rot}\emptyset \quad\quad\quad \sigma_a = \text{grad}A$
(2.7) $\quad\quad\quad\quad \beta_a = \text{grad}u \quad\quad\quad \beta_i = \text{rot}Z$

where u is called the displacement and $\emptyset$ is called the stress function of first order. Neither A nor Z seem to have names. It follows that

(2.8) $$\text{div}\sigma_i = \text{rot}\beta_a = 0$$

but there can be sources to the other two components

(2.9) $\quad\quad\quad\quad \text{div}\sigma_a = -f = \text{div}\sigma$
(2.10) $\quad\quad\quad\quad \text{rot}\beta_a = \alpha = \text{rot}\beta$

Classical elasticity is characterized by the existence of displacements u and the absence of dislocation densities α, while the so-called theory of internal stresses as developed by Kroener is usually performed for the absence of body forces f. As a matter of fact a very symmetric developement allowing for both to be present is possible. The symmetry between σ and β, f and α and other quantities will become obvious. According to Collonetti's theorem the cross terms between the internal stresses and the external ones vanish and there remains only

$$(2.11) \quad \hat{W} = \int_V [\sigma^i_{ij} \beta^i_{ij} + \sigma^a_{ij} \beta^a_{ij}] \, d^3x$$

With the internal fields present the theorem of work and energy is then

$$(2.12) \quad \hat{W} = \frac{1}{2} \int_V [\varepsilon_{rsp} \beta_{mp} \partial_s \phi_{mr} + \sigma_{mp} \partial_p u_m] \, d^3x =$$

$$= \frac{1}{2} \{ \int_S -\bar{\alpha}_{mr} \phi_{mr} \, d^2x - \int_V \alpha_{mr} \phi_{mr} \, d^3x + \int_S t_m u_m \, d^2x + \int_V f_m u_m \, d^3x \}$$

where S is the surface of the body V. The definitions

$$(2.13) \quad t_m = \sigma_{mp} n_p \qquad \bar{\alpha}_{mr} = -\varepsilon_{rsp} n_s \beta_{mp}$$

are used for the tractions t and the surface dislocation densities $\bar{\alpha}$. Defining the elastic potential

$$(2.14) \quad \hat{H} = \hat{W} - \int_V [f_i u_i - \alpha_{ij} \phi_{ij}] d^3x - \int_{S_1} t_i u_i d^2x + \int_{S_3} \bar{\alpha}_{ij} \phi_{ij} d^2x$$

where t_i is prescribed on S_1 and $\bar{\alpha}_{ij}$ is prescribed on S_3, we can take the variation of this with the forces f, the tractions t, the dislocation density α and the surface dislocation density $\bar{\alpha}$ held constant.

$$(2.15) \quad \delta\hat{H} = \int_V \sigma^a_{ij} (\delta\beta^a_{ij}) d^3x \quad - \int_V f_i (\delta u_i) d^3x \quad - \int_{S_1} t_i (\delta u_i) d^2x$$

$$+ \int_V (\delta\sigma^i_{ij}) \beta_{ij} d^3x \quad + \int_V \alpha_{ij} (\delta\phi_{ij}) d^3x \quad + \int_{S_3} \bar{\alpha}_{ij} (\delta\phi_{ij}) d^2x$$

$$= \int_V \sigma^a_{ij} \partial_j (\delta u_i) d^3x \quad - \ldots$$

$$+ \int_V [\varepsilon_{psj} \partial_s (\delta\phi_{ip})] \beta_{ij} d^3x + \ldots$$

$$= \int_V \partial_j [\sigma^a_{ij} (\delta u_i)] d^3x \quad - \int_S (\partial_j \sigma^a_{ij}) (\delta u_i) d^3x \quad - \ldots$$

$$+ \int_V \varepsilon_{psj} \partial_s \beta_{ij} (\delta\phi_{ip})] d^3x \quad - \int_S (\varepsilon_{psj} \partial_s \beta_{ij}) (\delta\phi_{ip}) d^3x + \ldots$$

With Gauss and the fact that $\delta u_i = 0$ on the complement S_2 of S_1, and the fact that $\delta\phi_{ij} = 0$ on the complement S_4 of S_3, it follows that (2.9), (2.10) and the two equations (2.13) are the variational equations that make H an extremum. The prescription of $\bar{\alpha}$ on S_3 is equivalent to the prescription of the displacement on S_3, so that $S_2 = S_3$ and $S_1 = S_4$. This fact is very much exploited in boundary integral equation methods.

Multiplication of (2.10) gives a more advantageous form

(2.16) $$\partial_n \beta_{mr} - \partial_r \beta_{mn} = \varepsilon_{rnt} \alpha_{mt}$$

From the definition (2.10) it also follows that the dislocation density, so to say the source of internal distorsions, is divergence free in the second index

(2.17) $$\partial_t \alpha_{mt} = 0$$

while no such differential condition has to be obeyed by the force density f which is, so to say, the source of the external stresses. This means that forces can be arranged at free will, but dislocations cannot, a fact that will become important when the forces of interaction between forces and dislocations and dislocations and forces is studied. For forces the connection between the displacements $u_k(x)$ and $f_i(x')$ is given by the Green tensor

(2.18) $$u_k(x) = \int G_{ki}(x,x') f_i(x') d^3x'$$

Practically this formula is only of use for an infinite homogeneous medium, where G depends only on the difference $|x-x'|$ and (2.18) becomes a convolution

(2.19) $$u_k = G_{ki} * f \qquad \beta_{ks} = \partial_s G_{ki} * f_i$$

which allows use of the convenient rules for differentiation of convolutions

(2.20) $$\partial_s [g*h] = (\partial_s g)*h = g*(\partial_s h)$$

The Green function has to be determined from the coupled set of partial differential equations

(2.21) $$\partial_i C_{ijkl} \partial_k G_{jn}(x,x') + \delta_{jn} \delta(x-x') = 0$$

For any variational we have in a linear elastic solid

(2.22) $$\delta\hat{W} = \frac{1}{2} \delta \int C_{abij}(x) \varepsilon_{ab}(x) \varepsilon_{ij}(x) d^3x = \int \sigma_{ji}(\delta\beta_{ji}) d^3x + \frac{1}{2}\int \varepsilon_{ab} \varepsilon_{ji} \delta C_{abji} d^3x$$

§3. TRANSLATIONAL VARIATION, ENERGY-MOMENTUM-TENSORS

The variation δ is arbitrary. By specifying this variation in one or the other way, various physical quantities and conservation theorems result. When this idea was proposed by Emmy Noether 65 years ago, it was quite a novelty. Today it is a standard tool of field theorists.

In a magnificent series of papers Eshelby [5, 6, 7, 8, 9, 10] introduced the concept of the energy momentum tensor to elasticity. Though he formulated the theory in order to find the force on a defect, he never allowed the presence of body forces associated with the defect, nor did he allow for calculation of the force felt by part of the defect. Being interested in a symmetric formulation of the theory, we will allow for the presence of forces and the presence of continuous distributions of dislocations, so that no displacement may be definable anywhere. This will make it possible to find the force felt by a volume within which dislocations and body forces are present. Moreover, dislocations and spatial distributions of forces might actually cut through the surface of the volume under consideration. This will allow application of the theory to self-stress problems.

In this section we want to consider forces and must, therefore, use the translational variation

(3.1) $$\delta = \delta x_k \partial_k$$

By applying (3.1) to β and C in (2.22) we get

(3.2) $$\delta\hat{W} = \int \{\sigma_{ji}\partial_k \beta_{ji} + \tfrac{1}{2}\epsilon_{ab}\epsilon_{ji}\partial_k C_{abji}\}\delta x_k \, d^3x =$$
$$= \int \{\sigma_{ji}[\partial_k \beta_{ji} - \partial_i \beta_{jk}] + \tfrac{1}{2}\epsilon_{ab}\epsilon_{ji}\partial_k C_{abji} + \sigma_{ji}\partial_i \beta_{jk}\}\delta x_k \, d^3x$$

The second equation follows from the first by addition and subtraction of the same term. The last term can be rewritten to yield

(3.3) $$\delta\hat{W} = \int \sigma_{ji}[\partial_k \beta_{ji} - \partial_i \beta_{jk}]\delta x_k d^3x + \tfrac{1}{2}\int \epsilon_{ab}\epsilon_{ji}\partial_k C_{abji} \delta x_k \, d^3x$$
$$+ \int \partial_i(\sigma_{ji}\beta_{jk})\delta x_k d^3x - \int \beta_{jk}[\partial_i \sigma_{ji}] \delta x_k d^3x$$

The square brackets of the first and the fourth integral are transformed with (2.9) and (2.16), and the total differential of the third term is moved to the left. Moreover, the variation of the total energy $\hat{W}$ is the integral over the variation of the local energy density w

(3.4) $$\delta\hat{W} = \int \delta w \, d^3x = \int (\partial_i w)\delta_{ik}\delta x_k \, d^3x$$

If the terms that are a pure divergence and can be transformed to surface integrals over the boundary of the volume under consideration are collected at one side, and the terms that involve the sources f_j and α_{jt} at the other side

(3.5) $$\int [\epsilon_{ikt}\sigma_{ji}\alpha_{jt} + f_j \dot\beta_{jk} + \tfrac{1}{2}\epsilon_{ab}\epsilon_{ji}\partial_k C_{abji}] \, \delta x_k \, d^3x =$$
$$\int \partial_i[w\delta_{ik} - \sigma_{ji}\beta_{jk}] \qquad \delta x_k \, d^3x =$$
$$\int \qquad\qquad F_k \qquad\qquad \delta x_k \, d^3x$$

- 374 -

One concludes that there must be a physical meaning to the integrands, because the first one refers to the sources and the second one to the surface. It is commonly called F_k, has the dimension of a force and is called the configurational force. The variations δx_k being arbitrary there follows the identity

$$(3.6) \quad F_k = \varepsilon_{ikt}\sigma_{ji}\alpha_{jt} + f_j\beta_{jk} + \frac{1}{2}\varepsilon_{ab}\varepsilon_{ji}\partial_k C_{abji} =$$

$$= \partial_i[w\delta_{ik} - \sigma_{ji}\beta_{jk}]$$

for any volume in the body. The first part of (3.6) is a generalized form of the Peach-Koehler **formula** that describes the configurational force felt by a dislocation in presence of a stress field. Indeed for $f_j=0$ and constant C and $\alpha_{jt} = b_j t_t$ the familiar Peach-Koehler formula

$$(3.7) \quad F_k = \varepsilon_{ikt}\sigma_{ji}b_j t_t$$

is obtained. Here b is the Burgers vector and t the tangent line element of the dislocation. A slight modification is necessary if not only dislocation glide but also climb is to be allowed for. In climb there is an additional volume change

$$(3.8) \quad \delta V = \varepsilon_{ikt}\alpha_{it}\delta x_k$$

which under the hydrostatic pressure $p = \sigma_{ss}/3$ does the external work

$$(3.9) \quad p\delta V = \varepsilon_{ikt}\alpha_{it}\delta x_k = \sigma_{ss}\varepsilon_{ikt}\alpha_{it}\delta x_k/3$$

On the left hand side of (3.2) one must consider the enthalpy $\hat{W}+pV$ instead of the internal energy $\hat{W}$ alone. This leaves the second part of (3.6) unchanged, but the first part is modified to

$$(3.10) \quad F_k = \varepsilon_{ikt}[\sigma_{ji} - \sigma_{ss}\delta_{ji}/3]\alpha_{jt} + f_j\beta_{jk} + \frac{1}{2}\varepsilon_{ab}\varepsilon_{ji}\partial_k C_{abji}$$

Besides the Peach-Koehler force felt by a dislocation in the presence of stress, (3.6) also introduces the concept of the configurational force felt by a force in the presence of a distorsion. This was noted earlier by Cherepanov [11]

$$(3.11) \quad F_k = f_j\beta_{jk}$$

Additionally, (3.6) also contains the force felt by the inhomogeneity of the medium [5]

$$(3.12) \quad F_k = \frac{1}{2}\varepsilon_{ab}\varepsilon_{ji}\partial_k C_{abji} = -\frac{1}{2}\sigma_{ab}\sigma_{ji}\partial_k S_{abji}$$

where S is the compliance tensor.

Since the derivation started from the total stress and distorsion present (never mind external or internal sources) it is clear that in (3.6) the total stress and the total distorsion give rise to the force F_k, and that it does not matter if they are external or internal. The choice of the volume under consideration was arbitrary, therefore they can also be image stresses from a surface or self-stresses and strains and whatever. For image stresses and (3.7) this point was elaborated by Gavazza and Barnett [12] and Eshelby [13].

The more important fact is, however, that neither the pressure modification nor the inhomogeneity enter the second part of equs. (3.6). The square bracket there is called the energy-momentum tensor.

$$(3.13) \qquad P_{ki} = w\delta_{ik} - \sigma_{ji}\beta_{jk}$$

and has the property that

$$(3.14) \qquad \text{Trace } P = P_{ii} = w$$

Now, in any case

$$(3.15) \qquad \int F_k(x) d^3x = \int \partial_i P_{ki}(x) d^3x = \int P_{ki} n_i dS$$

where this is the total force acting on all sources α_{jt} and f_j and inhomogeneities $\partial_k C_{abji}$ present within the volume over which d^3x is integrated. If the total differential is used for a transformation to a surface integral, $P_{ki}n_i$ gives the configurational force acting upon, felt by, anything discernible within the inclosed volume, be it a dislocation, force density or inhomogeneity. There is no need for these to be in any way singular, they can be smoothly distributed. In this sense (3.6) gives the force felt by all the "defects" within the volume considered. In absence of forces and dislocations ($\alpha_{jt}=f_j=0$) but with an inhomogeneity present, the surface integral (3.15) can be contracted to the discontinuity of P_{ki} across the interface and is equal to the force felt by that interface (Eshelby [7]). If the medium is homogeneous and neither forces nor dislocations are present, there is nothing to feel a configurational force and in that case P_{ki} is divergence free in the second index.

$$(3.16) \qquad \partial_i P_{ki} = 0$$

Of course the surface S can be arbitrarily deformed by including regions where $\alpha_{jt} = f_j = 0$ so that because of (3.16) $n_i P_{ki}$ gives no additional contributions from that region. The derivation shows that just as there is no need to restrict the concept of the energy-momentum tensor to elastic singularities, the continuous distributions can cut through the surface of the volume under consideration.

The question arises how the configurational force F_k is to be interpreted. Since in the absence of deformation, when $\beta=0$, the equs. (3.6, 11,15) give $F_k=0$ even in the presence of a body force $f_j \neq 0$, one concludes that F_k cannot be the total force. One either has to add the body force f to the configurational force F to obtain the total force $F^* = F + f$, or one can write in the equations $(1+\beta)$ instead of β and the total force F^* instead of the configurational force F. This defines another energy momentum tensor

(3.17) $\quad P^*_{ki} = w\delta_{ki} - \sigma_{ji}(\delta_{jk} + \beta_{jk}) = P_{ki} - \sigma_{ki}$

The divergence of P^* is the total force F^*, the divergence of P is the configurational force F. The advantage of (3.15) over the Peach-Koehler formulation (3.6a) is that no singularities need to occur : S can be taken in such a way that P_{ki} remains well behaved, it need not be known where the defect is situated within the volume enclosed. This, of course, can be important for experiments. The force felt by a crack (which is the equivalent to a dislocation pile-up) is conveniently treated by using the energy-momentum tensor concept (Bilby and Eshelby [14]) or the equivalent J-integral [15] . The disadvantage is that the surface S is not easily contracted so far that self-stress problems can be tackled. It seems that the same divergencies occur as in the Peach-Koehler formulation, if self-force effects are to be handled [16].

The Peach-Koehler formula or the concept of the energy-momentum tensor are special cases of so-called Γ-integrals which can be used to derive forces acting on singularities (Cherepanov [17]). Another general remark concerns the fact that the source of the energy-momentum tensor is recognized from (3.5) to be the product of stress and dislocation density, or the product of distorsion and body forces, or, more generally, the product of sources and conjugate fields. This is similar to electrodynamics, where the source of the energy-momentum tensor is the product of the electromagnetic field and the current

§4. THE NONLINEAR HOMOGENEOUS CASE

In the above derivation for the linear case we did essentially the following: we started from a direct product in differential form (2.22)

(4.1) $\quad \hat{W} = \int \bar{T}_{ij} \delta(A_{ij} - \delta_{ij}) \, d^3X$

and we derived that, with the differential operators now taken with respect to the coordinates (capital) X one can obtain an expression that contains $\bar{T}$ and (A-1). The difference to (2.22) is the change from σ to $\bar{T}$ and from $\delta\beta$ to $\delta(A-1) = \delta A$. With this transcription (3.5) reads for the homogeneous case

$$\text{(4.2)} \quad \begin{aligned} &\int [\varepsilon_{ikt}\bar{T}_{ji}(\text{Rot}A)_{jt} - (\text{Div}\bar{T})_j (A_{jk}-\delta_{jk})] \; \delta X_k \; d^3X = \\ &\int \partial [W\delta_{ik} - \bar{T}_{ji}(A_{jk}-\delta_{jk})]/\partial X_i \quad \delta X_k \; d^3X = \\ &\int F_k \qquad\qquad\qquad\qquad\qquad\qquad \delta X_k \; d^3X \end{aligned}$$

But equ. (4.1) is the proper expression for nonlinear elasticity if $\bar{T}$ is the (nonsymmetric) first Piola-Kirchoff stress tensor

(4.3) $$\bar{T}_{ik} = \partial W/\partial A_{ik}$$

and A is the distorsion defined by

(4.4) $$dx_k = A_{km} dX_m$$

Here X are the (Lagrangian) coordinates in the reference state and x are the (Eulerian) coordinates in the current configuration. W is the energy density per reference volume. The energy-momentum tensors for the nonlinear theory are then

(4.5) $$P_{ki} = W\delta_{ik} - \bar{T}_{ji}(A_{jk}-\delta_{jk}) = W\delta_{ik} - \bar{T}_{ji}A_{jk} + \bar{T}_{ki} = \overset{*}{P}_{ki} + \bar{T}_{ki}$$

which is analogous to (3.17). If one looks for a Peach-Koehler type formula that should give the force on a dislocation density because of the presence of some stress, one has to try to transform the first part of (4.2) into a form containing one of the three distinct types of dislocation density defined in a nonlinear theory. Besides the true dislocation density $\bar{\alpha}$ there is also the local dislocation density α and Noll's dislocation density $\tilde{\alpha}$. They are related by [18]

(4.6) $$\alpha = A\bar{\alpha} = jA\tilde{\alpha}A^T$$

where, as (4.7) $\quad 1/j = J = \det A = d^3x/d^3X$

There are three stress tensors defined: Besides the (symmetric) Cauchy stress T there is also the Piola-Kirchoff stress of the first kind $\bar{T}$ and the (symmetric) Piola-Kirchoff stress of the second kind $\tilde{T}$. They are related by

(4.8) $$T = j\bar{T}A^T = jA\tilde{T}A^T$$

In the presence of dislocations the equilibrium condition in terms of the first Piola-Kirchoff stress $\bar{T}$ is modified [2, 19]. Starting from the equilibrium condition in terms of the Cauchy stress T

(4.9) $$\partial T_{jk}/\partial x_k + \rho b_j = 0$$

we find from the definition (4.8) that

(4.10) $$j\partial \bar{T}_{js}/\partial X_s + \bar{T}_{js}[\partial(jA_{ks})/\partial x_k] + b_j\rho = 0$$

The square bracket is found as follows: Since the determinant $|A^{-1}|=j$ is a linear function of its elements,

(4.11) $$j = A^{-1}_{\mu m} (\partial j/\partial A^{-1}_{\mu m})$$

(4.12) $$[\partial j/\partial A^{-1}_{\mu s}][\partial A^{-1}_{\mu s}/\partial x_1] = jA_{s\mu}[\partial A^{-1}_{\mu s}/\partial x_1] = \partial j/\partial x_1$$

On the other hand
$$\partial (jA_{1\lambda})/\partial x_1 = A_{1\lambda} \partial j/\partial x_1 + j\, \partial A_{1\lambda}/\partial x_1$$

and
(4.13) $$\partial (jA_{1\lambda})/\partial x_1 = jA_{1\lambda} A_{m\mu}[\partial A^{-1}_{\mu m}/\partial x_1 - \partial A^{-1}_{\mu 1}/\partial x_m] = -\varepsilon_{m1t}\bar{\alpha}_{\mu t} jA_{1\lambda} A_{m\mu}$$

so that, with (4.6)

(4.14) $$\partial (jA_{1\lambda})/\partial x_1 = jA_{1\lambda} \varepsilon_{1mt}\alpha_{mt} = j\varepsilon_{\lambda mt}\tilde{\alpha}_{mt}$$

where the last identity emerges after somewhat lengthy calculations. The equilibrium condition becomes, with $\rho_o = \rho J$

(4.15) $$-\rho_o b_j - \bar{T}_{js}\varepsilon_{sab}\tilde{\alpha}_{ab} = -\rho_o b_j - JT_{js}\varepsilon_{sab}\alpha_{ab} = \partial \bar{T}_{js}/\partial X_s$$

The RotA term in (4.2) has to be rewritten in a form that contains one of the familiar dislocation densities (4.6). The true dislocation density is defined

(4.16a) $$\text{rotA}^{-1} = -\bar{\alpha} \qquad \varepsilon_{rsm}\partial (A^{-1}_{kr})/\partial x_s = -\bar{\alpha}_{km}$$

Just as (2.10) implied (2.16) this equation implies

(4.16b) $$[\partial (A^{-1}_{kr})/\partial x_n] - [\partial (A^{-1}_{kn})/\partial x_r] = -\varepsilon_{rnt}\bar{\alpha}_{kt}$$

Now $(\text{RotA})_{mt} = \varepsilon_{pst}\partial A_{mp}/\partial X_s \underset{4}{=} \varepsilon_{pst} A_{as}\partial A_{mp}/\partial x_a = -\varepsilon_{pst} A_{as} A_{mx}[\partial A^{-1}_{xy}/\partial x_a]A_{yp} =$

$= -\varepsilon_{pst} A_{as} A_{mx}[\partial (A^{-1}_{xy})/\partial x_a - \partial A^{-1}_{xa}/\partial x_y]A_{yp} - \varepsilon_{pst} A_{as} A_{mx}[\partial A^{-1}_{xa}/\partial x_y]A_{yp} =$

$= -\varepsilon_{pst}\varepsilon_{yaz} A_{as} A_{mx}\bar{\alpha}_{xz} A_{yp} - \varepsilon_{pst} A_{mx}(\partial A^{-1}_{xa}/\partial X_p)A_{as} \underset{4}{=}$

$= -\varepsilon_{pst}\varepsilon_{yaz} A_{as} A_{mx}\bar{\alpha}_{xz} A_{yp} + \varepsilon_{pst}\partial A_{ms}/\partial X_p$

The last term on the right hand side is the negative of the left hand side. With (4.6) a form containing the local density α is found.

(4.17) $$(\text{RotA})_{mt} = \tfrac{1}{2}\varepsilon_{pst}\varepsilon_{yaz} A_{as}\alpha_{mz} A_{yp}$$

With (4.12) and (4.17) inserted into the integrand of (4.2) we find a nonlinear Peach-Koehler formula for the configurational force

(4.18) $\quad F_k = J\varepsilon_{yaz} T_{my} \alpha_{mz} A_{ak} + (\bar{T}_{js}\varepsilon_{sab}\tilde{\alpha}_{ab} + \rho_o b_j)(A_{jk} - \delta_{jk}) = \partial P^*_{ki}/\partial X_i + \partial \bar{T}_{ki}/\partial X_i$

Suppose now we had defined another tensor in terms of current coordinates, say

(4.19) $\quad\quad\quad\quad\quad \Sigma^*_{kl} = \partial w / \partial A^{-1}_{kl}$

An explicit form for this in terms of A and T is found as follows. Since

(4.20) $\quad\quad\quad\quad\quad \partial j / \partial A^{-1}_{kl} = j A_{lk}$

and

(4.21) $\quad\quad\quad\quad\quad \partial A_{mn}/\partial A^{-1}_{kl} = -A_{ln}A_{mk} \quad\quad \partial A^{-1}_{xy}/\partial A_{mn} = -A^{-1}_{xm}A^{-1}_{ny}$

we can write

(4.22) $\quad \Sigma^*_{kl} = \partial(jW)/\partial A^{-1}_{kl} = W \partial j/\partial A^{-1}_{kl} + j\partial W/\partial A^{-1}_{kl} = A_{lk}w - T_{ml}A_{mk}$

By inversion there follows an equation for T [20]

(4.23) $\quad\quad\quad\quad\quad T_{ad} = w\delta_{ad} - \frac{\partial w}{\partial A^{-1}_{xa}} A^{-1}_{xd}$

Had we now started with the variation appropriate for (4.19)

(4.24) $\quad\quad\quad\quad\quad \delta w = \int \Sigma^*_{kl} \delta(A^{-1}_{kl} - \delta_{kl}) d^3x$

we would have got, instead of (4.2)

(4.25) $\quad \int [\varepsilon_{ikt}\Sigma^*_{ji}(\text{rot}A^{-1})_{jt} - (\text{div}\overset{*}{\Sigma})_j (A^{-1}_{jk} - \delta_{jk})] \delta x_k \, d^3x =$

$\quad\quad\quad \int \partial [w\delta_{ik} - \Sigma^*_{ji}(A^{-1}_{jk} - \delta_{jk})]/\partial x_i \quad\quad \delta x_k \, d^3x =$

$\quad\quad\quad \int \quad\quad\quad\quad\quad \Psi_k \quad\quad\quad\quad\quad\quad \delta x_k \, d^3x$

say. This defines an energy-momentum tensor

(4.26) $\quad \Sigma_{ki} = [w\delta_{ik} - \Sigma^*_{ji}A^{-1}_{jk} + \Sigma^*_{ji}] \underset{4.23}{=} T_{ki} + \Sigma^*_{ki}$

so that (4.27) $\quad \partial \Sigma_{ki}/\partial x_i = \Psi_k$

With (4.22)

$$\Psi_k = -\varepsilon_{ikt}\Sigma^*_{ji}\bar{\alpha}_{jt} - (A^{-1}_{jk}-\delta_{jk})[\partial(A_{1j}w)/\partial x_1 - A_{mj}\partial T_{ml}/\partial x_1 - T_{ml}\partial A_{mj}/\partial x_1] =$$
(4.28)
$$= -\varepsilon_{ikt}A_{ij}\bar{\alpha}_{jt}w + \varepsilon_{ikt}T_{si}A_{sj}\bar{\alpha}_{jt} + (\delta_{jk}-A^{-1}_{jk})\{\rho b_m A_{mj} + [\partial(A_{1j}w)/\partial x_1 - T_{ml}\partial A_{mj}/\partial x_1]\}$$

The square bracket is transformed according to

$$[\ ] = W\partial(jA_{1j})/\partial x_1 + jA_{1j}\partial W/\partial x_1 - T_{ml}\partial A_{mj}/\partial x_1 =$$
$$ \qquad\qquad\qquad\qquad\qquad\qquad\qquad\qquad 4.16$$
$$= W\varepsilon_{jab}\tilde{\alpha}_{ab} + j[\partial W/\partial A_{kl}][\partial A_{kl}/\partial X_j] - j\bar{T}_{ms}\partial A_{kj}/\partial x_1 =$$
$$\qquad\qquad\qquad\qquad\qquad\qquad\qquad\qquad\qquad 4.21,13$$
$$= W\varepsilon_{jab}\tilde{\alpha}_{ab} + j\bar{T}_{kl}\varepsilon_{1jt}(RotA)_{kt} = W\varepsilon_{jab}\tilde{\alpha}_{ab} + T_{mj}\varepsilon_{yaz}\alpha_{mz}A_{aj}$$

so that the Peach-Koehler formula in current coordinates becomes

(4.29) $$\Psi_k = \varepsilon_{yaz}T_{my}\alpha_{mz}A_{ak} - \rho b_k + \rho b_m A_{mk}$$
$$-\varepsilon_{ikt}\alpha_{it}w - W[\varepsilon_{jab}A^{-1}_{jk} - \varepsilon_{kab}]\tilde{\alpha}_{ab}$$

If we compare now F_k and Ψ_k we find

(4.30) $$J\Psi_k - F_k = P_{ks}\varepsilon_{sab}\tilde{\alpha}_{ab}$$

This allows us to write instead of (4.28)

(4.31) $$\Psi_k = \varepsilon_{yaz}T_{my}\alpha_{mz}A_{ak} + b_j(A_{jk}-\delta_{jk}) + (jA^T\bar{T} + P^*)_{js}\varepsilon_{sab}\tilde{\alpha}_{ab}$$

§5. LAGRANGIAN AND EULERIAN FORM

A comparison of the forces in both cases shows that

(5.1) $$(Jdiv\Sigma - DivP)_k = P_{ks}\varepsilon_{sab}\tilde{\alpha}_{ab}$$

or, if transformed to surface integrals,

(5.2) $$\int\Sigma_{kn}ds_n - \int P_{kn}dS_n = \int P_{ks}\varepsilon_{sab}\tilde{\alpha}_{ab}\,d^3X$$

The equation of equilibrium (4.17) was

(5.3) $$(JdivT - Div\bar{T})_k = \bar{T}_{ks}\varepsilon_{sab}\tilde{\alpha}_{ab}$$

or, (5.4) $$\int T_{kn}ds_n - \int\bar{T}_{kn}dS_n = \int\bar{T}_{ks}\varepsilon_{sab}\tilde{\alpha}_{ab}\,d^3X$$

By addition according to (4.5) and (4.26) it follows that

(5.5) $$(Jdiv\Sigma^* - DivP^*)_k = P^*_{ks}\varepsilon_{sab}\tilde{\alpha}_{ab}$$

or, (5.6) $$\int\Sigma^*_{kn}ds_n - \int P^*_{kn}dS_n = \int P^*_{ks}\varepsilon_{sab}\tilde{\alpha}_{ab}\,d^3X$$

Equation (5.2) is at variance with equations (48) and (6.1) of Eshelby (1970, 1975), respectively, who has zero on the right hand side. The inhomogeneous forms (5.1) to (5.6) arise because the presence of dislocations is allowed for. It seems that indeed the force felt by a volume element d^3x is Ψ_k, and by the volume element d^3X is F_k. The difference between the two, (4.30) is attributable to the dislocation density $\tilde{\alpha}$, which vanishes only when α and $\bar{\alpha}$ vanish and displacements are defined.

Altogether P^* is conjugate to the Cauchy stress T

(5.7) $\quad P^*_{1j} = W\delta_{1j} - [\partial W/\partial A_{ij}]A_{i1} \qquad T_{1j} = w\delta_{1j} - [\partial w/\partial A^{-1}_{ij}]A^{-1}_{i1}$

and the first Piola-Kirchoff stress $\bar{T}$ is conjugate to Σ^*

(5.8) $\quad \bar{T}_{kl} = \partial W/\partial A_{kl} \qquad\qquad\qquad \Sigma^*_{kl} = \partial w/\partial A^{-1}_{kl}$

but P and Σ are conjugate

(5.9) $\quad P_{1j} = W\delta_{1j} - [\partial W/\partial A_{ij}](A_{i1}-\delta_{i1}) \qquad \Sigma_{1j} = w\delta_{1j} - [\partial w/\partial A^{-1}_{ij}](A^{-1}_{i1}-\delta_{i1})$

References

[1] E. Kroener: Kontinuumstheorie der Versetzungen und Eigenspannungen, Springer, Berlin, 1958.
[2] W. Noll: Archive for Rational Mechanics and Analysis 27 (1967) 1.
[3] B.K.D. Gairola: Nonlinear Elastic Problems, in: Dislocations in Solids, F.R.N. Nabarro, ed., North Holland, Amsterdam-New-York-Oxford, vol.1, p. 223, 1979.
[4] E. Noether: Goettinger Nachr.(Math.-Phys.Klasse) (1918) 235.
[5] J.D. Eshelby: Phil. Trans. A 244 (1951) 87.
[6] J.D. Eshelby: in Progr. in Solid State Physics, F. Seitz and D. Turnbull, eds., Academic Press, New York, p.79, vol.3, 1956.
[7] J. D. Eshelby: in Inelastic Behaviour of Solids, M.F. Kanninen, W.F.Adler, A.R. Rosenfeld and R.I. Jaffee, eds., Mc Graw-Hill, New York, p.77, 1970.
[8] J.D. Eshelby: in Prospects of Fracture Mechanics, G.C. Shih, ed., Noordhoff, Leyden, p. 69, 1975.
[9] J.D. Eshelby: J. Elasticity 5 (1975) 321.
[10] J.D. Eshelby: in Proceedings of the Third International Symposium on Continuum Models of Discrete Systems, Freudenstadt, E. Kroener and K.H. Anthony, eds., University of Waterloo Press, p. 651, 1980.

[11] G.P. Cherepanov: Engin. Fract. Mech. 14 (1981) 39.

[12] S.D. Gavazza and D.M. Barnett: Scripta Metall. 9 (1975) 1263.

[13] J.D. Eshelby: Boundary Problems, in: Dislocations in Solids, F.R.N. Nabarro, ed., North Holland, Amsterdam-New York- Oxford, vol.1, p.168, 1979.

[14] B.A. Bilby and J.D. Eshelby: in Fracture, H. Liebowitz, ed., Academic Press, New York, vol.1, p. 99, 1968.

[15] J. Rice: in Fracture, H. Liebowitz, ed., Academic Press, New York, vol.2, p. 191, 1968.

[16] H.O.K. Kirchner: Phil. Mag. A43 (1981) 1393.

[17] G. P. Cherepanov: Mechanics of Brittle Fracture, Mc Graw-Hill, New York, 1979.

[18] C. Teodosiu: Elastic Models of Crystal Defects, Springer, Berlin-Heidelberg-New York, 1982.

[19] C. Teodosiu and A. Seeger: Non-Linear Dynamic Problems for Anisotropic Elastic Bodies in the Continuum Theory of Dislocations, in: Fundamental Aspects of Dislocation Theory, J.A. Simmons, R. deWit and R. Bullough, eds., NBS, Washington, Spec. Publ. 317, II, p. 877, 1970

[20] P. Chadwick: J. Elasticity 5 (1975) 249.

SIMULATION OF KINKS AND JOGS IN DISLOCATIONS USING POINT FORCE ARRAYS

J.-P. J. Georges* and C. S. Hartley**

*Formerly Graduate Student, Department of Engineering Science and Mechanics, University of Florida, Gainesville, Florida, 32611

**Professor, Materials Group, Department of Mechanical Engineering, Louisiana State University, Baton Rouge, Louisiana 70803

INTRODUCTION

Atomic displacements associated with the presence of point defects in crystals have been accurately simulated by an harmonic lattice model in which an array of forces are applied to first and second nearest neighbors of the defect [1]. The success of this model led to the construction of a non-local force model for a vacancy in a continuum [2]. In this construction forces are imposed on points in the continuum corresponding to the initial positions of atoms in the vicinity of the defect. When the forces are chosen to give the same strength as an equivalent defect in the lattice model, displacements at points in the continuum corresponding to the initial positions of atoms in the perfect lattice agree well with those obtained from the more detailed model. Models of extended defects consist of the superposition of force arrays corresponding to point defects.

Local continuum theory permits the synthesis of various configurations of dislocations by the superposition of arrays of infinitesimal loops consisting of displacement dipoles or the corresponding force multipoles [3-5]. A similar construction results when dislocations in crystals are formed by arrays of primitive loops, i.e. hypothetical point defects in the lattice having the long-range displacement field of infinitesimal dislocation loops. Two basic types of primitive loops suffice to describe all possible dislocation arrays: the prismatic loop, consisting of a vacancy collapsed in a direction normal to the plane of the loop, and the shear loop, consisting of an array of forces which create a state of pure shear. In each case the area of the loop, δS, is chosen so that the magnitude of its product with the burgers vector of the loop equals one atomic volume. Force arrays forming primitive prismatic loops have been obtained for isotropic simple cubic [6] body-centered and face-centered cubic lattices [7]. Corresponding models for shear loops have been constructed for isotropic simple cubic [6] and body-centered cubic lattices [7].

Energies and displacement fields associated with dislocations formed from primitive loops contain terms which depend on force constants, relating forces to the displacement of their points of application. The displacement field, $u_k(\underline{r})$, due to a point force, $F_m(\underline{r}')$, in a continuum is

(1) $\quad u_k(\underline{r}) = G_{km}(\underline{r} - \underline{r}')F_m(\underline{r}'),$

where $G_{km}(\underline{r} - \underline{r}')$ represents the symmetric Green's tensor giving the displacement at $\underline{r}$ due to a unit point force at $\underline{r}'$. Determination of the displacement of the point at which the force is applied requires definition of Green's function at $\underline{r} = \underline{r}'$. An averaging procedure results in the definition of a "point force core," R_o, as the radius of a sphere centered on the point at which the force is applied. For an isotropic material,

(2) $\quad u_k(\underline{r}') = F_k(\underline{r}')/4\pi\mu R_o = F_k(\underline{r}')/\alpha$

where μ represents the shear modulus. The quantity $4\pi\mu R_o$ can be interpreted as an interatomic force constant, α, when the force arises from the gradient of an interatomic potential.

The relationship between the force constant and the elastic constants follows from the theory of metallic cohesion [8], which gives

(3) $\quad \dfrac{\beta\Omega}{2} = \dfrac{1}{2}\left(\dfrac{\partial^2 W}{\partial \varepsilon^2}\right)$

where β, Ω, W and ε represent the bulk modulus, atomic volume, interatomic potential energy and dilatation, respectively. Differentiating equation 1, using the isotropic Green function and equation 2 yields[1]

(4) $\quad \varepsilon = u_{k,k} = -\alpha u/8\pi\mu R_o^2 = -2\pi\mu u/\alpha$

whence

(5) $\quad \dfrac{\partial^2 W}{\partial \varepsilon^2} = \left(\dfrac{\alpha^2}{4\pi^2\mu^2}\right)\left(\dfrac{\partial^2 W}{\partial u^2}\right).$

For an harmonic potential, $\alpha = \partial^2 W/\partial u^2$, so equations 3 and 5 yield

(6) $\quad \beta\Omega = \alpha^3/4\pi^2\mu^2 = 2\mu(1 + \nu)\Omega/3(1 - 2\nu)$

or

(7) $\quad (\alpha^3/\mu^3\Omega) = 8\pi^2(1 + \nu)/3(1 - 2\nu).$

For a simple cubic structure having $\nu = 1/3$, $(\alpha/\mu a) = 4.72$ and $(R_o/a) = 0.375$. This relationship between force constants and elastic constants removes the singularity in the displacement field due to a point force and permits a complete calculation of the atomic displacements due to an array of forces, subject to the approximation of an harmonic potential.

This paper describes the application of these concepts to the calculation of kinks and jogs in screw and edge dislocations in an isotropic, simple cubic lattice. The next section reviews concepts associated with primitive loops. A description of the construction of rectangular glide and prismatic loops follows, succeeded by an illustration of the construction of

---

[1] Summation from 1 to 3 over repeated subscripts is implied and ,k refers to partial differentiation with respect to x_k.

a rectangular glide loop. Finally, kinks and jogs on the straight dislocations will be simulated by adding suitable arrays of primitive loops. In some of the preceding cases, energies and displacement fields for extended defects will be presented.

PRIMITIVE LOOPS

An infinitesimal dislocation loop in a continuum constitutes a center of plastic strain having the form [4]

$$(8) \quad \varepsilon_{ij}^P = Q_{ij}/|\underline{b}||\underline{\delta S}|$$

where

$$(9) \quad Q_{ij} = (b_i n_j)^S \delta S$$

with $(b_i n_j)^S$ representing the symmetric part of the dyadic product of the burgers vector, $\underline{b}$, and the normal, $\underline{n}$, to the plane of a loop having an area δS. The plastic stress source, P_{ij}^P, defines the associated force dipole:

$$(10) \quad P_{ij}^P = C_{ijkl}\varepsilon_{kl}^P = P_{ij}/|\underline{b}||\underline{\delta S}|$$

where P_{ij} represents the strength of the force dipole and C_{ijkl} is the tensor of elastic constants.

The force dipoles constituting a primitive loop result from placing point forces at the initial positions of atoms corresponding to the nearest neighbors of the loop. Since

$$(11) \quad P_{ij} = F_i h_j$$

defines the strength of a dipole consisting of equal and opposite forces, F_i, applied to points separated by a vector h_j, knowledge of the strength of the double force tensor and the points of application of the forces permits determination of the forces,

$$(12) \quad F_i = P_{ij}h_j/|\underline{h}|^2,$$

which lead to the displacement field of the defect,

$$(13) \quad u_m(\underline{r}) = \sum_{n=1}^{N} G_{mk}(\underline{r} - \underline{r}'_n)F_k(\underline{r}'_n),$$

for N forces $F_k(\underline{r}'_n)$, applied at points $\underline{r}'_n$ from the origin.

Figure 1 illustrates a primitive prismatic loop on an {100} plane in a simple cubic lattice. In this case the burgers vector, $b_i = a\delta_{i3}$, and the loop normal, $n_j = \delta_{j3}$. Forces applied to the atomic positions surrounding the loop are

$$(14) \quad F_1 = F_2 = \lambda a^2/2; \quad F_3 = (\lambda + 2\mu)a^2/2.$$

The corresponding shear loop is shown in Figure 2. In this case the forces are

$$(15) \quad F_2 = F_3 = \mu a^2; \quad F_2' = -F_3' = \sqrt{2}\mu a^2/2$$

for $b_i = a\delta_{i2}$ and $n_j = \delta_{j3}$. The following section illustrates how rectangular dislocation loops can be constructed by superposition of these primitive loops.

FINITE LOOPS

The superposition of primitive loops lying on appropriate crystallographic planes simulates finite dislocation loops. Figure 3 illustrates a rectangular prismatic loop and Figure 4, a rectangular shear loop, each formed by arrays of primitive shear loops and prismatic loops, respectively, lying on {100} planes of a simple cubic crystal. Summation of the displacement fields of the individual point forces gives the displacement field for each loop. In the case of the shear loop

$$(16) \quad u_m(x_1, x_2, x_3) = \left\{ \frac{\mu a^2}{2} \sum_{p=-(\frac{R}{2})}^{R/2} \left[\left(\sum_{q=-L/2}^{L/2} + \sum_{q=-(L/2-1)}^{L/2-1} \right) \right. \right.$$

$$G_{2m}(x_1 - pa, x_2 - qa, x_3 - a/2) - G_{2m}(x_1 - pa, x_2 - qa, x_3 + a/2)$$
$$- G_{3m}(x_1 - pa, x_2 + La/2, x_3 - a/2) - G_{3m}(x_1 - pa, x_2 + La/2, x_3 + a/2)$$
$$+ G_{3m}(x_1 - pa, x_2 - La/2, x_3 - a/2) - G_{3m}(x_1 - pa, x_2 - La/2, x_3 + a/2)] \}$$

where the summation on q applies only to terms of the form $G_{2m}(\underline{R})$. Portions of the loop composed of pure screw dislocations correspond to $x_1 = -Ra/2 + \varepsilon_1$; $x_2 = \varepsilon_2$ and $x_1 = Ra/2 - \varepsilon_1$; $x_2 = \varepsilon_2$ where $\varepsilon_1 \ll Ra$ and $\varepsilon_2 \ll La$. Edge dislocations correspond to $x_1 = \varepsilon_1$; $x_2 = -La/2 + \varepsilon_2$ and $x_1 = \varepsilon_1$; $x_2 = La/2 - \varepsilon_2$. Equation 16 reduces to the displacement fields of single dislocations in the above regions. A similar summation gives the displacement field of the prismatic loop.

The self-energy of the loop arises from three sources: the self energy of the point forces; the interaction energy of the point forces; a correction term accounting for the fact that the points of application of the forces have moved sufficiently far that the energy of the resulting array must be based on the distance between neighboring atomic positions in their final configuration rather than the initial configuration. Requiring this energy to have the same form as the self energy of the corresponding edge and screw dislocations in these limiting cases leads to values of the effective force constant which depend on the details of the force array. This situation arises because the force array displaces each atomic position from its equilibrium location at the point of minimum interatomic energy. Subsequent application of a force to this atomic position results in a response influenced by the anharmonic nature of the interatomic potential. This changes the effective force constant at an atomic location surrounded by an array of forces. For the pure screw dislocation obtained from the rectangular shear loop the effective force constant, α_2, becomes [9].

$$\text{(17)} \quad \frac{\alpha_2}{\mu a} = \frac{4\pi}{2\pi - A}$$

where

$$\text{(18)} \quad A = \frac{3 - 4v}{8\pi(1 - v)} \left\{ \frac{2}{(3 - 4v)} \sum_{q=1}^{\infty} \frac{1}{(q^2 + 1)} + \sum_{q=1}^{\infty} \left[\ln\left(\frac{q^2 + 1}{q^2}\right) + \frac{1}{q} - \frac{1}{\sqrt{1 + q^2}} \right] - \frac{1}{2} \right\}.$$

This choice of force constant results in a self energy per unit length of

$$\text{(19)} \quad E = (\mu a^2/4\pi)\ln(R/0.263)$$

for the screw dislocation.

The edge dislocation presents somewhat greater complications due to the extra row of forces acting in the x_3 direction on atoms lying along the dislocation line. Since these forces act in a direction orthogonal to the forces distributed across the slip plane, their effect on the effective force constant corresponding to atomic displacements in the x_3 direction should be different from that for displacement in the x_2 direction. This circumstance leads to the result

$$\text{(20)} \quad E = \frac{\mu a^2}{4\pi(1 - v)} \left[\ln L - \left(\frac{4.327 - 6.730v + 2.540v^2}{1 - 2v} \right) + (1 - v)\left(\frac{\mu a}{\alpha_2} - \frac{\mu a}{\alpha_3} \right) \right]$$

where the force constants α_2 and α_3 correspond to atomic displacements in the x_2 and x_3 directions, respectively. This form results from choosing α_2 as for the screw dislocation, equation 17, but does not permit an independent determination of α_3. Despite this complication, the energy per unit length of the edge dislocation has the form

$$\text{(21)} \quad E = [\mu a^2/4\pi(1 - v)]\ln(L/r_o)$$

with the only uncertainty in the core parameter, r_o arising from the unknown force constant, α_3. A similar construction for the edge dislocation from prismatic loops results in the determination of an effective force constant for atomic displacements normal to the extra half plane, which has a numerical value close to α_2, but no satisfactory result for the effective force constant for atomic displacements in the direction of the slip plane normal.

KINKS AND JOGS

Kinks and jogs in edge and screw dislocations result when appropriate primitive loops are added to the segments of the finite rectangular loop corresponding to edge and screw dislocations. Figures 5 and 6 illustrate the formation of single and double kinks in a screw dislocation by addition of an array of shear loops. The displacement field and energy of these configurations are found as before. The largest relative atomic displacements occur along the line of the kink segment, but the far-field results are identical with the unkinked dislocation. Energies of single and double kinks are taken to be the difference in energies between the kinked configuration and the straight dislocation. In the following expressions for energy, the correction term corresponding to excess strain energy in the volume occupied by the kink itself has been neglected. When the dislocation is much longer than a double kink of length 2Na, the energy of the double kink becomes

$$(21) \quad (W/\mu a^3) = 2N \left\{ \frac{\mu a}{\alpha_2} + \frac{A}{4\pi} - \frac{1}{4\pi} \sum_{2N}^{\infty} \left[2\left(\frac{1}{q} - \frac{1}{\sqrt{(q^2+1)}}\right) + \frac{1}{2(1-\nu)(q^2+1)^{3/2}} \right] \right\}$$

$$- \left(\frac{\mu a}{\alpha_2} - \frac{\mu a}{\alpha_3}\right) + \frac{1}{32\pi(1-\nu)} - \frac{1}{2\pi} \sum_{q=1}^{2N-1} \left[1 - \frac{1}{\sqrt{(q^2+1)}} + \frac{1}{2(1-\nu)(1+q^2)^{3/2}} \right]$$

$$- \frac{1}{32\pi(1-\nu)} \left[\frac{(7-8\nu)}{\sqrt{(4N^2+1)}} + \frac{4N}{(4N^2+1)^{3/2}} \right] .$$

Determination of the appropriate correction energy, W_c, as for the straight dislocations leads to a result which can be written

$$(22) \quad W_{kink} = 2W_s + W_{int} ,$$

where W_s is the self energy of a simple kink and W_{int} represents the interaction energy. Terms in W_c which are linear in N will combine with the coefficient of N in braces; the force constant α_2 can then be chosen to make this coefficient vanish in order to give the proper form for energy of a double kink [10]. Then the self energy becomes

$$(23) \quad W_s = \frac{\mu a^3}{4\pi(1-\nu)} \left\{ \frac{1}{16} - \sum_{q=1}^{2N-1} 2(1-\nu) \left[\left(1 - \frac{q}{\sqrt{(1+q^2)}}\right) + \frac{q}{(1+q^2)^{3/2}} \right] \right\}$$

$$+ \left(\frac{\mu a}{\alpha_2} - \frac{\mu a}{\alpha_3}\right) + W_c',$$

where W_c' represents those terms in W_c which are independent of N, and the interaction energy,

$$(24) \quad W_{int} = \frac{-\mu a^3}{32\pi(1-\nu)} \left[\frac{(7-8\nu)}{\sqrt{(4N^2+1)}} + \frac{4N}{(4N^2+1)^{3/2}} \right] + W_c'',$$

where W_c'' represents terms in the correction energy which are $O(N^{-1})$. Note that, to first order in $(2N)^{-1}$, W_{int} has the same form as that determined by Hirth and Lothe using a local continuum model. Neither the proper correction energy nor the appropriate force constant, α_3, have been determined, although the proper procedure has been described [9].

Single and double kinks in an edge dislocation are illustrated in Figures 7 and 8. In these illustrations the defects have been formed by the superposition of shear loops on a portion of an edge dislocation line. The procedure for obtaining the displacement fields and energies of the kinked configurations are identical to those used for the screw dislocation. However it has not yet been possible to determine the appropriate correction energy and final expressions for kink energies await these calculations.

Primitive prismatic loops added to the boundaries of the finite loop simulate jogs in the same way that shear loops simulate kinks. Procedures for obtaining displacement fields and energies are also identical. No calculations of this nature have yet been attempted.

CONCLUSIONS

Displacement fields and energies of dislocation configurations in crystals can be obtained by the superposition of point force arrays which form primitive loops. Expression for displacement fields and energies match those obtained by the local continuum method when suitable choices are made for the effective atomic force constraints. These constructions can provide values of atomic displacements in the vicinity of dislocation cores which are more accurate than those obtained from the local linear continuum model but which require less computational effort than discrete lattice models.

ACKNOWLEDGEMENTS

This work is based on research supported by Metallurgy Program of the U.S. National Science Foundation and was submitted by one of the authors (J.-P.J.G.) to the Graduate School of the University of Florida in partial fulfillment of the requirements of the Doctor of Philosophy degree in Engineering Science. The authors are also grateful to Dr. R. A. Johnson for a critical reading of the manuscript.

REFERENCES

/1/ Bullough R., Hardy J. R.: Phil. Mag. 17 (1968) 833.

/2/ Bullough R., Norgett M., Webb: J. Phys. F. 1 (1971) 345.

/3/ Kröner E.: Kontinuumstheorie der Versetzungen and Eigenspannungen, Ergeb. der Angew. Math., v. 5, Springer-Verlag, Berlin 1958.

/4/ Kroupa F.: Czech. J. Phys. B 12 (1962) 191.
/5/ Simmons J. A., Bullough R.: Fundamental Aspects of Dislocation Theory, NBS Spec. Pub. 317, v. 1, Washington, D.C., (1970) 89.
/6/ Hartley C. S. and Bullough R.: J. Appl. Phys. 48 (1977) 4557.
/7/ Georges J.-P.J: Simulation of Dislocations by Point Force Arrays, M.S. Thesis, University of Florida, Gainesville, Florida 1970.
/8/ Mott N. F., Jones H.: The Theory of the Properties of Metals and Alloys, Dover Publications, New York 1958.
/9/ Georges J.-P.J.: Simulation of Defects in Crystals by Point Force Arrays, Ph.D. Dissertation, University of Florida, Gainesville, Florida 1972.
/10/ Hirth J. P., Lothe J.: Theory of Dislocations, McGraw-Hill, New York 1970.

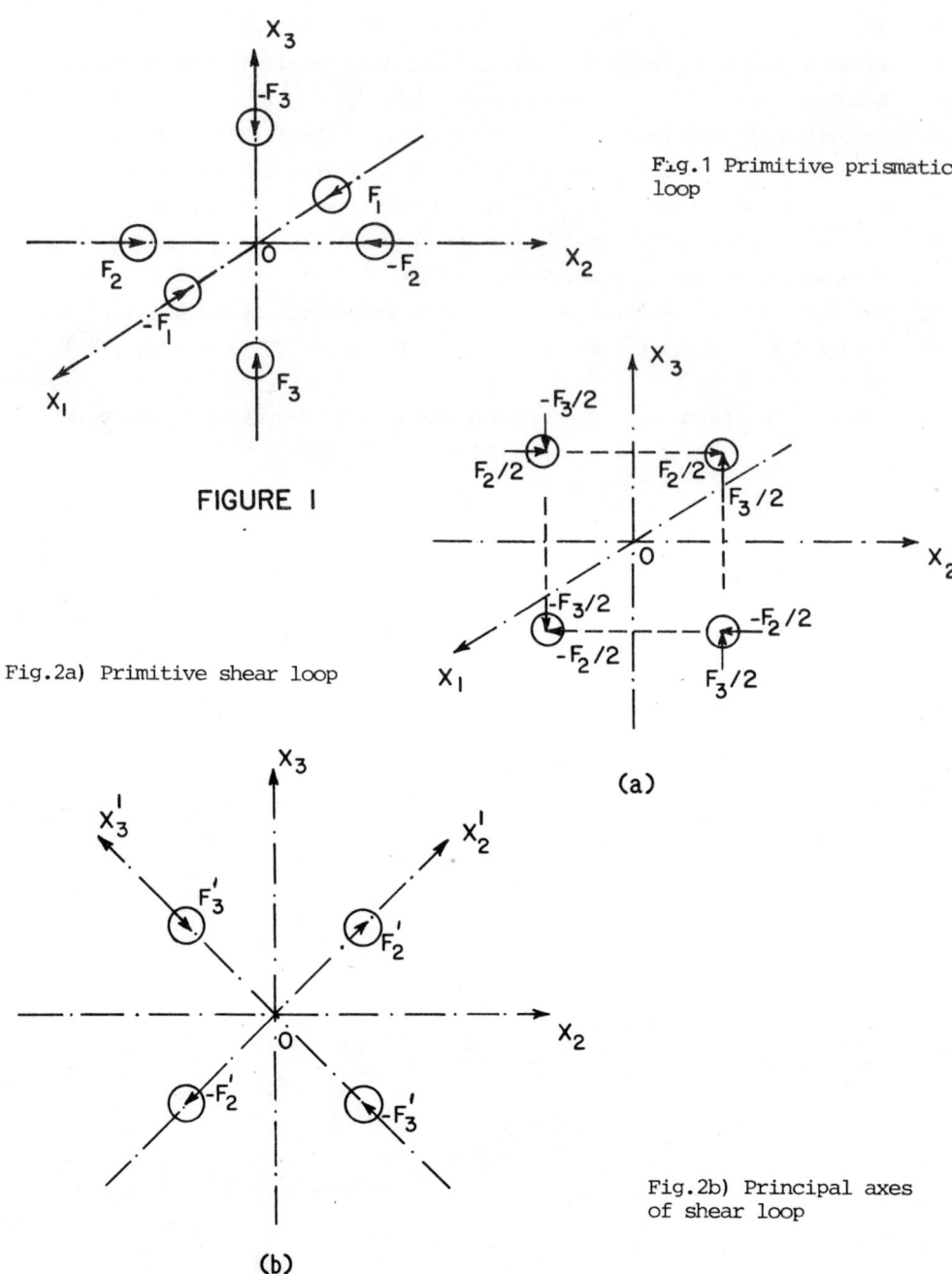

FIGURE 1

Fig.1 Primitive prismatic loop

Fig.2a) Primitive shear loop

(a)

Fig.2b) Principal axes of shear loop

(b)

FIGURE 2

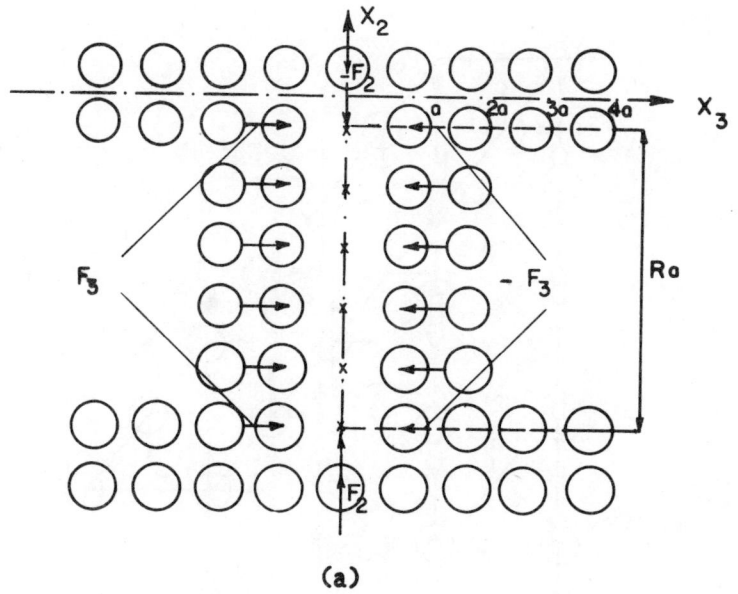

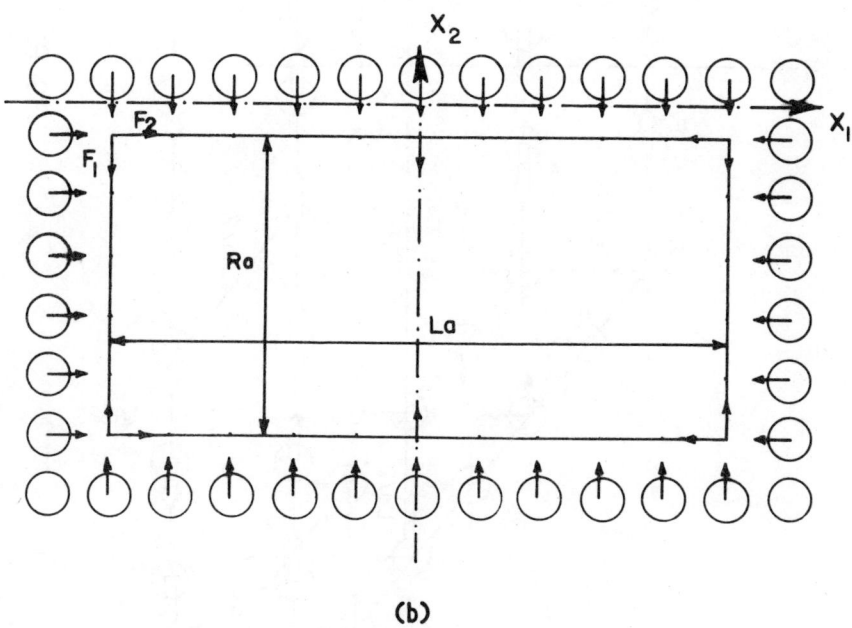

FIGURE 3

Fig.3 Finite prismatic loop

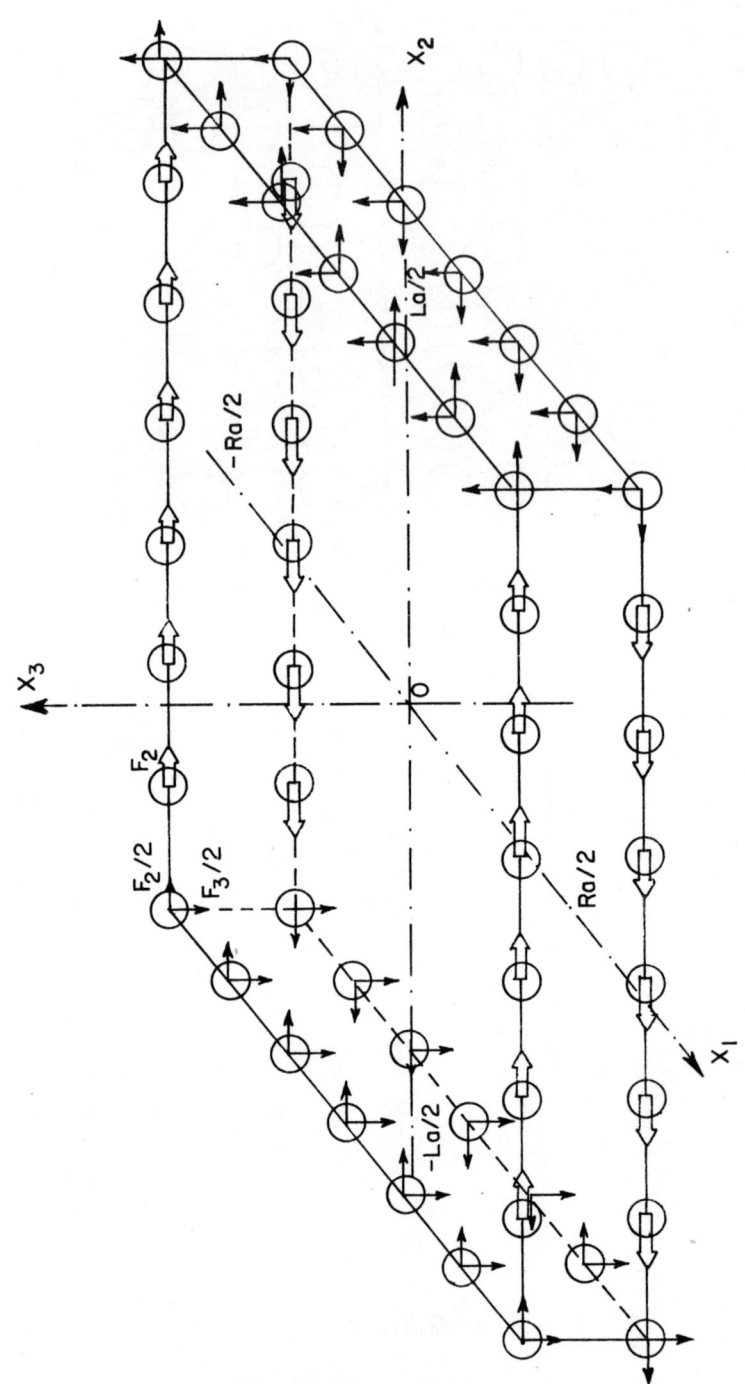

FIGURE 4

Fig.4 Finite glide (shear) loop

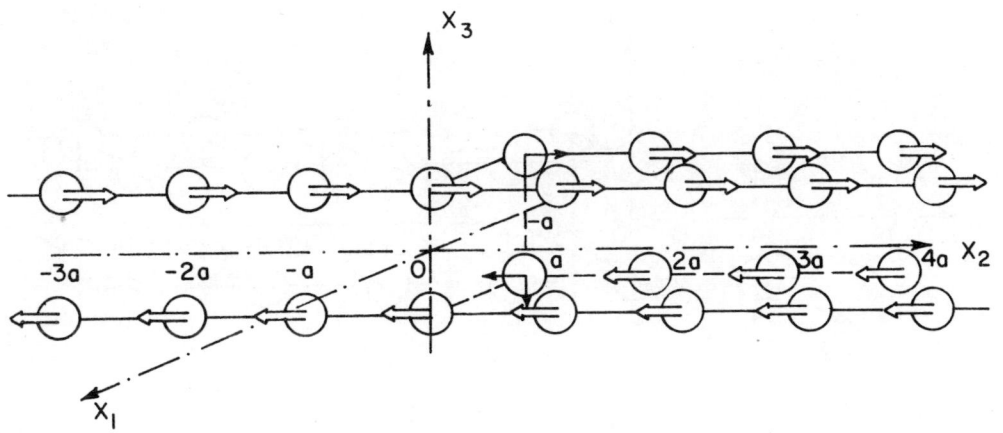

FIGURE 5

Fig.5 Single kink in screw dislocation

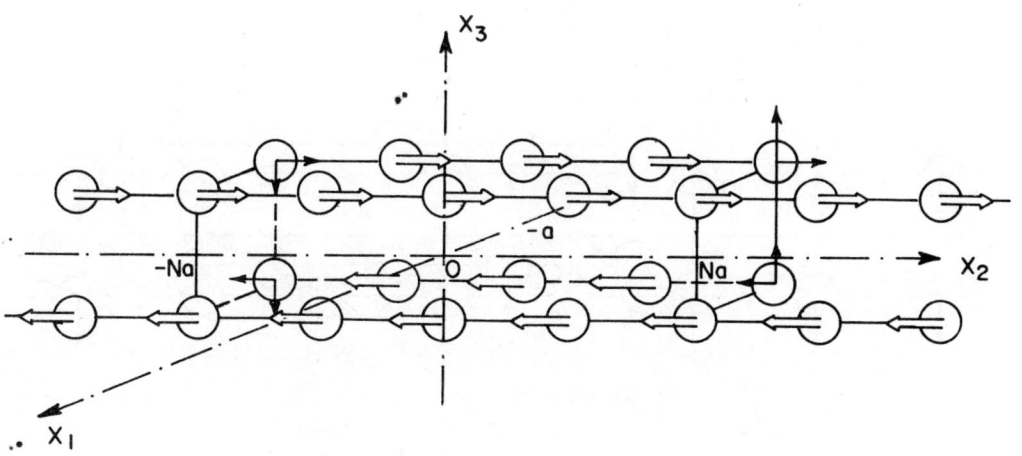

FIGURE 6

Fig.6 Double kink in screw dislocation

- 395 -

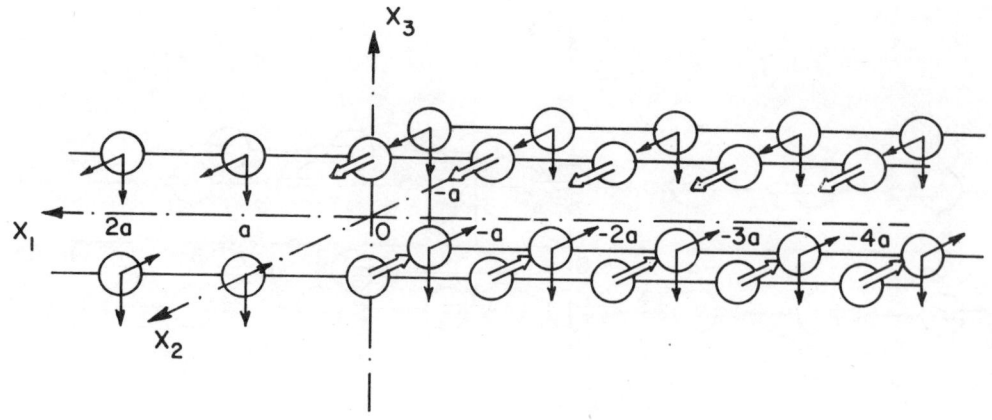

FIGURE 7

Fig.7 Single kink in edge dislocation

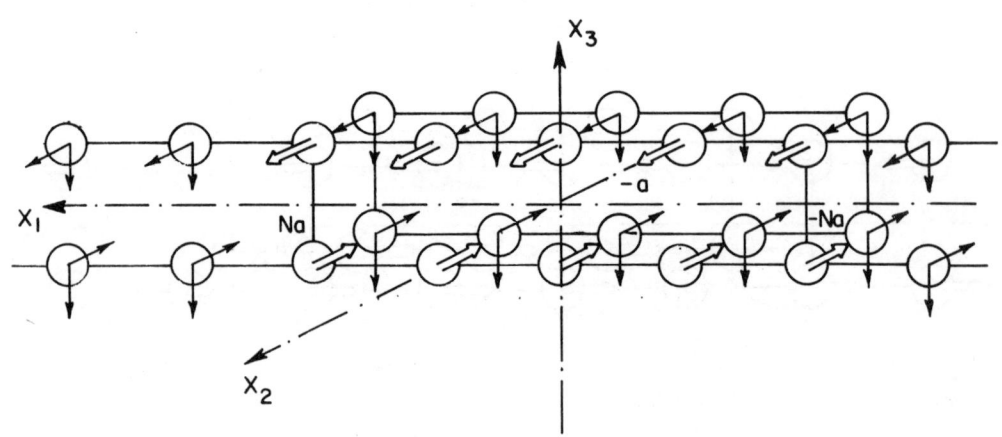

FIGURE 8

Fig.8 Double kink in edge dislocation

INTERACTION OF DISLOCATION WITH CRYSTAL SURFACE AND EMERGENCE OF DISLOCATION ON SURFACE

A.M. Kosevich and Yu.A. Kosevich

Institute for Low Temperature Physics and Engineering, Ukr.SSR Academy of Sciences, 47, Lenin Avenue, Kharkov, 310164, USSR

A complete system of dynamic equations describing deformation of solids subject to allowance for surface (capillary) phenomena is derived in Ref. 1, and several examples of application of such a system are given. In the present paper we shall determine more accurately the nature of changes in the boundary conditions of bulk dimensional equations of equilibrium on the surface of a solid resulting from capillary effects, and also the explicit dependence of the surface free energy on the strain. Further examples will be given of the application of the resultant equations to problems of formation of a step on the surface of a crystal as a result of quasistatic emergence of an edge dislocation from the bulk and of the elastic interaction of point defects and dislocations with the surface of a stacking fault.

DISCUSSION OF THE SURFACE ENERGY AND BOUNDARY CONDITIONS

It is shown in Ref. 1 that the density of the surface free energy α of an arbitrary two-dimensional defect (including a free surface of a crystal) separating media 1 and 2 obeys, at a given temperature, the following thermodynamic identity:

$$(1) \quad d\alpha = g_{\mu\nu} du_{\mu\nu} + \sigma_{in} d\Delta_i; \quad \mu,\nu = 1,2; \quad i,k = 1,2,3.$$

Here, u_{ik} is the strain tensor; σ_{ik} is the bulk stress tensor; $\sigma_{in} = \sigma_{ik} n_k$; $n_i = \delta_{i3}$ is the unit vector along the normal to the interface directed from medium 1 to medium 2. The indices μ and ν label the coordinate axes in a plane tangential to the defect surface. In Eq.(1) the quantity $g_{\mu\nu}$ is the symmetric tensor of surface elastic stresses and $\Delta_i = u_i^{(2)} - u_i^{(1)}$ is an abrupt change in the displacement vector u_i on the surface of a defect.

We shall describe $g_{\mu\nu}$ and Δ_i by the following linear expansions /1/:

$$(2) \quad g_{\mu\nu} = g_{\mu\nu}^{(0)} - a_{i\mu\nu}\sigma_{in} + h_{\mu\nu\gamma\delta} u_{\gamma\delta}, \quad \Delta_i = a_{i\mu\nu} u_{\mu\nu} + c_{ik}\sigma_{kn},$$

where $g^{(0)}_{\mu\nu}$, $a_{i\mu\nu}$, C_{ik}, $h_{\mu\nu\gamma\delta}$ are independent parameters representing the elastic properties of the surface of a two-dimensional defect.

The thermodynamic relationship (I) and the expansion (2) allow us to find α as a function of its independent variables $u_{\mu\nu}$ and Δ_i:

$$\alpha(u_{\mu\nu},\Delta_i) = \tfrac{1}{2} g^{(0)}_{\mu\nu}\left(\frac{\partial u_\mu}{\partial x_\nu} + \frac{\partial u_\nu}{\partial x_\mu} + \frac{\partial u_l}{\partial x_\mu}\frac{\partial u_l}{\partial x_\nu}\right) +$$
$$(3) + \tfrac{1}{2}\left(h_{\mu\nu\gamma\delta} + \bar{C}^{-1}_{pq} a_{p\mu\nu} a_{q\gamma\delta}\right) u_{\mu\nu} u_{\gamma\delta} + \tfrac{1}{2} C^{-1}_{ik}\Delta_i \Delta_k - C^{-1}_{lm} a_{l\mu\nu} u_{\mu\nu} \Delta_m ,$$

where C^{-1}_{ik} is a tensor which is the reciprocal of the tensor C_{ik}. Equation (3) represents in fact an expansion of the surface energy of a two-dimensional defect in terms of independent invariants (scalars) composed of quadratic combinations of variables describing the state of the surface: $u_{\mu\nu}$ and Δ_i.

The first term in the expansion (3) appears because on the surface of a crystal (or at an interface between two crystals) in equilibrium there are definite residual tangential stresses $g^{(0)}_{\mu\nu} = g^{(0)}_{\mu\nu}(T)$ independent of bulk strains /2/ (T is the absolute temperature). In the expansion of the surface energy the surface strain tensor $g^{(0)}_{\mu\nu}$ obtained in the linear theory of elasticity corresponds to the invariant

$$g^{(0)}_{\mu\nu} u_{\mu\nu} = \tfrac{1}{2} g^{(0)}_{\mu\nu}\left(\frac{\partial u_\nu}{\partial x_\mu} + \frac{\partial u_\mu}{\partial x_\nu} + \frac{\partial u_l}{\partial x_\mu}\frac{\partial u_l}{\partial x_\nu}\right).$$

In terms quadratic in respect of the strain it is usual to assume that

$$u_{\mu\nu} = \tfrac{1}{2}\left(\frac{\partial u_\mu}{\partial x_\nu} + \frac{\partial u_\nu}{\partial x_\mu}\right).$$

The boundary conditions at an interface can be found by varying with respect to the displacement vector u_i the total bulk and surface free energy F. Application of the identity (I), of the definition of the vector Δ_i, and of the generally valid (in accordance with the above discussion) relationship for a surface

$$\delta u_{\mu\nu} = \tfrac{1}{2}\left(\frac{\partial \delta u_\mu}{\partial x_\nu} + \frac{\partial \delta u_\nu}{\partial x_\mu} + \frac{\partial u_l}{\partial x_\mu}\frac{\partial \delta u_l}{\partial x_\nu} + \frac{\partial u_l}{\partial x_\nu}\frac{\partial \delta u_l}{\partial x_\mu}\right),$$

yields the following boundary conditions:

$$(4) \quad -\left(\frac{\delta F}{\delta u_i}\right)_T = \nu_o \ddot{u}_i = \sigma^{(2)}_{in} - \sigma^{(1)}_{in} + \frac{\partial}{\partial x_\mu} g^*_{i\mu}.$$

Here, ν_0 is the density of the excess surface mass and
$$g^*_{i\mu} = g_{\mu\nu}(\delta_{i\nu} + \partial u_i/\partial x_\nu).$$
In the adopted approximation, we have

(5) $$g^*_{i\mu} = g_{\mu\nu}\delta_{i\nu} + g^{(0)}_{\mu\nu}\partial u_i/\partial x_\nu.$$

We shall now consider the boundary conditions on a plane free surface (ignoring the capillary phenomena so that $\sigma_{in}=0$). If a crystal surface is perpendicular to a sixfold symmetry axis (isotropic model), then the following relationships apply:

(6) $$g^{(0)}_{\mu\nu} = g\delta_{\mu\nu}, \quad c_{ik} = c_1\delta_{i\mu}\delta_{\kappa\mu} + c_2 n_i n_k,$$
$$a_{i\mu\nu} = an_i\delta_{\mu\nu}, \quad h_{\mu\nu\gamma\delta} = h_1\delta_{\mu\nu}\delta_{\gamma\delta} + h_2(\delta_{\mu\gamma}\delta_{\nu\delta} + \delta_{\mu\delta}\delta_{\gamma\nu}).$$

If the z axis is directed along the outer normal to the undeformed surface $z=0$, then the static boundary conditions (4) subject to Eqs.(2), (5) and (I6) assume the following form for a free surface:

(7) $$\sigma_{zz} = g\frac{\partial^2 u_z}{\partial x^2_\mu}, \quad \sigma_{\mu z} = h_1\frac{\partial}{\partial x_\mu}u_{\nu\nu} + 2h_2\frac{\partial}{\partial x_\nu}u_{\mu\nu} + g\frac{\partial^2 u_\mu}{\partial x^2_\nu}.$$

The components of the tensor $g^*_{i\mu}$ are subject to uncertainty typical of surface quantities: this uncertainty is due to the doubts about the correct selection of the position of the interface between two media. We shall assume that the initial free surface is displaced in the direction of the normal $\vec{n}$ by a small (of the order of the interatomic) distance ζ. We can show /I/ that $g^*_{i\mu}$ is transformed in the following way to $\langle g^*_{i\mu}\rangle$ for the new surface:

(8) $$\langle g^*_{i\mu}\rangle = g^*_{i\mu} - \zeta\sigma_{i\mu}.$$

In the adopted principal (in respect of the surface parameters) approximation we can calculate $\sigma_{i\mu}$ in Eq.(8) on the assumption that $\sigma_{in}=0$.

Since the tensor $g^{(0)}_{\mu\nu}$ is the zeroth term of the expansion of the tensor $g^*_{i\mu}$ in terms of strains, it cannot change as a result of the assumed displacement of the interface and, therefore, it is independent of the selection of the interface. In other words, the tensor $g^{(0)}_{\mu\nu}$ is a unique characteristic of the surface tension forces. For a planar problem ($u_y=0, \partial/\partial y=0$), we obtain

$$\langle g^*_{xx}\rangle = g+(g+h_1+2h_2)u_{xx}-\zeta\sigma_{xx}, \quad \langle g^*_{zx}\rangle = g^*_{zx}$$

Using Hooke's law subject to $u_{yy}=\sigma_{zz}=0$, we find that

$$\sigma_{xx} = \frac{E}{1-\sigma^2}u_{xx}$$

where σ is the Poisson ratio and E is the Young modulus. We can see that a suitable selection of the position of the interface(i.e., of ζ) can ensure that the coefficient in front of u_{xx} in the expansion for g^*_{xx} can vanish. We are then left with

(9) $$\langle g^*_{xx}\rangle = g, \quad \langle g^*_{zx}\rangle = g\frac{\partial u_z}{\partial x}.$$

Consequently, it is clear from Eqs.(7) and (9) that in a static planar problem in the theory of elasticity we can define a homogeneous boundary surface in such a way that it is free of tangential forces of capillary origin.

EMERGENCE OF AN EDGE DISLOCATION TO THE SURFACE

One of the main extended surface defects is a growth step frequently discussed in connection with the problem of crystallization. Recrystallization waves predicted in Ref. 3 and detected in Ref. 4 on the surface of a quantum crystal have drawn special attention to growth steps as objects whose motion may be responsible for the motion of a crystallization-melting front. The special feature of the motion of discrete steps influences the dynamic properties of a vibrating surface and it makes a contribution to the dispersion law of recrystallization waves /5/.

However, a step on a crystal face may form not only in the process of crystallization but also because of emergence of an edge dislocation parallel to the surface (positions I and 2 in Fig. I illustrate the cases when a dislocation is in the bulk and on the surface). On the other hand, an edge dislocation can, in principle, be created in the bulk of a crystal by applying a load that suppresses a surface step. Therfore, there should be a definite correspondence between the properties of an edge dislocation and a surface step, both being sources of elastic stresses in a crystal. It is shown in Refs. I and 2 that, because of the surface tension forces, steps should create elastic stresses in the bulk. We shall demonstrate below that these stresses are governed by the properties of an edge dislocation that could create such a step by emerging on the surface /8/.

We shall seek the solution of the bulk equilibrium equations in the form

$$u_i = u_i^0 + u_i^1, \quad \sigma_{ik} = \sigma_{ik}^0 + \sigma_{ik}^1,$$

where u_i^0 and σ_{ik}^0 represent the solutions obtained without allowance for the capillary phenomena, i.e., the solutions obtained subject to the boundary condition $\sigma_{in}^0 = 0$. The fields u_i^1 and σ_{ik}^1 can be found by the method of successive approximations without exceeding the adopted degree of accuracy. In the case of planar problem corresponding to $u_y = 0$, $\partial/\partial y = 0$ the boundary conditions (7) for σ_{ik}^1 subject to Eq.(9) assume the following form on a free surface ($z = 0$):

(10) $$\sigma_{zz}^1 = g \frac{\partial^2 u_z^0}{\partial x^2}, \quad \sigma_{zx}^1 = 0.$$

We shall rewrite the right-hand side of the first condition (10) in terms of σ_{ik}^0. On a free surface $z = 0$, we have

(11) $$\frac{\partial^2 u_z^0}{\partial x^2} = -\frac{1-\sigma^2}{E} \frac{\partial \sigma_{xx}^0}{\partial z}$$

We shall consider an edge dislocation parallel to a free surface $z = 0$ located on the line $x = 0$, $z = -l$ (Fig. I) and characterized by a Burgers vector $\vec{b}$ (0, 0, b) perpendicular to the surface. If an explicit expression for σ_{xx}^0 is substituted in Eq.(11) (see, for example, Sec. 3-5 in Ref. 6), the first condition in Eq.(10) becomes

(12) $$\sigma_{zz}^1 = -gb\frac{8}{\pi} \frac{l^3 x}{(l^2+x^2)^3}.$$

We shall be interested in fields at distances r from a dislocation much greater than l ($r \gg l$). This is equivalent to going to the limit $l \to 0$ in Eq.(12). In this limit the boundary condition (12) becomes

$$\sigma_{zz}^1 = gb\frac{\partial}{\partial x} \delta(x),$$

where $\delta(x)$ is the Dirac δ-function. The field σ_{ik}^0 disappears in the limit $l = 0$ and, therefore, the bulk elastic fields created by a newly formed step are subject to the following boundary conditions:

$$(I3) \quad \sigma_{zz}|_{z=0} = gb\frac{\partial}{\partial x}\delta(x), \quad \sigma_{zx}|_{z=0} = 0.$$

The density of the forced normal to the surface $P_z = \sigma_{zz}$ under the conditions described by Eq.(I3) is equal exactly to the density obtained earlier /1, 2/ for a step of height b. This force characterized a step as a center of a dipole force with a moment. The problem of compensation of the moment of this force is eliminated by assuming that the emergence of a dislocation on the $X = Z = 0$ line is accompanied by the simultaneous emergence of a dislocation of the opposite sign on a surface at infinity $X = \infty$, $Z = 0$. Such a dislocation is associated with a second edge of an extraatomic layer carried to a given crystal face by an edge dislocation.

We shall study geometric changes in the surface in the limit $l \to 0$. When a dislocation emerges from a crystal, it gives rise to plastic deformation concentrated on its surface /7/:

$$\frac{\partial u_z^{pl}}{\partial z} = b\delta(z)\theta(x),$$

where $\theta(x)$ is the Heaviside unit function.

The part of the crystal surface above the glide plane of the dislocation ($X > 0$) experiences a residual plastic displacement by an amount equal to the Burgers vector:

$$u_z^{pl} = \begin{cases} b, & z=0, \; x>0; \\ 0, & z=0, \; x<0. \end{cases}$$

The residual displacement alters the shape of the surface creating a characteristic step of height b.

We shall now consider the emergence of a dislocation whose Burgers vector is parallel to the surface. We shall assume that this dislocation is located as before and that its Burgers vector is $\vec{b}(b, 0, 0)$. The elastic stress field σ_{ik}^o in the half-space $Z < 0$ can be described by a superposition of three fields: the field of a dislocation located on the line $X = 0$, $Z = -l$ in an infinite crystal, the field of an image dislocation on the $X = 0$, $Z = l$ line, and an additional field $\bar{\sigma}_{ik}$ ensuring that the boundary conditions $\sigma_{in}^o = 0$ are satisfied on the $Z = 0$ surface.

The stress function $\bar{\psi}(X, Z)$ describing the planar field $\bar{\sigma}_{ik}$ can be described by the following expression:

$$\bar{\psi}(x,z) = \frac{\mu b l}{\pi(1-\sigma)}\left\{\frac{z(l-z)}{x^2+(l-z)^2} + \frac{1}{2}\ln[x^2+(l-z)^2]\right\},$$

where μ is the shear modulus. A logarithmic divergence of $\bar{\psi}$ at high values of z does not give rise to any physical inconsistencies, because real fields σ_{ik} are governed by the second derivatives with respect to ψ.

If we now substitute σ_{xx}^0 in Eq. (II), we find that the first condition of Eq. (10) becomes

$$\sigma_{zz}^1 = P(x,l) \equiv gb\frac{2l^3(3x^2-l^2)}{\pi(x^2+l^2)^3}.$$

We shall consider the properties of the function $P(x,l)$ in the limit $l \to 0$, i.e., we shall find $P(X, 0)$. We note that

$$P = 0 \quad \text{for } l=0, \; x\neq 0,$$
$$\int_{-\infty}^{\infty} P(x,l)\,dx = 0 \quad \text{for } l\neq 0.$$

Therefore, we should assume that $P(X, 0) = 0$. Therefore, both fields σ_{ik}^0 vanish in the limit $l = 0$. Hence, it follows that after emergence of a given dislocation on the surface there are no residual elastic stresses in a crystal.

This result is quite self-evident from the physical point of view. We shall consider plastic deformation which appears in a crystal as a result of emergence of such a dislocation on the surface. This plastic deformation can be assumed to be concentrated in the $x = 0$ plane perpendicular to the free plane:

$$\frac{\partial u_x^{pl}}{\partial x} = b\,\delta(x)[1-\Theta(z+l)].$$

After the emergence of a dislocation on the surface ($l=0$) half a crystal experiences a homogeneous residual displacement along the x axis by the vector $\vec{b}$. There is no change in the physical state of the crystal and there are no residual elastic stresses.

In view of the linearity of the theory, these results can be generalized to the case when a step is formed by emergence of an edge dislocation with a Burgers vector $\vec{b}$ making an arbitrary angle with the normal $\vec{n}$ to the surface. The elastic fields in the bulk of a crystal are subject to the following boundary conditions:

$$\sigma_{nn} = g\vec{b}\vec{n}\frac{\partial}{\partial x}\delta(x) \quad , \quad \sigma_{nx} = 0.$$

Here the X axis is drawn on the surface at right-angles to the dislocation line in such a way that $\vec{b}\vec{n} > 0$ and $b_x > 0$ are satisfied simultaneously. Consequently, the resultant step with $\vec{b}\vec{n} > 0$ can be called positive, whereas that with $\vec{b}\vec{n} < 0$ may be called negative.

It is worth noting that an edge dislocation regarded as a lattice defect in the bulk does not carry to the surface a zero-moment dipole force, introduced phenomenologically in Refs. 1 and 2. This may be associated with a change in the dislocation core as a result of its transformation from a lattice into a surface defect, and a calculation of such a force requires an appropriate microscopic analysis.

References

/1/ Andreev A.F., Kosevich Yu.A.: Zh. Eksp. Teor. Fiz. 81 (1981) 1435 /Sov. Phys. JETP 54/.

/2/ Marchenko V.I., A.Ya. Parshin; Zh. Eksp. Teor. Fiz. 79 (1980) 257 /Sov. Phys. JETP 52 (1980) 129.

/3/ Andreev A.F., Parshin A.Ya.: Zh. Eksp. Teor. Fiz. 75 (1978) 1511 /Sov. Phys. JETP 48 (1978) 763.

/4/ Keshishev K.O., Parshin A.Ya., Babkin A.V.: Pis'ma Zh. Eksp. Teor. Fiz. 30 (1979) 63 /JETP Lett. 30 (1979) 56.

/5/ Kosevich A.M., Kosevich Yu.A.: Fiz. Nizk. Temp. 7 (1981) 809 /Sov. J. Low Temp. Phys. 7/.

/6/ Hirth J.P., Lothe J.: Theory of Dislocations, McGraw-Hill, New York, 1968 (Russ. Transl., Atomizdat, M., 1972).

/7/ Kosevich A.M.: Dislokatsii v teorii uprugosti (Dislocations in the Theory of Elasticity), Naukova Dumka, Kiev, 1978.

/8/ Kosevich A.M., Kosevich Yu.A.: Fiz. Nizk. Temp. 7 (1981) 1347 /Sov. J. Low Temp. Phys. 7/.

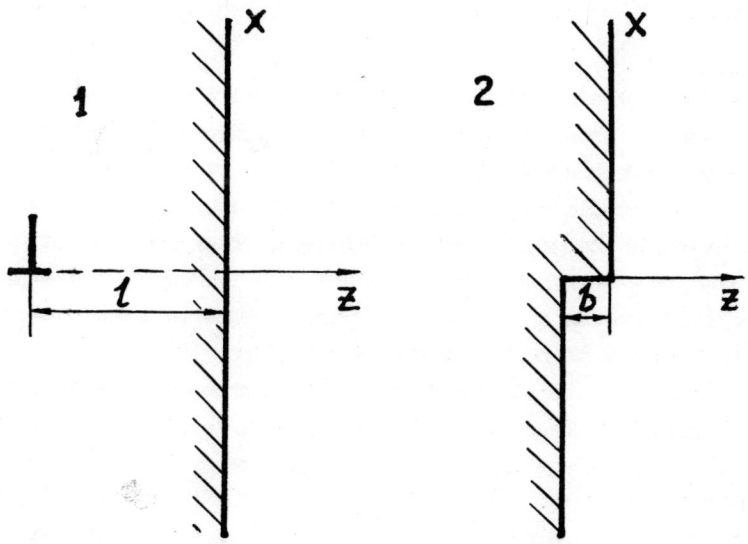

Fig. 1

CONTINUUM MECHANICS AND COLLECTIVE BEHAVIOUR OF DISLOCATIONS

B. Pegel

Zentralinstitut für Festkörperphysik und Werkstofforschung Dresden
der Akademie der Wissenschaften der DDR
DDR 8027 Dresden

1. Introduction

The appearance of distinct macroscopic dislocation structures during a deformation process is, when considered at level of individual dislocations, is clearly a co-operative phenomenon. A particular case of structure formation in deformed metals is locatlization of plastic deformation, i.e. the observation that in a macroscopic homogeneous (or smoothly variable) deformation field, further deformation concentrates into narrow zones. Eventually, localized plastic flow can appear as the primary deformation mode in a homogeneous situation, i.e. without a preceding homogeneous deformation.

Localization of inelastic flow is a universal phenomenon in so far as i) it is found in many different material classes, e.g. metal single crystals, polycrystals, metallic glasses, polymers, geological materials (rocks, soils); ii) it is observed at scales differing in several orders of magnitude, and iii) the localization zones appear in typical and phenomenologically similar forms independent of the micromechanisms of inelastic deformation which are quite different in different material classes. E.G. there is a striking similarity between slip line patterns in b.c.c. single crystals /1/ and sand stones /2/ or between kink band formations in hexagonal metal single crystals and oriented crystalline polymers /3/.

In the spirit of synergetics (the science of co-operative behaviour) co-operative modes of behaviour should be governed by universal principles /4/. A particular principle, clearly holding in the present case, is symmetry breaking: by localization of plastic flow the initial symmetry of the deformation field is reduced. The evolution of structures by co-operative action of dislocations requires the deformation system to attain certain critical conditions and can be described at two different levels. On the macroscopic level, collective modes appear as fluctuations under critical conditions. Once established they prescribe the behaviour of individual dislocations at the microscopic level. On the oné hand, macroscopic order "slaves" individual dislocations while on the other hand it cannot exist without them. Thus, a strict reductionism (explaining collective dislocation behaviour from micromechanical events alone) does not seem to be an adequate concept. E.g. collective dislocation modes in single crystals may be essentially governed by mechanical principles while individual dislocation behaviour is strongly coupled to the crystallography. Then, the orientation of deformation bands is not simply and directly related to crystallographic slip systems. It is, therefore, more reasonable to look for a general framework comprising relevant features of dislocation behaviour and general mechanics of solids which can be used for analyzing the instability of structures and processes in deforming solids.

In a fundamental paper /6/ Rice studied a unifying continuum mechanical concept for understanding deformation localization as a mechanical instability of (macroscopic) homogeneous deformation. Thereby localization is explained by pre-localization constitutive properties (relating stress increments to strain increments) of the material, i.e. it is assumed that the constitutive law of the homogeneous deformation can be continued beyond the instability point. In other words, it is assumed that localization is not connected with a principle change in the deformation mechanism. The onset of localization is then interpreted as a bifurcation from the homogeneous deformation state which loses its uniqueness at some critical point in the homogeneous deformation history (the bifurcation point). The analysis revealed relevant features of the constitutive description of inelastic material behaviour and of the pre-localization stress field on which the critical bifurcation conditions may depend. Considering rate independent and thermally decoupled constitutive models such important features are: i) deviations from plastic "normality" which in single crystal plasticity is equivalent to any departure from Schmid's law, ii) a "vertex" on the yield surface corresponding to the presence of two or more active slip systems in single crystal plasticity.

Strain localization in single crystals was theoretically analyzed in detail by Asaro and Rice /6/, Asaro /7/ and Pegel et al. /8/ and studied experimentally in /8,9/. Some results will be presented in section 3 after a discussion of the general concepts of stability and bifurcation of deformable in section 2.

2. Mechanical instability of homogeneous deformation

Clearly conceptions such as "homogeneous", "localization", formation of "structures" are meaningfully applied only at a level of description beyond the atomistic one. Therefore, the adequate concept for describing collective modes of dislocation behaviour is classical continuum mechanics dealing with suitable averages of physical properties. In the framework of continuum mechanics the stability of a deformation process can be analysed by means of a virtual perturbation, $\delta v_i(r)$, of the velocity field applied to any actual state whose stability is to be examined. Assuming rate-independent forces a stability criterion can be formulated by means of a functional, S, defined by (e.g. /10/)

(1) $$S = - \int dv (\delta \dot{n}_{ik,i}) \delta v_k$$

where $\delta\dot{n}_{ik}$ is the virtual perturbation of the nominal stress rate tensor corresponding to the virtual perturbation of the velocity field. The integration is over the actual (deformed) volume of the body. The nominal stress rate, $\dot{n}_{ik}$, is defined by $(D/Dt)(df_i \sigma_{ik}) = df_i \dot{n}_{ik}$ with D/Dt the convective time derivative and df_i a convected surface element. σ_{ik} is the true (Cauchy) stress tensor. $\delta\dot{n}_{ik}$ can be represented as

(2) $\quad \delta\dot{n}_{ik} = \delta(\frac{D}{Dt}\sigma_{ik}) + (\delta v_{1,1})\sigma_{ik} - (\delta v_{i,1})\sigma_{1k}$.

Starting from a stability analysis for mechanical systems with a finite number of degrees of freedom the meaning of the functional (1) can be clearly understood /11/. Depending on the sign of S and actual deformation field is stable or unstable against the virtual perturbation:

(3) $\quad S \gtreqless 0$: stable / unstable

Evidently, the limiting case, S = 0, is realized by a perturbation field which satisfies (besides the boundary conditions of the deformation system considered) the conditions

(4) $\quad \delta\dot{n}_{ik,i} = 0$

expressing continued mechanical equilibrium. Such a field represents a real possibility for the deformation process. If it exists the deformation problem has no unique solution. The loss of uniqueness of the deformation field is called a bifurcation and marks the transition between stable and unstable deformation regimes. Bifurcation analyses by means of (2) and (4) require the knowledge of incremental constitutive equations

(5) $\quad (D/Dt)\sigma_{ik} = F_{ik}(v_{1,m})$.

If F_{ik} is a linear function it follows from (2) that $\dot{n}_{ik}$ is a homogeneous linear function of the gradient of the bifurcation field:

(6) $\quad \delta\dot{n}_{ik} = C_{iklm}(\vec{r})\delta v_{m,1}$.

Taking the reference state (whose stability is to be analysed) to be a homogeneous deformation field the tensor C_{iklm} is constant and (4) becomes a system of linear differential equations with constant coefficients. For elastic-plastic solids the incremental constitutive equations are strongly non-linear for states on the yield surface. But Rice and Rudnicki /12/ have shown that discontinuous bifurcations with elastic unloading outside the zones of incipient localization are not possible before continuous bifurcations with further plastic deformation inside and outside the localization zone. Thus, critical bifurcation conditions can be obtained by restricting the analysis to the plastic branch of the constitutive law and thereby to a linear relation (5).

The central issue in bifurcation analysis is clearly a proper selection of localization modes. Here the clue is given by experimental experience. There are two broad classes of localization modes, namely

i) modes connected with geometrical softening, i.e. local stress concentrations by a change of the external shape of deformed bodies. Well known examples are simple necking in bars, multiple necking in fibre composites, or combined necking-shearing modes in sheet specimens.

ii) modes excluding geometrical softening which are due to internal or material instabilities. Probably all kinds of macro scopic deformation bands and some kind of microscopic shear bands belong to this class. (Localization zones forming layers in the material appear as bands on external or internal surfaces and are generally called deformation bands.)

From the mathematical point of view both classes represent different mathematical problems. In the case of internal instabilities we can ignore external body shapes and consider infinitely extended bodies. If the bifurcation of a homogeneous deformation field into a deformation band is to be analysed we proceed as follows. The virtual perturbation is written in the form

(7) $\quad \delta v_i = g_i f(n_k x_k) \, , \quad g_i g_i = n_i n_i = 1$

where n_i is the unit normal of the deformation band and f = const. outside the band. g_i is a direction vector of unit length. With (6) and (7) the bifurcation conditions (4) yield

(8) $\quad \delta \dot{n}_{ik,i} = f'' n_i C_{iklm} n_l g_m = f'' T_{km} g_m = 0 \, .$

Assuming $f'' \neq 0$ the existence of non-trivial solutions of (8) requires the determinant of T_{km} to vanish:

(9) $\quad |T_{km}| = |n_i C_{iklm} n_l| = 0 \, .$

The bifurcation analysis is now reduced to an algebraic problem raising the following questions:

- Do there exist real solutions n_i of eq. (9)? The existence of real solutions n_i requires the system of differential equations (4) to be of hyperbolic character.
- Since the fourth rank tensor C_{iklm} contains parameters describing constitutive properties (elastic moduli, hardening rates) and stress state the existence of bifurcation modes depend on these parameters which change during the

deformation. Those parameter combinations for which the bifurcation conditions are first met in deformation history are called critical conditions. The main tasks of analysis are to elucidate the relevant features of dislocation behaviour on which the critical conditions depend, to find the band orientation n_i, and to deter mine the stress distribution of the critical localization mode.

When the system of differential equations (4) is of elliptic character the proper mathematical problem is a boundary value problem: the bifurcation field must satisfy (homogeneous) boundary conditions at the body surface. This is typical for the first class of bifurcation modes with changes of the external shape of the deformed body. These boundary value problems lead to eigenvalue problems which have physical solutions only in certain areas of parameter space of the constitutive equations. The critical bifurcation modes are typically diffuse necking modes (in tension) or buckling modes (in compression) and will not be further discussed in the present paper. For ductile single crystals the bifurcation conditions (9) for internal instabilities depend typically on the parameters σ/G and h_i/G with G denoting the order of magnitude of a representative elastic modulus, σ a representative stress level, and h_i the hardening rate of the i-th active slip system. For metals σ/G is clearly a small quantity. But also the parameters h_i/G turn out tl be small quantities near the bifurcation point. Then, eq. (9) can be expanded in a series with terms of rising order of these small parameters. Corresponding to the terms retained in the series we shall speak about a theory of order zero, order one, etc. Let the quantities corresponding to the theory of order zero be designated by a superscript o. Then, in single crystal plasticity the determinant $|T^o_{km}|$ is positive semidefinite function of n_i. Usually, there exist discrete orientations n^o_i for which it vanishes. The corresponding solutions g^o_m of (8) are then fully defined. The discrete band orientations, n^o_i, are crystallographically determined and are only slightly modified in the theory of order one. In special situations involving multiple slip, however, the bifurcation conditions $T^o_{km} g^o_m = 0$ determine neither n^o_i nor g^o_m but are identically satisfied for certain subspaces of n^o_i and g^o_m. In these cases the band orientations will be found only in the next approximation. Such situations are particularly suspect of instability and will be discussed in section 3.2.

3. Deformation localization and collective dislocation modes in single crystal plasticity

In this section the formation conditions and structures of deformation bands are reviewed in connection with experimental observations. Although it is only conditionally admissible to compare observations on well developed deformation bands with predictions of bifurcation analysis which, by its very spirit, is concerned with the incipient process of localization, experimental results often fir remarkably well to the theory.

3.1 Single slip orientations

The simplest rate-independent constitutive model of single crystal plasticity is based on slip theory and Schmid´s law. Let us consider $\vec{G}$ and $\vec{N}$ to be the unit vectors of the slip direction and slip plane normal, respectively. Then, the theory of order zero yields two different bifurcation modes corresponding to ordinary slip bands of primary slip and kink bands, respectively (e.g. /6/):

(10) $\vec{g}^o = \vec{G}$, $\vec{n}^o = \vec{N}$ (slip band); $\vec{g}^o = \vec{N}$, $\vec{n}^o = \vec{G}$ (kink band)

The theory of order zero yields no information on the conditions of localization, which are determined by the first order theory:

(11) $h \leq 0$ (slip bands); $h \leq \vec{N} \underline{\sigma} \vec{N} - \vec{G} \underline{\sigma} \vec{G}$ (kink bands)

where h is the hardening rate of the slip system and $\underline{\sigma}$ the stress tensor. The equality signs in (11) designate critical conditions. While slip band formation requires the hardening rate to be smaller than or equal to zero (actual material weakening or at least ideal plasticity) kink band formation should be possible with positive hardening rates. The specific condition for kink band formation is due to a geometrical effect caused by a lattice rotation inside the band with respect to the surrounding matrix. Since the slip system is crystallographically fixed to the lattice the resolved shear stress is changed by the rotation. Thereby, depending on the orientation of the band with respect to the stress axes, either a promotion or a suppression of further deformation is achieved. In the paper /6/ by Asaro and Rice this effect was overlooked. (The term analogous to eq. (3.45) of that paper does not vanish if $\vec{m}$ is replaced by $\vec{s}$.)

For an uniaxial stress state with a stress axis $\vec{a}$ and stress level σ (positive in tension and negative in compression) the condition for kink band formation becomes

(12) $h \leq \sigma F$, $F = (\vec{N}.\vec{a})^2 - (\vec{G}.\vec{a})^2$.

Fig.1 shows curves of constant F in the standard orientation triangle for f.c.c. crystals. Let us assume that the hardening rate is monotonically decreasing during homogeneous deformation. Then, for axis orientations in the area $F > 0$ kink band formation is favoured against slip band formation in tension ($\sigma > 0$). This is in general accordance with observations on f.c.c. single crystals, namely that strong kink bands appear for orientations of the tensile axis near the circle $\langle 100 \rangle - \langle 110 \rangle$ /13,14/. In unaxial compression orientations of the stress axis in the area $F < 0$ should be favourable for kink band formation.

If we take the slip systems of b.c.c. crystals to be of type $\{110\}, \langle 111 \rangle$ the factor F changes only in sign. Then we expect for axis orientations near $[111]$ favoured kink band formation in tension and suppressed kink band formation in compression. Exactly that was found by Flewitt and Crocker /15/ for Nb single crystals deformed at room temperature. Moreover, the single slip system partaking in kink band formation was identified as (101), $[11\bar{1}]$. Axis orientations near $[110]$ are predicted to be easy orientations for kinking in compression. However, no kink bands were observed by Flewitt and Crocker at these orientations. Though the actual slip system was (112), $[11\bar{1}]$ in this case the calculation yields also $F < 0$ so that there would be no qualitative change of the expectation. A simple calculation shows, however, that the critical bifurcation condition was not achieved during the compression experiment. The deformation was stopped at a stress level of 118 MPa and a hardening rate $d|\sigma|/d\varepsilon$ = 900 MPa while the critical condition for kink band formation would require the hardening rate to fall below +77 MPa at the same stress level.

The bifurcation conditions (11) may be essentially modified by small departures from the Schmid law. Such non-Schmid effects, in the sense that other stress components than the resolved shear stress of the active slip system may effect the shear strain of this system, were theoretically investigated by Asaro and Rice /6/ as well in a general and elegant form as well as specifically for a constitutive model of cross slip. Let us consider p to be a small dimensionless parameter describing any non-Schmid effect. Then the general result is that the critical hardening rates (11) are shifted to positive values by terms of the order $p^2 G$ with G the elastic shear modulus. For example, when the departure from Schmid's law is caused by a pressure dependence of the critical resolved shear stress, the non-Schmid effect may be described by the "strength differential" $p = 2(\sigma_c - \sigma_t)/(\sigma_c + \sigma_t)$, i.e. the relative difference between the yield strengths in unaxial compression (σ_c) and in unaxial tension (σ_t).

3.2 Double slip orientations

If slip is proceeding simultaneously on two or more slip systems a bifurcation of homogeneous deformation into a shear band can occur at positive hardening rates even without non Schmid effects. This has been shown theoretically for plane double slip models by Asaro /7/ and Pegel et al. /8/ and will be roughly explained below. While Asaro studied a simplified model assuming, besides elastic isotropy, also elastic incompressibility the results (13) to (19) are obtained without the latter restriction. Let $\vec{G}^{(i)}$ and $\vec{N}^{(i)}$ be the slip direction and slip plane normal of the i-th slip plane normal of the i-th slip system

($i = 1,2$) and consider a symmetric configuration shown in Fig 2. The resolved shear stresses of both systems are $\tau^{(1,2)} = \frac{1}{2}(\sigma_{11} - \sigma_{22})\sin 2\varphi \pm \sigma_{12}\cos 2\varphi$. Fig.3 shows the yield locus in a two-dimensional stress space. At $\sigma_{12} = 0$, due to the equivalence of both slip systems in this stress state, the yield locus has a vertex. At the vertex the plastic deformation rate is undetermined since the total plastic deformation may be arbitrarily distributed among the slip systems. The bifurcation field can make use of this freedom to induce premature instability.

The relevant constitutive parameters describing double slip are the hardening rates of direct and latent hardening defined by $d\tau_c^{(i)} = \sum_k h_{ik} d\gamma^{(k)}$ where $d\tau_c^{(i)}$ and $d\gamma^{(i)}$ are increments of resolved shear stress and of plastic shear, respectively, of the i-th slip system. The diagonal components of h_{ik} represent direct hardening rates and the non-diagonal components latent hardening rates. In the theory of order zero the bifurcation condition (9) yields merely the statements $n_3^0 = 0$, $\vec{n}^0 \cdot \vec{g}^0 = 0$. Taking $h_{11} = h_{22} = h$, $h_{12} = h_{21} = qh$, eq. (9) reads in first order theory:

$$(13) + \frac{2h}{\sin^2 4\varphi}\left\{1 + q\cos 4\varphi - (1+q)\cos^2 2\varphi (n_1^2 - n_2^2)^2 - 4\sin^2 2\varphi (1-q)n_1^2 n_2^2\right\}$$
$$+ \sigma_{11}(n_1^2 - \tfrac{1}{2}) + \sigma_{22}(n_2^2 - \tfrac{1}{2}) + 2\sigma_{12} n_1 n_2$$
$$+ \frac{1}{2\cos 2\varphi}\left\{(\sigma_{11} - \sigma_{22})(1 - 4n_1^2 n_2^2) - 4n_1 n_2 (n_1^2 - n_2^2)\sigma_{12}\right\} = 0$$

(not valid in the particular case $\varphi = 45°$ of Fig.2). Let us consider the uniaxial stress state $\sigma_{12} = \sigma_{22} = 0$, $\sigma_{11} = \sigma$. Introducing the effective hardening rate $h_1 = 2h(1+q)/\sin^2 2\varphi$ for uniaxial deformation and the angle, χ, between the band and the stress axis ($n_1 = \sin\chi$, $n_2 = -\cos\chi$) the bifurcation condition (13) can be written as

$$(14)\ \frac{h_1}{\sigma} = F(\chi) = \frac{2\cos 2\varphi \cos 2\chi (1+q)(\cos 2\varphi + \cos 2\chi)}{(1+q)\cos^2 2\varphi \sin^2 2\chi + (1-q)\sin^2 2\varphi \cos^2 2\chi}$$

Assuming that $h_1/|\sigma|$ is monotonically decreasing during a homogeneous deformation history its critical value is defined by

$$(15)\ \left(\frac{h_1}{|\sigma|}\right)_c = \max \frac{\sigma}{|\sigma|} F(\chi) \equiv \frac{\sigma}{|\sigma|} F(\chi_c).$$

As a condition of consistency the plastic shear strain rates, $\delta\dot\gamma^{(1)}$, $\delta\dot\gamma^{(2)}$, of the bifurcation field must be positive semidefinite. This leads to the condition $|\tan 2\chi| \geq |\tan 2\varphi|$. With this restriction (14) and (15) yield the critical orientations

(16) a) $\cos 2\chi_c = \cos 2\varphi$, $F(\chi_c) = \frac{2(1+q)\cos 2\varphi}{\sin^2 2\varphi}$

b) $\cos 2\chi_c = -\frac{\cos 2\varphi}{q + \cos 4\varphi}(1 + q - \sqrt{2(1+q)}\sin 2\varphi)$, $F(\chi_c) = \cos 2\chi_c$

The difference of lattice rotation rates inside and outside the deformation band, $\delta\vec\omega$, is given by

(17) $\delta\vec{\omega} = \delta\dot{\gamma}\,(\vec{n}^{\,0} \times \vec{g}^{\,0})\,(1 + \frac{\cos 2\chi}{\cos 2\varphi})$

with $\delta\dot{\gamma}$ the localized shear strain rate in the band. The deformation bands are not strict shear bands. The condition for a pure shear, $\vec{n}.\vec{g} = 0$, holds true only in the lowest approximation while the first order theory yields

(18) $\vec{n}.\vec{g} = \frac{1-2\nu}{G}\,\frac{\sigma}{|\sigma|}\,\frac{\sin 2\chi}{2}\,\left\{ h_1 \frac{q+\cos 4\varphi}{1+q}\,\frac{\cos 2\chi}{2\cos^2 2\varphi} + \sigma\,(1+\frac{\cos 2\chi}{\cos 2\varphi}) \right\}.$

An interesting consequence of this deviation from pure shear is that additional stresses arise inside the band. This can be shown by calculating, for example, the excess hydrostatic stress rate

(19) $\frac{D}{Dt}\,\delta p = -\frac{2}{3}\,\frac{(1+\nu)}{(1-\nu)}\,G\,f^{\,\prime}(\vec{n}.\vec{r})\,\vec{n}.\vec{g}$

which is proportional to $\vec{n}.\vec{g}$ and vanishes outside the band where $f^{\,\prime} = 0$. The relation of such excess stresses with departures from pure shear can be well conceived in a dislocation model (Fig.4). Dislocations moving on slip planes not strictly parallel to the band edges must stop and pile up at the edges. The resulting dislocation walls of opposite sign create an internal stress component along the band. Assuming elastic incompressibility, i.e. putting $\nu = 1/2$ in eq. (18), the deformation bands become strict shear bands and the excess stresses must escape attention as was the case in Asaro´s paper /7/. The bifurcation conditions (13) or (14), not containing the Poisson ratio ν, are not sensitive to the incompressibility assumption in first order theory.

In /8/ a particular vertex situation, realized by uniaxial tension of b.c.c. Mo single crystals with a $\langle 110 \rangle$ tensile axis, was studied. This corresponds to $\varphi = 54.7°$ ($\tan\varphi = \sqrt{2}$) in Fig.2. Observing $\cos 2\varphi = -1/3$ the critical band orientation for tension is obtained from (15) and (16b). It is only weakly dependent on the ratio, q, of latent and direct hardening. E.g. $\chi_c = 40.9°$ at q = 0 and $\chi_c = 39.7°$ at q = 2. Thus the assumption q = 0 of paper /8/ is not relevant with respect to observations which fit remarkably well to theory.

An experimental study of shear localization in Al-2.8% Cu single crystals /9/ showed that macroscopic deformation bands were related with the occurence of double primary-conjugate slip. But the plane double slip model on which the authors based their discussion is not strictly valid for primary-conjugate slip. Generally, during non-symmetric double slip the localization modes are already determined by the theory of order zero to be crystallographic slip (or kink) bands of the primary and conjugate system and the specific vertex effect (non-crystallographic band orientations and positive hardening rates) are absent as was also mentioned in review /16/. In copper-titanium single crystals with coherent precipitates a sudden burst of intense localized flow occured as the tensile axis rotated to the vicinity of the $\langle 100 \rangle \langle 111 \rangle$ symmetry boundary

/17/. This phenomenon is also suspect of being related to the onset of double slip.

4. Conclusion

Bifurcation analysis is often complicated by several competing localization modes. Shearing modes may be preceded by necking modes /16,19/. Shear bands form more abruptly and are more distinct the stronger the crystal. This was verified by a numerical analysis of post-bifurcation behaviour of single crystals /16/ and seems to be a general tendency in materials /19/. In /18/ this tendency was attributed to the "gradient" $(d/d\varepsilon)(h/|\sigma|)$ of the stability parameter $h/|\sigma|$ at the bifurcation point. The more rapid by the critical point is crossed by the deformation path the more abruptly the corresponding deformation mode will form.

Since the bifurcation conditions in single crystals depend on subtle features in the description of material behaviour, u.e. non-Schmid effects, a careful formulation of mechanics is needed. But there is a certain arbitrariness in the definition of stress rates in continuum mechanics. The use of different stress rate measures will lead, in principle, to different first order terms in bifurcation theory. However, all terms by which the various admissible measures may differ fortunately cancel out in the (first order) bifurcation conditions. This was proved in general form for single slip models /6/ and for plane double slip models and elastic isotropy /20/. A general proof is not yet known. Summarizing it can be stated that, apart from crystallographic features, the relevant parameters governing the appearance of collective modes are flow stresses and hardening rates. Independently of the real micromechanisms by which these parameters are determined, the critical localization modes appear in phenomenologically similar forms which are governed by mechanical principles. The bifurcation concept has been successfully applied to localization phenomena in various materials and has proved remarkably useful in problems of single crystal plasticity.

References

/1/ Sestak B., Seeger A.: Z. Metallkunde 69 (1978), 195
/2/ Aydin A., Johnson A.M.: Pageoph. 116 (1978), 931
/3/ Kurokawa M., Ban T.: J. Appl. Polymer Sci. 8 (1964), 971
/4/ Haken H.: Naturwiss. 67 (1980), 121
/5/ Rice J.R.: Proc. 14th IUTAM Congr., North-Holland Publ. Comp., Amsterdam 1977, p. 207
/6/ Asaro R.J., Rice J.R.: J. Mech. Phys. Solids 25 (1977), 309
/7/ Asaro R.J.: Acta Met. 27 (1979), 445
/8/ Pegel B. et al.: Scripta Met. 29 (1980), 47

/9/ Chang Y.W., Asaro R.J.: Acta Met. 29 (1981), 241

/10/ Hill R.: Problems of Continuum Mechanics (eds: M.A. Lavrentev et al.), Soc.Ind.Appl. Maths., Philadelphia 1961, p. 155

/11/ Pegel B.: Wiss. Ber. ZFW 18 (1979), 59

/12/ Rice J.R., Rudnicki J.W.: Int. J. Solids and Struct. 16 (1980), 597

/13/ Seeger A.: in S. Flügge (ed.), Encyclopedia of Physics, VII, 2 Springer-Verlag, Berlin, Göttingen, Heidelberg 1958, p. 76

/14/ Kirch F.: Dissertation (1970), TH Aachen

/15/ Flewitt P.F.J., Crocker A.G.: Phil. Mag. 34 (1976), 877

/16/ Peirce D., Asaro R.J., Needleman A.: Acta Met. 30 (1982), 1087

/17/ Greggi J., Soffa W.A.: Scripta Met. 12 (1978), 525

/18/ Pegel B., Richter J.: Neue Hütte 26 (1981), 473

/19/ Richter J., Pegel B.: Neue Hütte 26 (1981), 286

/20/ Pegel B.: unpublished

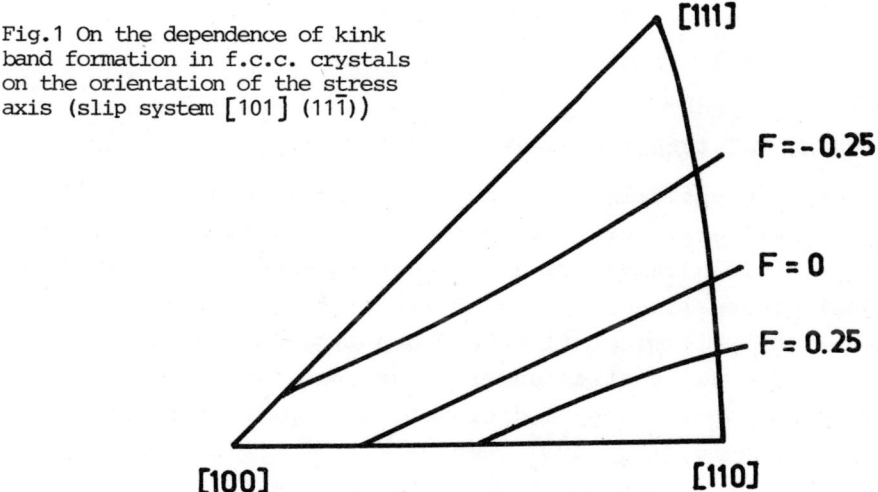

Fig.1 On the dependence of kink band formation in f.c.c. crystals on the orientation of the stress axis (slip system $[101]$ $(11\bar{1})$)

Fig.2 Plane double slip configuration with the x_1-x_3-plane as a mirror plane

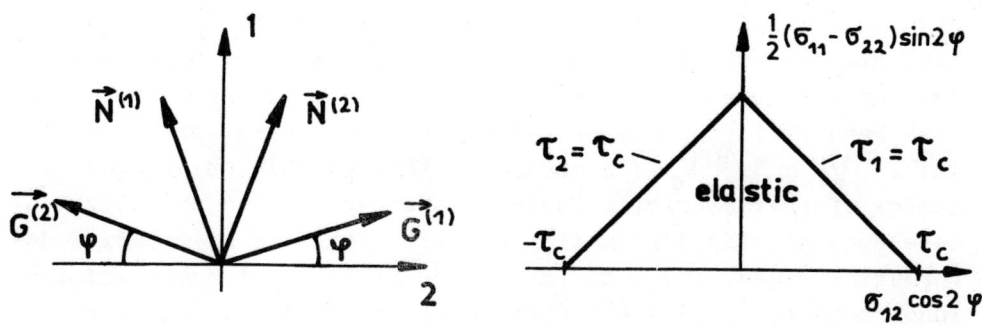

Fig.3 Yield locus with vertex at symmetric double slip. τ_c is the critical resolved shear stress corresponding to the Schmid law and taken to be equal for both slip system.

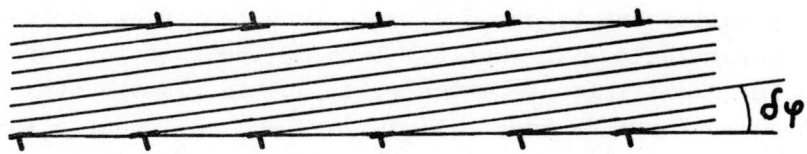

Fig.4 Dislocation model of excess stress in a deformation band.
$\vec{n}.\vec{g}. = \sin\delta\varphi \approx \delta\varphi$

- 417 -

DISCLINATION PHYSICS OF PLASTIC DEFORMATION

A.E. Romanov, V.I. Vladimirov

A.F. Ioffe Physico-Technical Institute, Academy of Sciences of the USSR, Polytechnicheskaya 26, 194021 Leningrad, USSR

At the present time the theory of plastic flow at small strains is well developed. It is not much more than platitude to claim that small strains are direct consequences of the glide of individual dislocations. Such a motion of dislocations can be compared with the laminar flow in hydraulic. An elementary event responsible for deformation under these conditions consists in a pair of kinks formation by a dislocation. A pair of kinks characteristic volume is: $V_s \leq 10^3 V_o$, where $V_o = b^3$ is an elementary cell volume. The magnitude of V_s determines a characteristic scale for the small strains in question.

As the amount of strain ($\varepsilon > 0.1$) increases, the scale becomes larger. Now the elementary event is a result of correlated displacement of big dislocation groups. Here are formed and come into play so-called mesoscopic defect structures. Correspondingly, there occurs displacement or rotation of large volumes V_ℓ with respect to the neighbouring ones. The scale for large strains is $V_\ell \approx 10^{10} V_o$. Alongside with the scale enlargement a number of characteristic features are peculiar to the stage of developed plastic deformation: i) - the arising of rotation deformation modes, ii) - the growth of internal stresses and their inhomogeneity, iii) - the dominant role of dinamic recovery, iv) - tendency to strain localization, v) - microcrack nucleation an so on.

The arising of the rotation (disclination) modes of plastic deformation is the most important feature of the process. Deformation progress due to the reciprocal rotations of the volumes of the matter can be compared with turbulent flow in liquids. This paper deals with physical laws of the rotation deformation.

Important role of matter rotations in plastic strain was pointed out by A.F. Ioffe /1/ as far back as in early thirties. Later some on studying re-orientation phenomena in plastic deformation were reported /2/. However, most interesting experiments in this area were run with the aid of high-voltage electron microscopy during last two decades. Thus a phenomenon of fragmentation /3/ was discovered which appeared to be characteristic for all metals at large strains in active deformation. It is reported in this and other numerous works that in certain stage of plastic flow takes place a fragmentation of a material into mutually rotated microvolumes, the further deformation progressing preferentially by micro-rotations.

Physical carriers of the plastic rotations in solids are linear defects of rotational type: disclinations. A review of studied properties of disclination-type defects is given, for example in /4/. In an elastic continuum an individual disclination defect is given by a spatial position of the defect line, the magnitude and direction of the rotation pseudovector $\vec{\omega}$ (the Frank vector) as well as the rotation axiy displacement with respect to the line. Disclinations can be also defined with the help of continuously distributed densities. Dislocation and disclination densities are introduced as magnitudes compensating for the violation of the deformation compatibility condition /5/.

Earlier theories of plastic deformation regarded disclinations to be of no importance in real crystalline specimens. It was connected with logarithmic divergence of elastic stresses and strains performed by individual disclinations at large distances from their lines. Such straight line defects (wedge disclinations, for instance) are characterized by a square energy dependence on the Frank vector modulus ω as well as a characteristic body size L /4/. Only decreasing the enrgy of disclination systems to magnitudes comparable with the external force work makes possible to regard them as real physical objects. Such a decrease in the energy of disclination defects can be reached by two ways: by decreasing disclination Frank vector $\vec{\omega}$ or by formation of screened disclination systems. The former is responsible for the origin of disclinations, the rotation angle of which does not correlate with the lattice symmetry. Such disclinations are partial: they are connected with the "stacking fault" surface (mis-orientation boundary), Fig.1. The later way uniting disclinations in dipoles (Fig.1,a), loop configurations (Fig.1,b) and other multipoles (Fig.1,c). The screening can be performed by different interfaces (Fig.1,d) or by the sources of elastic fields of non-disclination nature, the dislocation cloud, for instance (Fig.1,e). Thus, the physical basis of rotational deformation is, in essence, a theory of screened systems of partial disclinations.

With the aid of a three-dimensional net of mutually screened disclinations naturally one can describe the geometry and find the stresses in sub-grain and fragment structures /6/. Of great importance here is studying of intrinsic elastic fields of typical screened disclination systems. Main results obtained for circular disclination loops and dipoles by seventies are reported in /4/. Recently, a variety of other screened defects have been investigated: rectangular loops (Fig.1,b) /7/ and straight line disclinations at a free surface (Fig.1,d) /8/. Introduction of the rectangular defects permits to analyze the dependence of loop properties on their shape (i.e. dependence on the shape parameter $p = c/d$) and considerably simplifies calculations as compared with circular loops. In the case of disclinations free surface possesses much stronger screening effect as compared with dislocations /8/. For straight line disclinations at a free surface the characteristic screening parameter is not the body size L but a distance d between the defect line and the surface. Finally, the wedge disclination self energy turns out to be proportional to d^2, which increases the probability of disclination nucleation in the deformed sub-surface layer. In these terms can be explained experimental data on the subgrain structure mis-orientation average angle growth near the surface.

Rotational plasticity development passes through the stages of the nucleation of disclination deformation centers and the successive motion and multiplication of disclination configurations. At microscopic and mesoscopic levels the arising of rotational instability means that co-operative effects come into play in the dislocation ensemble. The possibility of cooperative effects is determined by an excessive dislocation density $\Delta\rho$ for dislocations of opposite signes, i.e. dislocation charge density. As a criterion for the inception of co-operative effects the equality between the external stress and the dislocation charge long-range field can be taken. A certain amount of previous plastic strain ε is necessary for increasing deformation inhomogeneity, only. Eventually, the deformation inhomogeneity aids in accumulating powerful dislocation charges. In the case of nucliation of disclination defects there occurs a relaxation of a portion of the dislocation charge long-range elastic fields due to the elastic stress moment $\vec{M}(\Delta g)$. The elastic stress moment $\vec{M}$ can be connected not only with dislocation charges, but with non-uniform external fields too, which explaines the heightened tendency of polymers and composites to the development of disclination plasticity modes. Essential in the nucliation of disclination defects is the rotation axis position, the possibility of its shifting with regard to a relatively immobile disclination line. In this case a considerable contribution into the energy balance of the process of disclination nucleation and motion is made (alongside with the non-uniform elastic field) by a certain average stress level. Therefore the rotational plasticity is not an obligatory relaxation process. It can be also an active one, i.e. a process going under the action of constant external forces.

Motion of disclination defects results in the rotation of some singled out micro-volumes with respect to the surrounding matter. A simplest picture illustrating the rotation contribution into shear deformation is given in Fig.2. The shear of the upper part of the spacimen with regard to the lower one can be performed due to a cut on the rolls (Fig.2,a) or moving the partial disclination wedge dipole (Fig.2,b). The motion of such a dipole is macroscopically equivalent to the displacement of an edge dislocation with Burgers vector $B = \omega a$ (Fig.2,c). The micromechanism of the disclination dipole movement at small misorientation angles $\omega \leq 0.2$ consists in the dislocation density ρ_0 re-distribution (separation of dislocation charges) in front of the dipole (Fig.3). There are limitations for the possibility of operation of such a mechanism. These limitations determine the range of the existence of the mobile dipoles (in coordinates the initial dislocation density ρ_0, the power ω, the arm a, the external stress σ) capable to fragmentize the crystal. Calculation of critical values ρ_{0c}, ω_c, a_c are in good agreement with experimental data /3/ on the observation of partial disclination dipoles. In order to evaluate the strain rate $\dot{\varepsilon}$ due to the dipoles moving with velocity v_d the following relation was used: $\dot{\varepsilon} = \Theta a \omega v_d$, Θ being the disclination dipole density.

It has been noted above that the disclination modes are peculiar to large plastic strains. Other characteristics (enumerated in the beginning of this paper) can be related, under certain conditions, to the development of the deformation rotational modes too. Fig.3 shows the interrelationship between the current and rotational instabilities of plastic deformation. The rotational instability is connected with secondary slip system operation. In the primary slip system dislocation charge separation is able to cover large distances. This leads to formation of a dislocation avalanche (light dislocations) sweeping forward a dislocationless channel. Crystal lattice in the channel interior turns out to be mis-orientated with respect to the surrounding matter, which is proved experomentally. Thus, the plastic flow localization in the form of the current instability and the development of disclination plasticity can be interrelated.

Disclination systems appeared due to some relaxation process are the sources of strong elastic fields. It means the connexion between progress of disclination modes and the accumulation during the developed deformation of high and inhomogeneous internal stresses. At the intermediate stage of deformation there arize situations when the number of disclination defects is relatively small. The plasticity being determined by dislocation motion, the disclination configurations become effective barriers for dislocations (Fig.4). Corresponding disclination models show qualitative and quantitative agreement with experiments. One can describe, for example, the hardening law at the third stage of BCC metals deformation, determining a linear dependence of the deforming stress σ_d on mis-orientation angle $\sigma_d \sim G\omega$, G being shear modulus. Under conditions of active disclination plasticity hardening is connected with latent elastic energy of disclination defects.

Availability of stress concentration in the vicinity of disclination defects results in interrelationship between the deformation rotational modes and the processes of micro-fracture. As is shown in /9/ under the disclination fault can occur a forced crack opening. In composites the development of kink bands and the torsional disclination modes is accompanied by failure and stratification of fibers. The connexion between the deformation mechanisms and fracture can acquire an inverse sense when stress relaxation in the plastic zone in front of the crack tip goes in a rotational way (Fig.5).

In conclusion, it should be noted that disclination mechanisms of plastic deformation play the dominant role in such macroscopic phenomena as kink band formation, Luders deformation, twinning and so on. The process of sub-grain re-orientation in creep can be also described in succession within the framework of disclination concept.

Further progress in disclination theory is connected with theoretical calculation or experimental study of partial disclination mobility. Of great importance here is also the analysis and observation of defect structures equivalent to disclination systems. The result of solution of these and other problems of experimental and theoretical physics will be building practical theories for different kinds of mechanical treatment of materials.

References

/1/ Ioffe A.F.: Physics of crystals, GIZ, Moscow-Leningrad 1929.
/2/ Müller H.: Z. Metallk. 50 (1959) 351.
/3/ Vergazov A.N., Likhachev V.A., Rybin V.V.: Fizika Metallov i Metallovedenie 42 (1976) 146.
/4/ Likhachev V.A., Khairov R.Yu.: Introduction to the theory of disclinations, Izd. LGU, Leningrad 1975.
/5/ De Wit R.: Continual theory of disclinations, Mir, Moscow 1977.
/6/ Vladimirov V.I., Zukowskii I.M.: Fizika Tverdogo Tela 17 (1975) 1196.
/7/ Vladimirov V.I., Romanov A.E.: Fizika Tverdogo Tela 23 (1981) 3719.
/8/ Romanov A.E., Vladimirov V.I.: Phys. Stat. Sol.(a) 63 (1981) 109.
/9/ Rybin V.V., Zukowskii I.M.: Fizika Tverdogo Tela 20 (1978) 1929

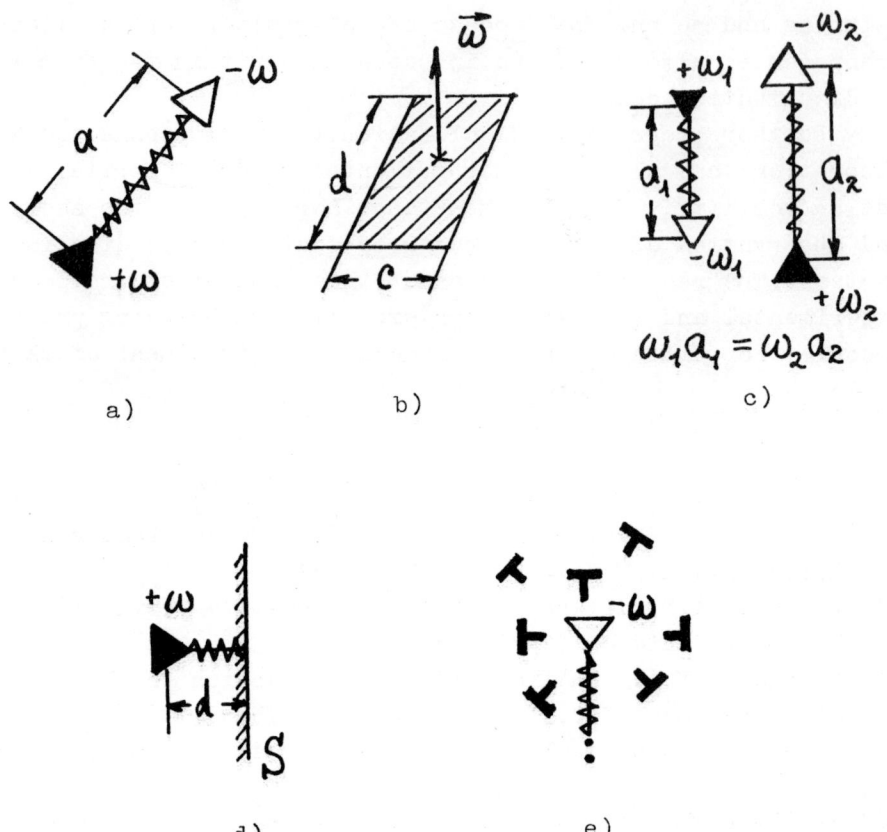

Fig.1. Screened disclination systems. The partial disclination "staking fault" Surfaces are shaded.

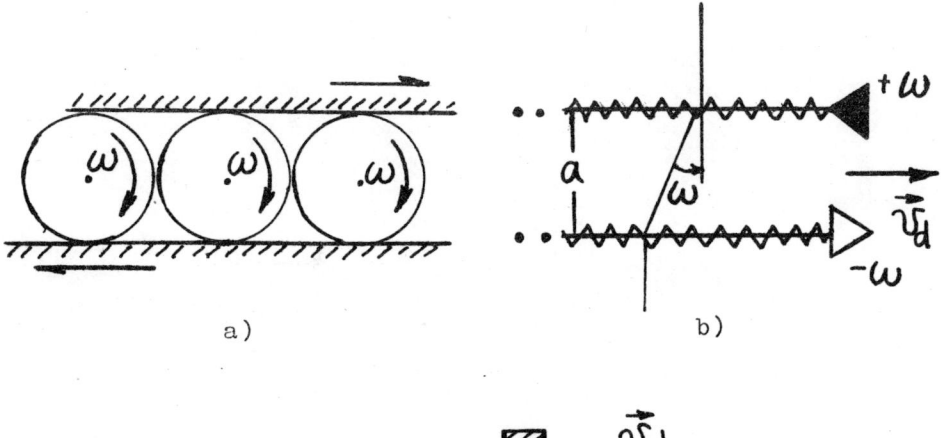

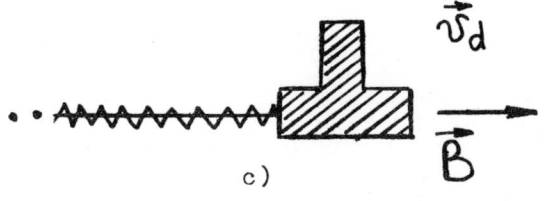

Fig.2. Contribution of rotations in plastic deformation.

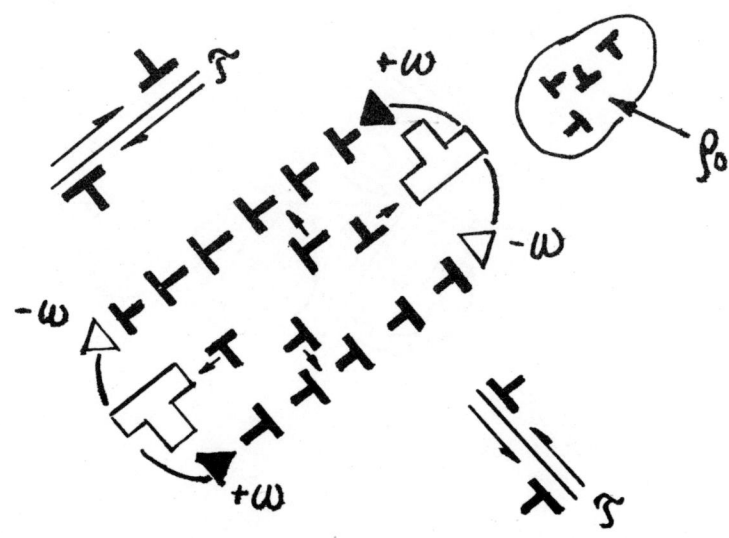

Fig.3. Current-rotation instability of plastic deformation.

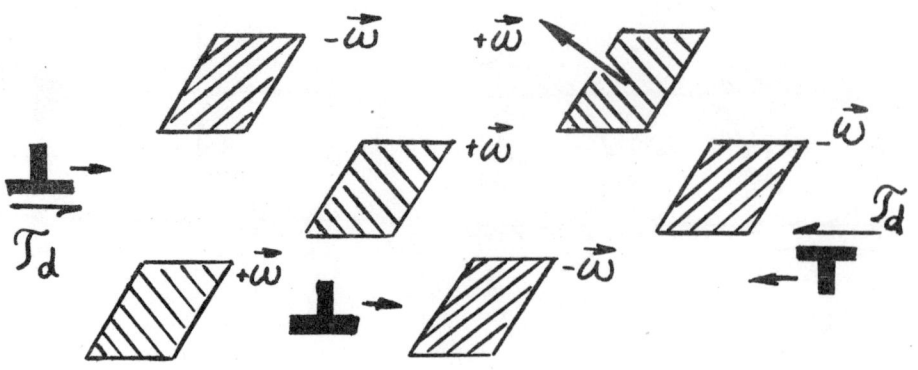

Fig.4. Disclination model of hardening in the intermediate stage of deformation.

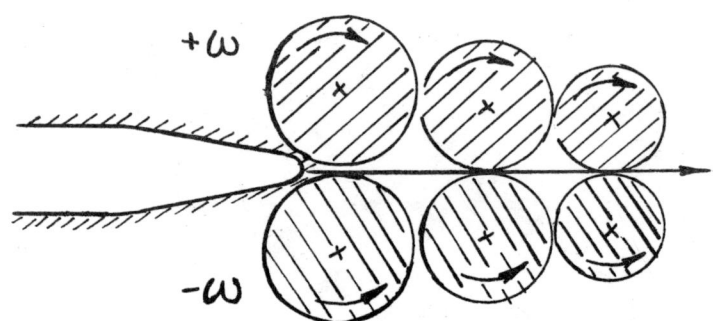

Fig.5. Relaxation in the plastic zone at a crack tip with the help of rotations.

EQUILIBRIUM CONFIGURATION OF DISLOCATIONS AROUND A CRACK TIP
G. Michot and G. CHAMPIER
Institut National Polytechnique de Lorraine - ENSMIM -
Parc de Saurupt, 54042 Nancy Cedex, France

1 - Introduction

Different models aiming at establishing a relation between the extension of the plastic zone developed at a crack-tip and the loading conditions of the specimen have been proposed, such as Dugdale's macroscopic approach [1] and Bilby, Cottrel and Swinden's microscopic approach [2]. The BCS model seems to lead to results which are very consistent with certain experimental observations [3-5]. However, it expects a dislocation density tending towards infinity on the crack tip and such a situation cannot occur physically. Recent works [6,7] allow for the existence of a "dislocation free zone" in the neighbourhood of the crack tip and this hypothesis does not result in an infinite dislocation density. Chang and Ohr [8] have modified the BCS model in this direction ; yet they have not taken into account the perturbation of the interaction of dislocations near the free surfaces [9-12]. Starting from the results obtained by Majumdar and Burns [10] we propose to characterize the distribution of the dislocations emitted in the vicinity of a crack as a function of the value of the applied stress intensity factor.

2 - Model

The calculation refers to an infinite solid containing a semi-infinite plane crack. The plane of the crack lies parallel to a slip plane of the solid and the crack tip is parallel to a glide direction in this plane. A force is applied to each face of the crack along a line that is parallel to the crack tip and in the same direction (Fig.1) ; the mode of application of the stress is thus mode III, with the corresponding applied stress intensity factor K_σ.

For a given value of K_σ screw dislocations parallel to the crack tip are emitted in the slip plane considered above ; these constitue a configuration of dislocations distributed according the $\rho(x)$ law between abscissae a_1 and a_2 as measured from the crack tip (Fig.1). The calculation aims at determining the variations of the characteristics a_1, a_2 and $\rho(x)$ of this configuration as functions of the values of the applied stress intensity factor.

3 - Basic equations

There are two basic equations : on the one hand the elastic equilibrium equation and on the other the expression of the effective stress intensity factor K^*.

Assuming that the solid is isotropic, the elastic equilibrium equation at point x of the configuration is expressed by

$$(1) \quad \frac{K^*}{\sqrt{2\pi x}} - \frac{\mu b}{4\pi x} - \tau_y + \frac{\mu b}{2\pi} \int_{a_1}^{a_2} \sqrt{\frac{\xi}{x}} \frac{\rho(x)}{x-\xi} d\xi = 0$$

μ is the shear modulus and b the Burgers vector of the dislocations. The first term of relation (1) expresses the stress around the crack tip ; the second one represents the stress resulting from the image force ; the third one, τ_y, is the value of the shear stress in the slip plane beneath which the dislocation can no longer move ; as for the last term it expresses the interaction between dislocations in presence of a crack. We owe the expressions of the second and last terms to Majumdar and Burns [10].

The expression of the effective stress intensity factor takes into account the feedback effect of the dislocations already emitted

$$(2) \quad K^* = K_\sigma - \frac{\mu b}{\sqrt{2\pi}} \int_{a_1}^{a_2} \frac{\rho(x)}{\sqrt{x}} dx$$

We owe the second term of the right member to Majumdar and Burns [10].

4 - Solution of the basic equations

Equation (1) is expressed as :

$$(3) \quad \omega(x) + \int_{a_1}^{a_2} \frac{\sqrt{\xi}\, \rho(x)}{x-\xi} d\xi = 0 \quad \text{where} \quad \omega(x) = \frac{\sqrt{2\pi}K^*}{\mu b} - \frac{1}{2\sqrt{x}} - \frac{2\pi\tau_y\sqrt{x}}{\mu b}$$

According to Muskhelishvili [13] equation (3) for $\rho(x)$ can be solved if the following condition is fufilled :

$$(4) \quad \int_{a_1}^{a_2} \frac{\omega(\xi)}{\sqrt{(\xi-a_1)(a_2-\xi)}} d\xi = 0$$

Taking into account the expression of $\omega(\xi)$, the calculation leads to the relation

$$(5) \quad \sqrt{a_2'}\,(k^*,p) = \frac{k^*}{4E} \left[1 + \sqrt{1 - \frac{8EF}{k^{*2}}} \right]$$

$$a_2' = 2\pi a_2/a_0 \qquad a_0 = \mu b/\tau_y \qquad p = \sqrt{(a_2-a_1)/a_2}$$

$$k^* = \pi K^*/K_o \qquad K_o = \sqrt{\mu b \tau_y}$$

$$F = F(\pi/2) \text{ with } F(\varepsilon) = \int_o^\varepsilon [1 - p^2\sin^2\theta]^{-1/2} d\theta$$

$$E = E(\pi/2) \text{ with } E(\varepsilon) = \int_o^\varepsilon [1 - p^2\sin^2\theta]^{1/2} d\theta$$

If condition (4) is fulfilled, the dislocation density $\rho(x)$ is formulated as :

$$(6) \quad \rho(x) = \frac{1}{\pi^2} \sqrt{\frac{(x-a_1)(a_2-x)}{x}} \int_{a_1}^{a_2} \frac{\omega(\xi)}{(x-\xi)\sqrt{(\xi-a_1)(a_2-\xi)}} d\xi$$

By replacing $\omega(\xi)$ by its expression and integrating we obtain

$$(7) \quad \rho(x) = \frac{2F}{\pi a_o} \left[2\sqrt{\frac{(x-a_1)(a_2-x)}{a_2 x}} - Z\left(2 - \frac{a_o}{2\pi x}\right) \right]$$

$$Z = E(\varepsilon) - E \cdot F(\varepsilon)/F \qquad \text{with } \varepsilon = \tan^{-1}\sqrt{(a_2-x)/(x-a_1)}$$

If the function $\rho(x)$ is kept positive in the interval $[a_1, a_2]$ we get the inequation

$$(8) \quad a_2' \geq a_{2\ell}' \qquad \text{with } a_{2\ell}' = \frac{E-F(1-p^2)}{2(1-p^2)(F-E)}$$

The number of the emitted dislocations is calculated by integrating expression (7) :

$$(9) \quad N = \int_{a_1}^{a_2} \rho(x) dx$$

The calculation shows that this relation can be formulated as :

$$(10) \quad a_2'(N,p) = A/B$$

$$A = \frac{\pi^2 N}{p^2 F} + \int_o^1 \frac{Z}{1-(1-X)p^2} dX \qquad \varepsilon = \tan^{-1}\sqrt{(1-X)/X}$$

$$B = \frac{4}{3p^2}\left[(2-p^2)E - 2(1-p^2)F\right] - 2\int_o^1 Z \, dX$$

If in equation (2) K^* is replaced by its value as inferred from relation (5) and $\rho(x)$ by its expression (6), the calculation leads to :

$$(11) \quad \sqrt{a_2'(k_\sigma,p)} = \frac{k_\sigma}{4(2E-F\sqrt{1-p^2})}\left[1 + \sqrt{1 - \frac{8(5FE-2F^2\sqrt{1-p^2}-2E^2/\sqrt{1-p^2})}{k_\sigma^2}}\right]$$

$$k_\sigma = \pi K_\sigma/K_o$$

5 - Results

The solution of the basic equations has lead to three formulations of the extreme abscissa a_2 (or a_2') of the dislocation configuration : (5) as a function of k^* and of the parameter p ; (10) as a function of N and of p ; (11) as a function of k_σ and of p. Each of these relations permits to draw a group of curves in the plan $(p, \sqrt{a_2'})$, the second parameter, respectively k^*, N and k_σ keeping a fixed value. An outline of the curves thus obtained is given in figures 2,3 and 4.

On each of these figures the limit curve $\sqrt{a_{2\ell}'(p)}$, corresponding to relation (8), has also been drawn. On the graph we notice -and this is accurately checked by calculation- that the minimum of the curve drawn for a fixed value of k_σ is located at the intersection of this curve with the limit curve. Besides, the curve with a fixed k_σ and that with a fixed k^* passing at the previous minimum point are tangent.

6 - Discussion

The distribution law $\rho(x)$ of the dislocations as expressed by relation (7) assumes that the values of a_1 and a_2 are known. Now we only have relation (11) to assess these values and in order to carry on with our calculation we have to introduce a new hypothesis. We have actually pursued our calculation in two particular cases.

First case : it is assumed that in equilibrium the effective stress intensity factor K^* (or k^*) has a value that is characteristic of the material, that is K_o^* (or k_o^*). For a given value of the applied stress intensity factor K_σ, $K_\sigma \geq K_o^*$, dislocations are emitted until $K^* = K_o^*$. The values of a_2 and p are deduced from those of the coordinates of the intersection point of the curve $K^* = K_o^*$ with the curve K_σ (Fig.2 and 4) in the plane $(p, \sqrt{a_2'})$; there is a solution only for K_σ less than $K_{\sigma\ell}$ which is the value of K_σ on the limit curve $\sqrt{a_{2\ell}'(p)}$. The curve giving the variation of a_2/a_o as a function of K_σ/K_o^* can be plotted. In fact if we draw the curve giving the variation of $a_2/a_o \cdot k_o^{*2}$ as a function of K_σ/K_o^*, the curve remains practically unchanged (Fig.5) whatever the value of K_o^* (or that of k_o^*, ranging form 50 to 300) ; after simplification, we can put :

$$(12) \quad a_2 = \frac{\pi^2 K_o^{*2}}{\tau_y^2} \left\{ 0.0161 + 0.0251 \left[1 - \exp\left(-\left(\frac{K_\sigma - K_o^*}{0.224 K_o^*}\right)^{0.726}\right) \right] \right\}$$

As in the case of classic models, the extension of the plastically deformed zone, measured here by a_2, varies as the inverse of the square of the yield stress. In the same mamer the curve representing the variation of N/k_o^{*2} as a function of K_σ/K_o^* is practically unchanged (Fig.6) whatever the value of K_o^*; after simplification, we obtain:

$$(13) \quad N = 0.0538 \frac{\pi^2 K_o^{*2}}{\mu b \tau_y} \left[1 - \exp - \left(\frac{K_\sigma - K_o^*}{0.422 K_o^*}\right)^{1.23}\right]$$

We can also establish the following approached relation between a_2 and N:

$$(14) \quad N = 160.4 \frac{\pi^2 \tau_y^{3.312}}{\mu b \, K_o^{*2.312}} \left[a_2 - 0.0161 \frac{K_o^{*2}}{\tau_y^2}\right]^{2.156}$$

The curve illustring this relation is given in figure 7.

Second case: it is assumed that in equilibrium the effective stress intensity factor K^* (or k^*) has a minimal value. For a given value of the applied stress intensity factor K_σ, dislocations are emitted until K^* reaches its minimal value. The values of a_2 and p are inferred from those of the coordinates of the intersection point of the curve K_σ with the limit curve $\sqrt{a'_{2\ell}}(p)$ (Fig.4) in the plane $(p, \sqrt{a'_2})$; the problem can be solved for $K_\sigma > K_{\sigma m}$, $K_{\sigma m}$ being the value of K_σ associated to the intersection point of the limit curve $\sqrt{a'_{2\ell}}(p)$ with the $\sqrt{a'_2}$ axis (Fig.4); the corresponding value is a'_{2m} (or a_{2m}). The calculation leads to the relations: $K_{\sigma m} = \sqrt{2} K_o$ and $a_{2m} = a_o/4\pi$. Figures 8,9 and 10 represent respectively the variations of a_2/a_{2m}, $K^*/K_{\sigma m}$ and N as functions of $K_\sigma/K_{\sigma m}$. As soon as $K_\sigma/K_{\sigma m}$ is large enough, each of these values can be approximated through the expression obtained when $K_\sigma/K_{\sigma m}$ tends towards infinity. After simplifying, we obtain for these expressions:

$$(15) \quad a_2 = \frac{\pi}{32} \frac{1}{\tau_y^2} K_\sigma^2$$

$$(16) \quad K^* = \frac{1}{2} K_\sigma \qquad N = \frac{1}{8\mu b \tau_y} K_\sigma^2$$

Again, as in the case of classic models, the extension a_2 varies as the inverse of the square of the yield stress. By recombing relations (15) and (16) we obtain:

$$(17) \quad N = \frac{4}{\pi} \frac{\tau_y}{\mu b} a_2$$

It must be noted that expression (15),(16) and (17) are identical with those which might be deduced from the BCS model if the crack length is large compared with the extension a_2 of the plastic zone. The curves in figure 11 represent the variations of $\rho(x)/a_o$ as a function of x/a_{2m} for different values of $K_\sigma/K_{\sigma m}$. The limit value $K_{\sigma m}$ can be understood as a "nucleation barrier". In fact the minimal value of the applied stress intensity factor K_σ corresponding to the appearance threshold of the dislocations is much superior to $K_{\sigma m}$ in the case of some semi-brittle materials [14]. It can thus be assumed that the proposed model applies essentially to ductile materials. Another model that is better adapted to semi-brittle materials is being studied.

In practical cases, measuring (a_2, K_σ) or (a_2, N) and comparing with relations (12) and (14) or (15) and (17) should make possible to determine which of the two hypothesis previously introduced gives a better approach to reality.

7 - Conclusion

We have studied the distribution law of dislocations around a crack tip in a mode III stressed specimen. Two basic equations have been used : the first one is the expression of the elastic equilibrium ; the second one is the expression of the effective stress intensity factor. Besides the stress field due to the crack and the lattice resistance, we have taken into account the image force and the effect of the presence of free surfaces (crack faces) on the form of the interaction between dislocations.

In order to solve the problem an extra assumption has had to be introduced. In a first case it has been assumed that dislocations are emitted only when the effective stress intensity factor is larger than a value K_o^* which is a characteristic of the material ; K_o^* can be considered as a "nucleation barrier" for this material. In a second case it has been assumed that dislocations are emitted when the applied stress intensity factor is larger than a value $K_{\sigma m}$ due to the image force and until the effective stress intensity factor reaches its minimal value ; again $K_{\sigma m}$ can be considered as a "nucleation barrier". We might expect that the first assumption can be applied to a a semi-brittle material and the second are to a ductile material.

Two kinds of relations habe been obtained between the extension of the plastic zone a_2, the total number of dislocations N and the value of the applied stress intensity factor K_σ. The experiment should permit to decide which of the hypothesis previously introduced gives a better approach to reality.

In fact we have put a "nucleation barrier" in terms of stress intensity factor, perhaps it would be better to introduce this concept in terms of stress.

References

/1/ Dugdale D.S. : J. Mech. Phys. Solids 8 (1960) 100.
/2/ Bilby B.A., Cottrell A.H., Swinden F.R.S. and K.H. : Proc. Roy. Soc. A272 (1963) 304.
/3/ Ohr S.M., Narayan J. : Phil. Mag. : A41 (1980) 81.
/4/ Kobayashi S., Ohr. S.M. : Scripta Met. : 15 (1981) 343.
/5/ Ohr S.M., Kobayashi S. : J. Metals 32 (1980) 95.
/6/ Thomson R. : J. Mat. Sci. 13 (1978) 128.
/7/ Thomson R. : Atomistic Fracture, Proc. NATO Conf. Corsica 1981.
/8/ Chang S.J., Ohr S.M. : J.A.P. 52 (1981) 7174.
/9/ Louat N.P. : Proc. ICF1, Sendai, Japan (1965) 117.
/10/ Majumdar B.S., Burns S.J. : Acta Met. 29 (1981) 579.
/11/ Dai S.H., Li J.C.M. : Scripta Met. 16 (1982) 183.
/12/ Chu S.N.G. : J.A.P. 53 (1982) 12.
/13/ Muskhelishvili N.I. : Singular Integral Equations, Noordhoff, Groningen 1953.
/14/ Michot G. : Thesis, Institut National Polytechnique de Lorraine, Nancy 1982.

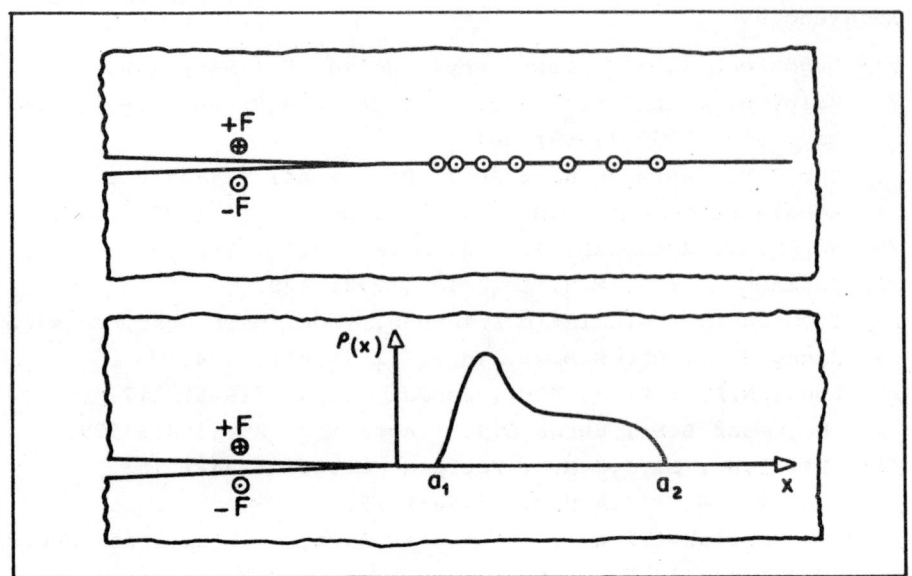

Fig.1 : Sketch of the crack ; definition of the abscissae a_1 and a_2 and of the distribution function of dislocation $\rho(x)$.

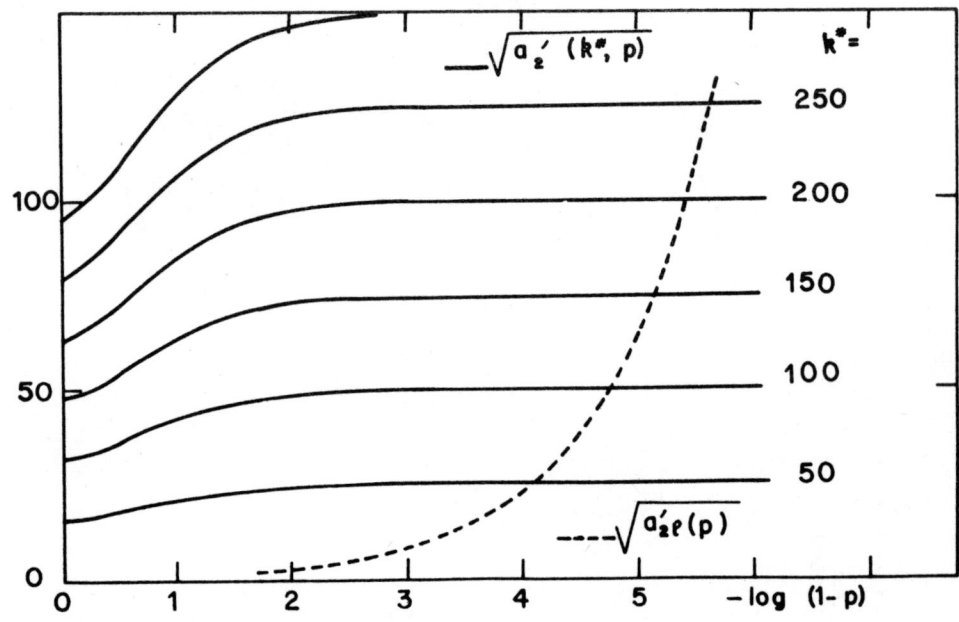

Fig.2 : Variation of $\sqrt{a_2'(k^*,p)}$ against p for different fixed values of k^*.

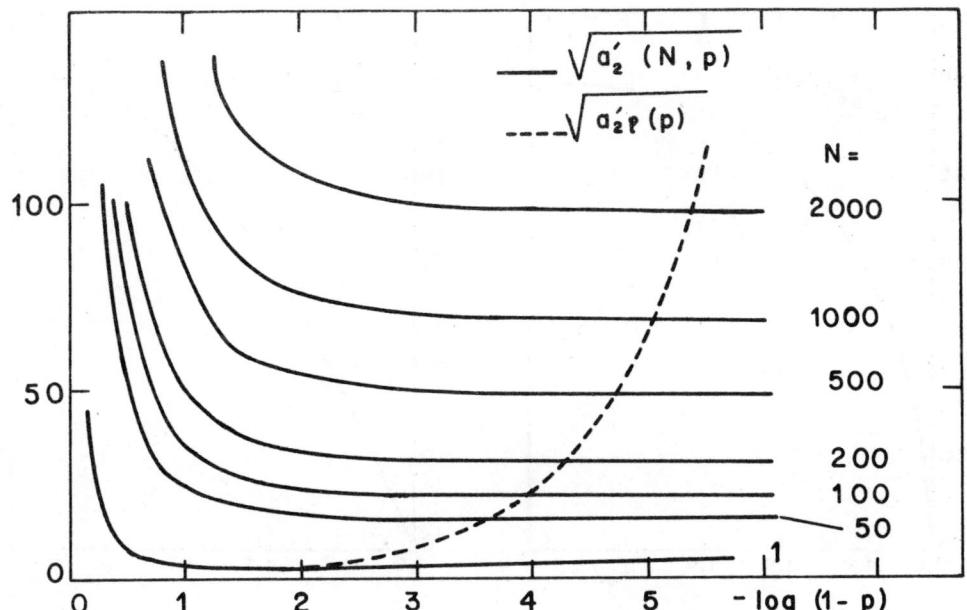

Fig.3 : Variation of $\sqrt{a_2'(N,p)}$ against p for different fixed values of N.

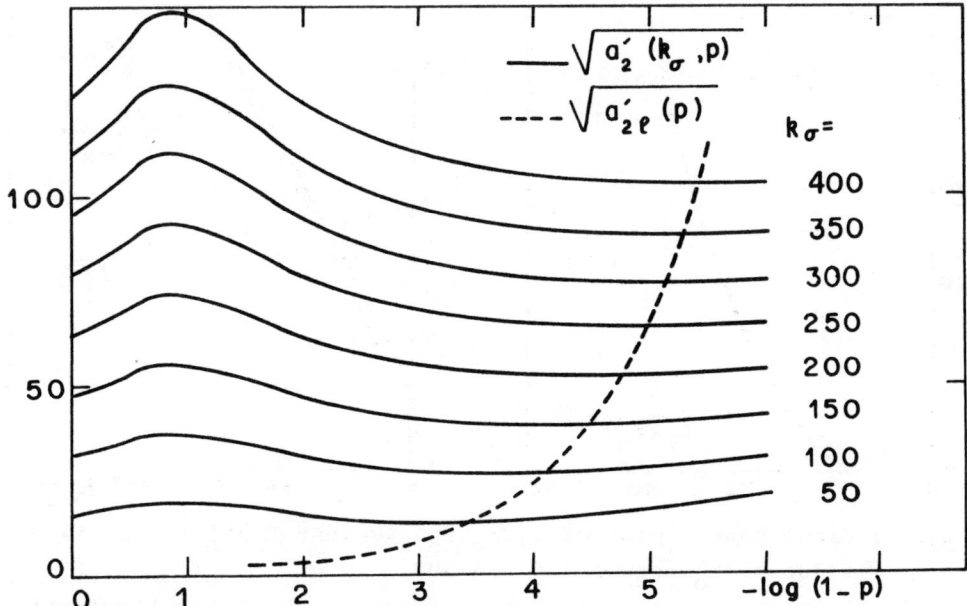

Fig.4 : Variation of $\sqrt{a_2'(k_\sigma,p)}$ against p for different fixed values of k_σ.

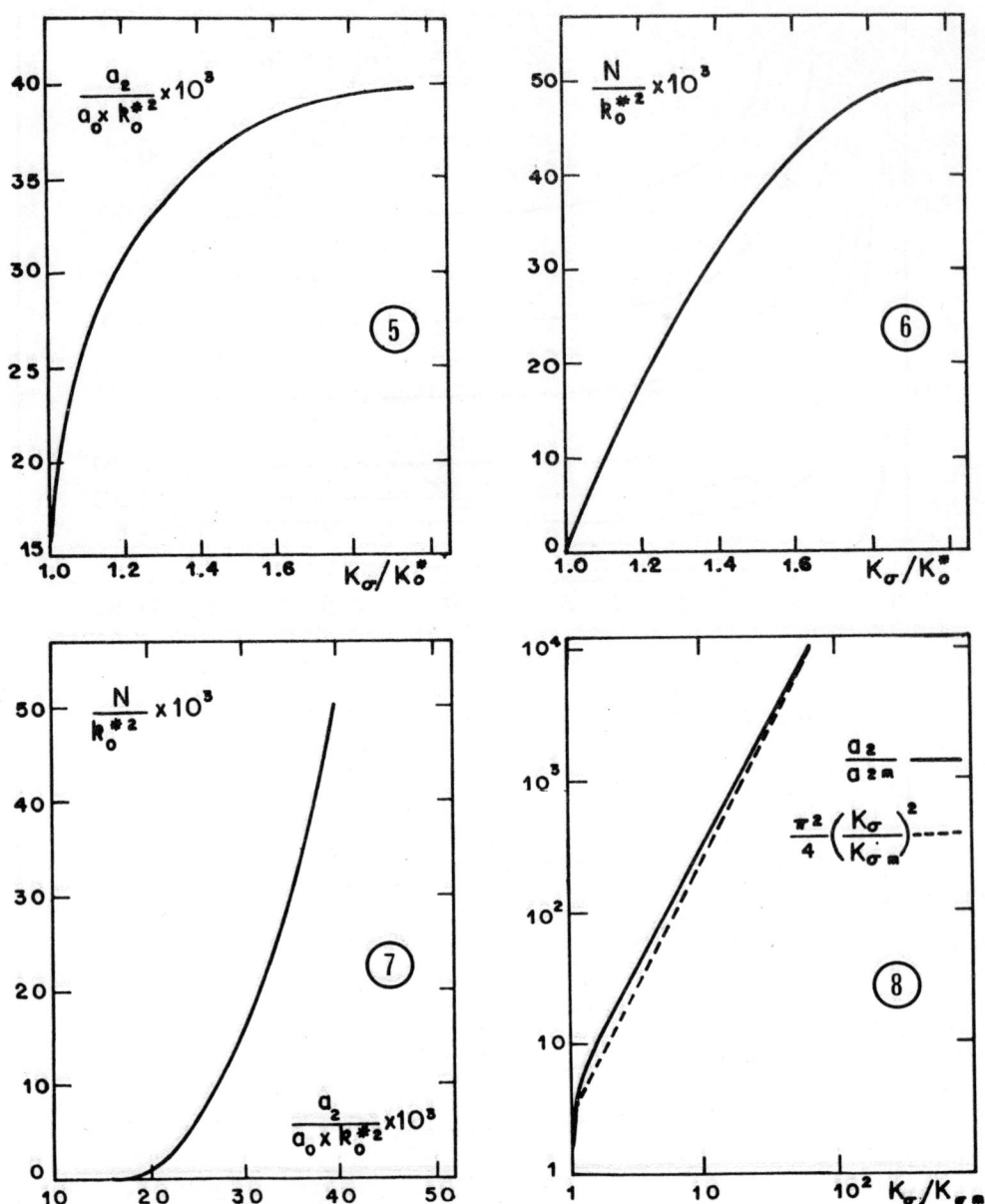

Fig.5 : First case : plot of $a_2/a_0 \cdot k_o^{*2}$ against K_σ/K_o^* for a fixed value of k_o^* between 50 and 300.

Fig.6 : First case : plot of N/k_o^{*2} against K_σ/K_o^* for a fixed value of k_o^* between 50 and 300.

Fig.7 : First case : plot of N/k_o^{*2} against $a_2/a_0 \cdot k_o^{*2}$ for a fixed value of k_o^* between 50 and 300.

Fig.8 : Second case : plot of a_2/a_{2m} against $K_\sigma/K_{\sigma m}$

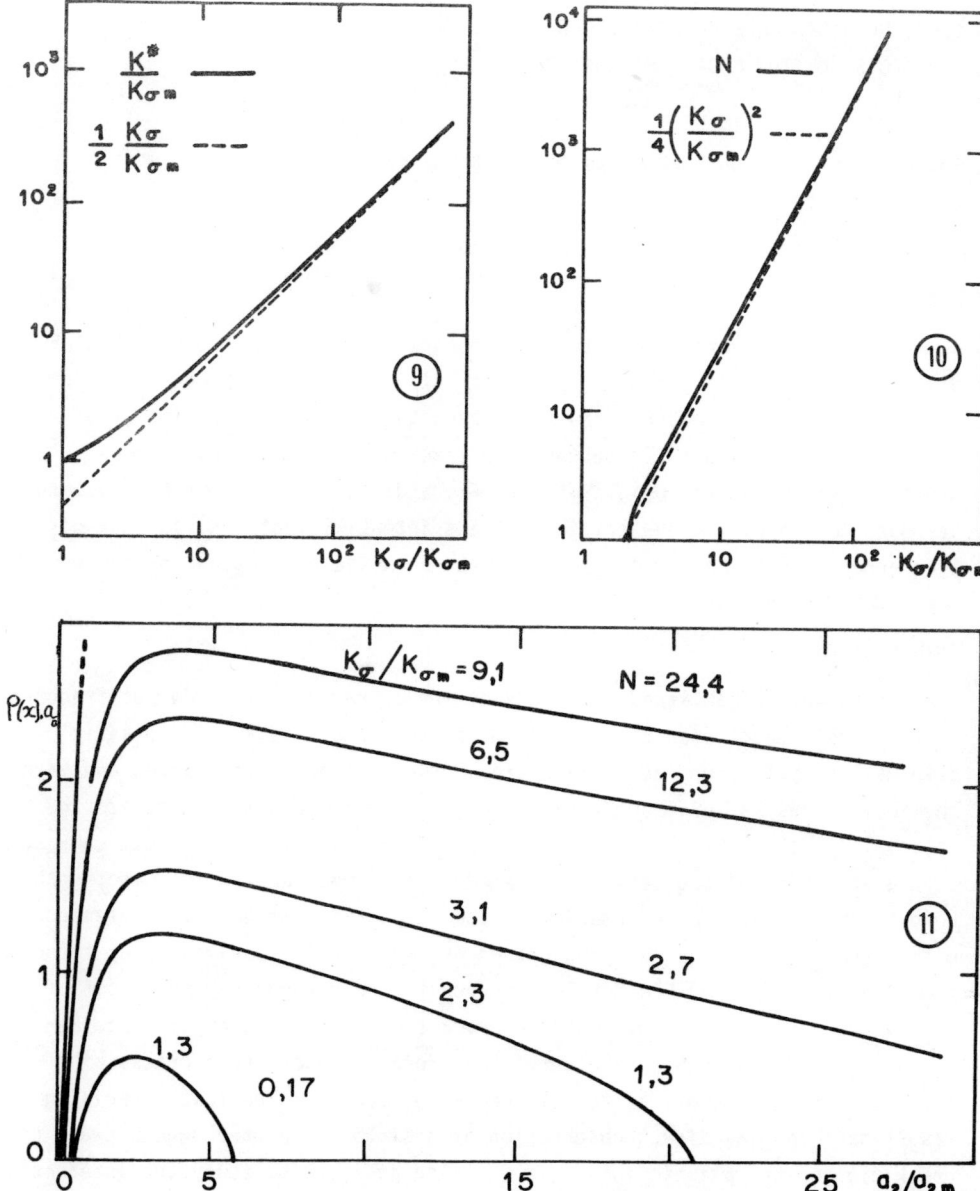

<u>Fig.9</u> : Second case : plot of $K^*/K_{\sigma m}$ against $K_\sigma/K_{\sigma m}$.

<u>Fig. 10</u> : Second case : plot of N against $K_\sigma/K_{\sigma m}$.

<u>Fig. 11</u> : Second case : plot of $\rho(x)/a_o$ against a_2/a_{2m} for different fixed values of $K_\sigma/K_{\sigma m}$.

ELECTRON MICROSCOPE OBSERVATION OF CRACK PROPAGATION
AND A DISLOCATION MODEL OF FRACTURE*

S. M. Ohr

Solid State Division, Oak Ridge National Laboratory
Oak Ridge, TN, U.S.A. 37830

ABSTRACT

This paper describes electron microscope observations of the emission and distribution of dislocations at the crack tip during in situ tensile deformation. The most interesting result has been the direct observation of a dislocation-free zone (DFZ) between the crack tip and the plastic zone. In order to understand the origin of the DFZ, a dislocation theory of fracture has been developed and the critical stress intensity factor K_g for the dislocation generation at the crack tip is proposed as the definition for the condition for crack tip deformation.

INTRODUCTION

It is well established that many of structural materials do not fracture at the stress level predicted by the Griffith formula because of plastic deformation that occurs at a crack tip. Under extreme temperatures and harsh chemical or nuclear environments however, crack tip deformation ceases and the materials fracture unexpectedly in a brittle manner. It is not well understood at present which of the material parameters are important in influencing the conditions for plastic deformation at the crack tip. We have made electron microscope studies of crack propagation and dislocation behavior near the crack tip of various fcc and bcc metals in order to understand the mechanisms of plastic deformation occurring at the crack tip. Depending on the specimen geometry, it was possible to observe the propagation of shear cracks of modes II and III as well as tensile cracks of mode I. The most surprising result has been the direct observation of a dislocation-free zone between the crack tip and the plastic zone. It was also possible to study the interaction between the cracks and grain-boundaries.

In order to understand the physical origin of the DFZ and its relationship to fracture criteria, a DFZ model of fracture was developed by considering the

---
*Research sponsored by the Division of Materials Sciences, U.S. Department of Energy under contract W-7405-eng-26 with the Union Carbide Corporation.

equilibrium between the crack and the dislocations in the plastic zone under stress. From the analysis it was possible to derive the relationship between the crack tip geometry, the local stress intensity factor K, and the number of dislocations in the plastic zone. It was shown that the DFZ is a manifestation of an impediment to the generation of dislocations at the crack tip and this was expressed in terms of the critical stress intensity factor K_g for dislocation generation. The present paper reviews some of the experimental results /1-5/ and the development of the DFZ model of fracture /6, 7/. Based on the DFZ model, a new micromechanical mechanism of ductile-brittle transition is presented.

EXPERIMENTAL RESULTS

Direct observations of crack tip deformation were made during tensile deformation in a Philips EM400T electron microscope using a specimen stage which was built specifically for this experiment. Sheet specimens (3 x 6.5 x 0.025 mm) were spark cut and an area about 2 mm in diameter was electropolished in a Struers Tenupol until perforation. As the stress was applied, cracks were nucleated at the edge of the polishing hole and propagated into the specimen. In thin areas of the specimen the mode of crack propagation was mode III. As the cracks moved into the thicker sections, the mode of fracture changed from mode III to predominantly mode I.

Figure 1 shows an electron micrograph of a crack tip area from a copper specimen deformed in tension. The crack was nucleated at the edge of the polishing hole and propagated into the specimen. The plastic zone consists of a linear array of dislocations on a plane which is coplanar with the crack. It was found that the (111) slip plane makes an angle of approximately 22° with the foil plane. Contrast analysis has shown that the dislocations are very close to screw orientation with the Burgers vector of $a/2[1\bar{1}0]$. This, along with the result of a stereoscopic observation, has shown that the mode of crack propagation is mode III. It can be seen that the region between the crack tip and the plastic zone is dislocation-free.

There are approximately 150 dislocations in the plastic zone and their total Burgers vector is nearly 400 A. The thickness of the specimen at the crack tip is found to be approximately 600 A. It can be seen that the contribution of the dislocations to the crack opening displacement (COD), i.e. the plasticity portion of the COD, is 2/3 of the total COD needed to propagate the crack. The final 1/3 of the COD is provided when the DFZ ruptures elastically. Thus, it may be concluded that the crack propagates by a combination of plastic and elastic processes.

Figure 2 shows the distribution of dislocations near a crack tip observed in a niobium single crystal. In this specimen, two slip systems were activated simultaneously on inclined planes. The slip bands are delineated by extinction contours and the slip systems were identified as $(231)/[1\bar{1}1]$ and $(011)/[11\bar{1}]$. The DFZ is again present between the crack tip and the plastic zone. The dislocations in the lower half of the plastic zone are not visible in this micrograph because $\underline{g} \cdot \underline{b} = 0$, where $\underline{g}$ is the diffraction vector and $\underline{b}$ is the Burgers vector. The two slip vectors are combined to give the crack opening displacement along the [100] direction, commonly recognized as the direction of cleavage fracture for bcc metals. The crack tip geometry observed is very similar to that predicted for mode I fracture.

Figure 3 shows a series of electron micrographs taken from a polycrystalline molybdenum specimen which was stressed in the electron microscope to study the growth of a crack and its interaction with a grain-boundary. In Fig. 3(a), the crack is nucleated at the edge of the polishing hole. Although the crack is at an early stage of propagation, it has emitted a number of dislocations at the crack tip and some of the dislocations have moved along their slip plane and are piled up at the grain-boundary. At this stage, no dislocation activity can be detected in the adjacent grain. By increasing the external stress, the crack was allowed to grow toward the grain-boundary and this is shown in Fig. 3(b). The dislocation activity in front of the crack tip has intensified and some of this activity was transmitted into the next grain.

As the external stress was increased further, a small crack was nucleated at the grain-boundary approximately 2 μm to the left of the main crack. This can be seen in Fig. 3(c). The growth direction of this new crack is nearly parallel to the main crack. As the stress was increased even further, the cracks were joined together by breaking of the ligament separating the two. This is shown in Fig. 3(d) where it can be seen that the crack has started to propagate in a zig-zag manner. As to the interaction between the crack tip dislocations and grain-boundaries, it was found that some of the dislocations entered the boundaries and were annihilated. In some instances, the grain-boundary emitted dislocations in the direction opposite to that of the crack-generated dislocations along the plane that was parallel to the plastic zone. The grain-boundary also emitted dislocations into the adjacent grain depending on the relative orientation of the two neighboring grains.

DISLOCATION-FREE ZONE MODEL OF FRACTURE

The distribution of dislocations ahead of the crack tip observed in the electron microscope is generally in good agreement with the model of a plastic zone proposed by Bilby, Cottrell, and Swinden (BCS) /8/. One of the experimental results not considered in the BCS theory is the presence of the DFZ. The DFZ implies that the crack tip area can remain elastic after plastic deformation has occurred and hence the stress field can be described in terms of a stress intensity factor K. We have extended the BCS theory of fracture by including the DFZ as a part of the equilibrium crack tip geometry. The results show that the local stress intensity factor can be defined as

$$K = \frac{2 \sigma_f}{\pi e} \left[\pi c(e^2 - c^2)\right]^{1/2} F(\pi/2, k) \qquad (1)$$

where σ_f is the flow stress, F is the complete elliptic integral of the first kind, 2c is the crack length, e-c is the length of the DFZ, $k^2 = (a^2 - e^2)c^2/(a^2 - c^2)e^2$, and a - e is the length of the plastic zone. It can be shown that when the DFZ vanishes the value of K approaches zero. This is the crack tip geometry treated by Bilby et al.

If the crack tip encounters little difficulty in generating dislocations, a sufficient number of dislocations will be generated and hence the DFZ will be eliminated. Therefore, the presence of the DFZ is a manifestation of an impediment to the generation of dislocations at the crack tip. In order to define explicitly this impediment to dislocation generation, we have to examine the physical processes associated with the emission of dislocations from a crack tip by extending the crack tip dislocation nucleation model of Rice and Thomson /9/ and the nonlocal elasticity theory of Eringen /10/. It was shown that this impediment can be expressed in terms of a critical stress intensity factor for the generation of dislocations given for mode III geometry by

$$K_g = \frac{\mu b}{(8\pi r_c)^{1/2}} + (2\pi r_c)^{1/2} \sigma_f \qquad (2)$$

where μ is the shear modulus, b is the Burgers vector, r_c is the core radius of a dislocation, and σ_f is the flow stress. The crack tip is expected to generate dislocations when the local stress intensity factor K is greater than K_g.

With this definition of K_g, it is possible to discuss the criteria of brittle versus ductile fracture. The discussion is based on the magnitude of K_g relative to K_c, the critical stress intensity factor for brittle fracture, which is given for mode III fracture as

$$K_c^2 = 4\mu\gamma \qquad (3)$$

where γ is the surface energy. As the stress is increased, the value of K at the crack tip increases. The manner in which the crack grows will depend on whether K reaches K_c or K_g first. If $K_c < K_g$, K reaches K_c first and the crack will grow in a brittle manner. If $K_g < K_c$, K reaches K_g before it reaches K_c and the dislocations are generated at the crack tip before the crack can grow. The material will fail in a ductile manner through necking and void growth.

The present model can also be extended to discuss a possible mechanism of the ductile-brittle transition (DBT) in metals. It can be seen from Eq. (2) that K_g is directly proportional to the flow stress σ_f. In many of the metals that exhibit the DBT, it is found that σ_f increases with decreasing test temperature. This means that K_g increases with decreasing temperature. When the value of K_g reaches K_c, dislocation generation at the crack tip ceases and the crack now grows in a brittle manner without crack tip deformation. The critical flow stress σ_f^c at which this transition occurs is given by

$$\sigma_f^c = \frac{K_c}{(2\pi r_c)^{1/2}} - \frac{\mu b}{4\pi r_c} \qquad (4)$$

This is a new micromechanical mechanism for the DBT. Following neutron irradiation, the flow stress is observed to increase over the entire range of test temperature. In neutron irradiated metals, therefore, the temperature at which the flow stress reaches the critical value σ_f^c is expected to be higher than that for unirradiated metals. When the DBT temperature increases beyond the reactor ambient temperature, the metal will fail in a brittle manner. Further development of the model is currently underway; it is expected that this model will explain one of the most puzzling and costly problems of material failure found in various energy and transportation systems.

References

/1/ Ohr, S. M., Narayan, J: Phil. Mag. A41 (1980) 81.
/2/ Kobayashi, S., Ohr, S. M.: Phil. Mag. A42 (1980) 763.
/3/ Kobayashi, S., Ohr, S. M.: Scripta Metall. 15 (1981) 343.
/4/ Horton, J. A., Ohr, S. M.: Scripta Metall. 16 (1982) 621.
/5/ Horton, J. A., Ohr, S. M.: J. Mater. Sci. 17 (1982) 3140.
/6/ Chang, S. -J., Ohr, S. M.: J. Appl. Phys. 52 (1981) 7174.
/7/ Ohr, S. M., Chang, S. -J.: J. Appl. Phys. 53 (1982) 5645.
/8/ Bilby, B. A., Cottrell, A. H., Swinden, K. H.: Proc. R. Soc. London A272 (1963) 304.
/9/ Rice. J. R., Thomson, R.: Phil. Mag. 29 (1974) 73.
/10/ Eringen, A. C.: Crystal Lattice Defects 7 (1977) 109.

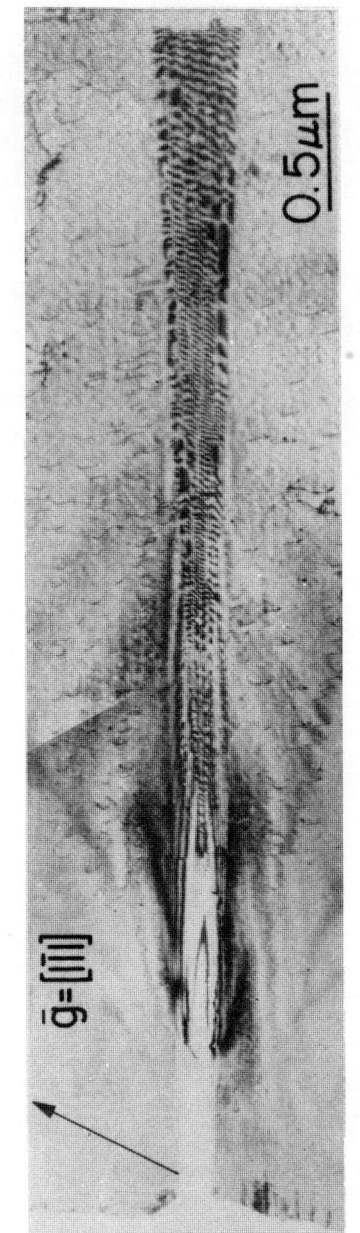

Fig. 1. Electron micrograph showing a shear crack of mode III type and its plastic zone in copper.

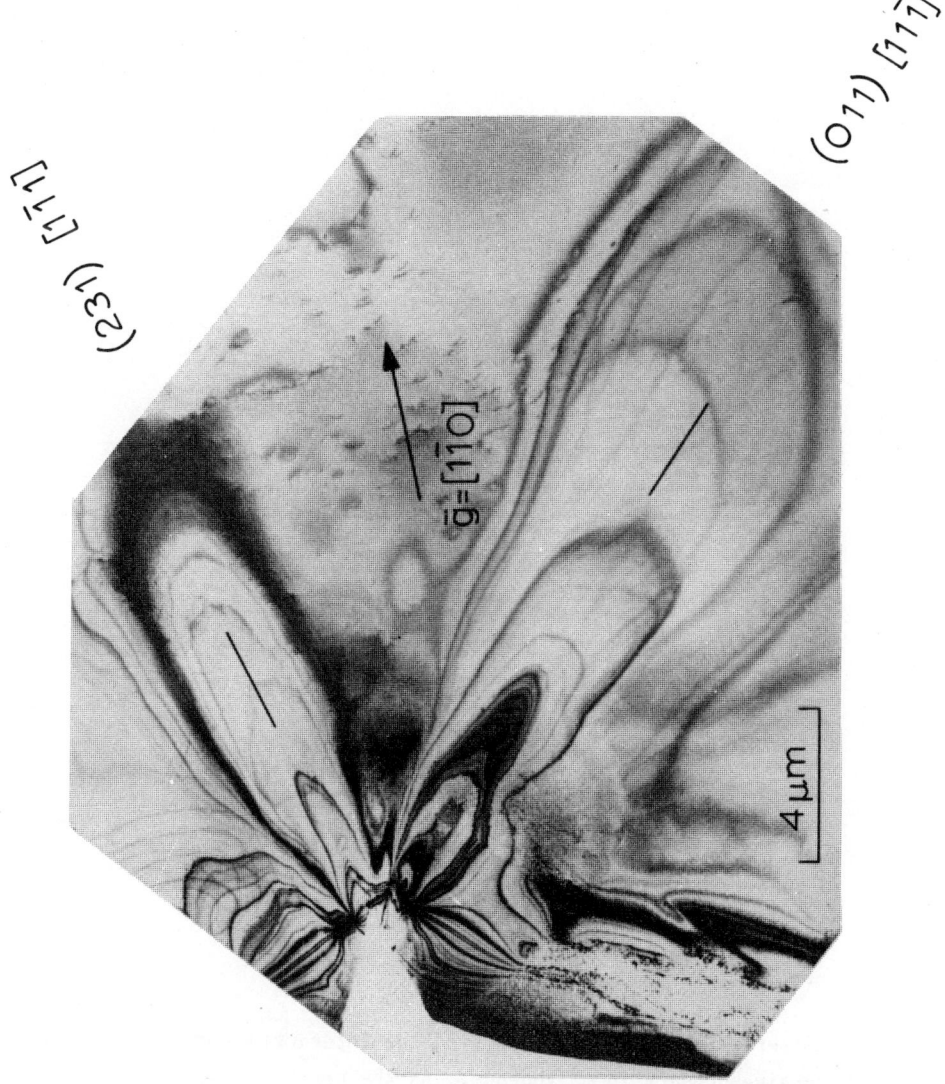

Fig. 2. Dislocation structure around a crack tip in niobium. The plastic zone contains two slip bands with two slip vectors on planes not coplanar with the crack.

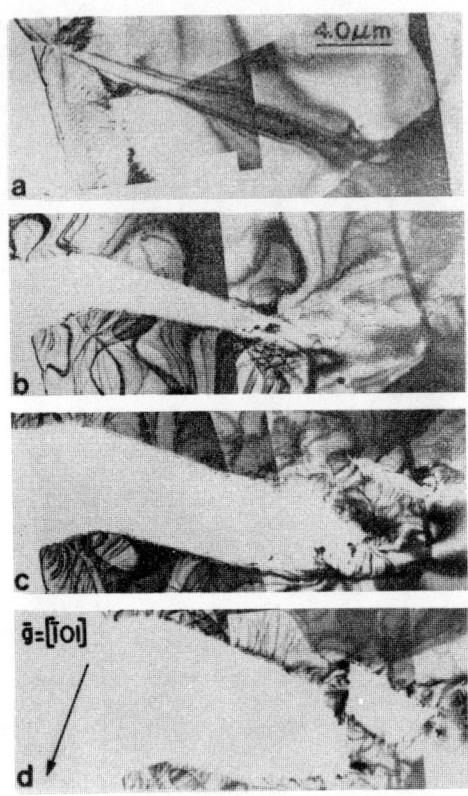

Fig. 3. A series of micrographs showing the interaction between a crack and grain-boundary in molybdenum. As the crack approached the boundary, a small crack was nucleated and eventually joined the main crack.

CREEP RATE AND MICROSTRUCTURE OF FCC METALS
D. Caillard* and J.L. Martin**
*Laboratoire d'Optique Electronique du CNRS, B.P. 4347, F-31055 Toulouse Cedex
**Ecole Polytechnique Fédérale de Lausanne, PHB-Ecublens, CH-1015 Lausanne

INTRODUCTION

Relationships between the creep rate and the microsctructure have been questioned for a long time and are the subject of several reviews [1][2]. Here, attention will be focused on the properties of the subboundaries, static as well as dynamic ones : What is their detailed geometry ? How do they behave under load ? How do they influence the deformation rate ? Recent description of subboundaries will be first reported, various dynamic observations of their properties will then be described. Finally in situ deformation experiments in the electron microscope will be summarized, related to the rate controlling mechanism in aluminium at intermediate temperatures.

STATIC PROPERTIES OF THE MICROSTRUCTURE

Chemical etching is the most ancient method used to reveal subgrains. Lacombe and Beaujard [3] evidenced rows of etch pits in aluminium deformed at high temperatures. These were later related to the presence of subboundaries made of periodic arrays of dislocations [4].

The first three dimensional observations of such substructures were performed, using the electron microscope in Al [5] and the decoration technique in NaCl and KCl for instance [6]. It was therefore possible to identify several types of subboundaries such as the pure tilt ones, the square grids of screw dislocation arrays, the hexagonal networks, and more complicated ones. Imperfections in the periodic networks became also evident : mesh distorsions, extrinsic dislocations, incomplete subboundaries. As will be stated below, these features are of importance for the understanding of the creep rate. It is not possible to list here all the descriptions of the creep substructure which were published since that time in various types of crystal. The influence of stress, temperature, strain and orientation was investigated [1][2], concerning the subgrain size, the misorientation between adjacent blocks, the existence of dislocation tangles or subboundaries, also in the case of single glide oriented crystals[7]. Essential features such as the state of equilibrium of the creep boundaries, and the dissociation of dislocations in their networks will now be reported.

a) <u>detailed geometry of subboundaries, long range stress fields</u> : Electron microscope observations in Al, W and Mo after creep [8] indicate that some of the subboundaries seem to be away from their equilibrium positions. However, a systematic study of numerous dislocation arrays after creep of aluminium plates at intermediate temperatures [9] shows that the subboundaries are made of 1, 2 or 3 dislocation families (out of the 6 possible ones) which are the most sensitive to the local stress. Conversely, the three dimensional network in the subgrains includes the six Burgers vectors in equal amounts. Weak beam observations of the dense networks (mesh size of the order of 150 Å) reveal that the dislocations segments are in the {111} sometimes {110} or {100} type glide planes. This feature controls the migration ability of the boundary. Detailed identification of the subboundary geometry indicates that the Frank criterion is approximately satisfied, i.e. that the long range stress field of the subboundaries, if any, is smaller than the applied stress. This agrees with observations on spinels[10] and differs from others on NiO [11]. However, one can notice that for large mesh networks, dislocation densities which deviate slightly from the Frank criterion do not create substantial long range stress fields. An example of creep subboundary in Al can be seen on fig. 1.

b) <u>dislocation dissociation in the subboundaries</u> : A close inspection of the network geometry indicates that the line tension equilibrium is not fulfilled at nodes. That is the case in Al [9] and in crystals for which the dissociation decreases the core energy by a larger amount than the increase of line energy.

At low angle boundaries in gold bicrystals [12], one of the dislocation families exhibits a serrated shape : the corresponding defects increase their length to dissociate onto different {111} planes.

Another type of dislocation dissociation has been evidenced in subboundaries of a Al-Zn-Mg alloy : some of the dislocation segments decompose on one or two{111} planes, Lomer Cottrell locks dissociating into strain-rod dislocations [13].

The resulting boundaries are not planar anymore, but exhibit "chairs".

High resolution observations of atomic columns in silicon bicrystals [14], indicate unusual subboundary dislocations with <111> or $\frac{1}{2}$<112> type Burgers vectors, which dissociate into three partial dislocations.

At last dissociation by climb has been reported in subboundaries of YIG single crystals after high temperature deformation [15].

The use of high resolution techniques has reevaluated the interest in the field of subboundaries. It has supplied complementary informations about their detailed geometry. These help to understand their dynamic properties which are of great importance for the rate controlling process of creep.

DYNAMIC PROPERTIES OF THE SUBSTRUCTURE

The local creep strain has two components [16][17]: the most significant one is bound to the motion of individual dislocations. The second one results from the migration of subboundaries. This two phenomena may not be completely unrelated and they are successively described below.

a) <u>movement of individual dislocations</u> : They can only be observed in the electron microscope because of the required resolution. Sometimes the high voltage electron microscope is used (HVEM) which enables thicker samples to be observed. In situ creep experiments in a HVEM [18] on an Al-1% Mg alloy at 300°C indicate, according to the authors, that 5% of the moving dislocations would contribute to strain and 95% to recovery processes. Other HVEM experiments on Al at 20°C [19] have shown that dislocation tangles form. They act as source and obstacle for mobile defects. The escaping of a dislocation from a subboundary has been observed in the case of the gold bicrystal [20]: the network consists of a square array of screw defects. During straining, dislocations escape on {111} planes leading to a partial destruction of the subboundary.

More recent HVEM studies [16][17] have been performed on precrept Al samples between 80°C and 200°C. Dislocations are originating from one ended sources located inside subgrains. They have to cross subboundaries to ensure a homogeneous strain, since sources are much less numerous than subgrains. Dislocation movements from one subboundary to the opposite are very fast and separated by large waiting times. This implies that the three dimensional network is a weak obstacle, long range stresses are lower than the applied stress and waiting times are due to subboundary crossing [17] . The latter mechanism is partially understood and illustrated on fig. 2. The dislocation waiting at the subboundary is AC which after extraction moves to A'C' by pencil glide (cross slip). Typical traces can be observed at the foil surface, from which the Burgers vector of AC can be deduced (one trace is straight, the other one is bent near the boundary, then straight). Such a glide geometry has been observed quite frequently. This is indication that cross slip operates during the cutting process of dislocations through subboundaries.

b) <u>subboundary migration</u> : Washburn and Parker optical observations [21] have proved that subboundaries were able to migrate in Zinc bicrystals. Later, this phenomenon has been reported several times under creep conditions, from etch-pitting experiments (in Al[22], LiF[23] and NaCl[24]). A systematic study was undertaken in Al between 400 and 600°C using X-ray topography [25]: the average migration distance is proportional to strain and the resulting strain rate to the total one. It exhibits the same stress and temperature dependance. This migration contributes to about a maximum of 1/4 of the total strain. At last a recent study by synchrotron radiation topography on thick samples of NaCl under creep conditions has shown that the migration rate is larger during stage I while the subgrain misorientation is weak [26]. In stage II, only the new created subboundaries are very mobile. All these experiments emphasize the importance of migration during creep. Nevertheless, the mechanisms proposed depend on the authors : glide, climb or cross slip.

The HVEM experiments on the creep mechanisms of aluminium have also described this process [16]. It plays an important role in the substructure evolution in stage II. Fig. 3 shows how it occurs due to the local stress only : no individual dislocation is seen to enter the subboundary between fig. 3a and 3b. Fig. 4 shows that the rate of migration is enhanced if dislocations are cutting through the boundary. Between fig. 4a and 4b, a group of dislocations has crossed the subboundary. At the place where intersection has occurred, migration is seen to be more pronounced. This seems to indicate a high stress sensitivity of the migration rate. To estimate it, a strain rate jump experiment has been performed in situ and is described below.

As already shown [17], local strains and strain rates can be evaluated by considering that each dislocation shearing a subgrain of size L provides an amount of strain $\varepsilon = b/L$ (b = Burgers vector). If dislocations cannot be unambiguously counted as a function of time, their slip traces can, and as an example of local creep curve (fig. 5) is shown, which could be established for the area of fig. 5. The strain rate appears to be rather constant before and after the jump and close to $3.7 \times 10^{-7} s^{-1}$ and $4.5 \times 10^{-6} s^{-1}$ respectively. Its stress sensitivity will be characterized by the usual exponent n (n' for the migration rate).

From the macroscopic creep data : $n_1 = d \log \dot{\varepsilon} / d \log \sigma = A\sigma b/kT$ where A is the activation area. If $A \simeq 200 \, b^2$ [9], $n_1 \sim 29$.

From the microscopic creep curve, a n_2 value can be derived as follows : the quantity $d\log \dot{\varepsilon}$ can be obtained from fig. 4 and $d\log \sigma = \Delta\sigma/\sigma$. If one notices that $\Delta\sigma/\sigma = \Delta R/R$, where R is the radius of curvature of any dislocation which can be measured on dislocation d of fig. 6, as an example, before and after the strain rate change. It comes out : $\Delta\sigma/\sigma \lesssim 10\%$ and $n_2 \gtrsim 1/0.04 = 24$. From these considerations, it appears that the stress exponent of the creep rate (n_1 or n_2) is of the same order of magnitude in microscopic and macroscopic experiments and ranges between 20 and 30. This means that at least for the problem investigated here, radiation damage and surface effects in the HVEM are not too disturbing.

For the migration rate, $n' = d\log(v_{migration})/d\log \sigma$. $d\log \sigma$ has been

[20] Balluffi
[21] Washburn
[22] Brunner H
[23] Smirnov B
      Sol. Stat
[24] Pontikis
[25] Exell S.F
[26] Fries E.,
[27] Caillard
[28] Dorn J.E.
[29] Luthy H.,
[30] Myshlyaev
[31] Sastry D.
[32] Sastry D.
[33] J. Friede
[34] J.P. Poir

Fig. 1 : A subbo
field - b) Dark
projection.

Fig. 2 : Interac
ment 200ºC. 1 Me
such as d, comin
the typical slip
c) Stereogram -
AC.

Fig. 3 : Subboun
riment as in fig
ary positions (c

Fig. 4 : Subboun
a) and b) are se
to fig. 3. ε : z

Fig. 5 : Local c
area of fig. 6.
formation states

Fig. 6 : Sequenc
a) b) c) are rep

Fig 7 : Measure
location d. The
rate jump- b) af

computed above and the velocity of migration can be measured on fig. 6. Micrographs 6a and 6b correspond to the slow regime of fig. 5 and 6c to the fast one. A comparison of the subboundary positions as a function of time on the sketch of fig. 5d shows that, by increasing approximately ten times the strain rate, the migration velocity gets amplified by a factor of 3 to 7. A value of n' ranging between 7 and 17 is found. As stated above, other experiments [25] show that n = n'. The value derived here for n' is probably underestimated because it is averaged over a too small number of subboundaries. Nevertheless, n' is definitely larger than 1 which should be the stress exponent of the migration rate provided it occurs by climb of some of the subboundary dislocation segments.

This experiments shows that climb is not the rate controlling process of subboundary migration.

DISCUSSION AND CONCLUSION

At least in the case of aluminium at intermediate temperatures, in situ deformation studies in the HVEM provide some hints for the understanding of the creep rate in relation with the microstructure. It is clear that a glide mechanism takes place, with the subboundaries as obstacles. The bypassing mechanism is not completely understood. It certainly requires high stresses larger than the applied stress [17] because of the necessity of recombining junctions in a small size network. The dislocation slip traces furnish some evidence of cross slip near the subboundaries. The high local stresses may be achieved at irregular points of the creep boundaries where the internal elastic stress can help the applied stress. The process of subboundary migration which occurs by glide of most of the network segments might help in concentrating the stress at irregular points of the boundaries where the periodicity of the structure is disturbed [27]. It also ensures a redistribution of network dislocations which move along the boundary plane, cross through the triple junctions and rearrange themselves in the neighbouring subboundaries [16]. An experiment performed in the microscope has shown that the stress dependance of migration is incompatible with a dislocation climb process.

Since Dorn experiments [28] which evidenced an activation energy typical of intermediate temperature regimes, conflicting mechanisms have been proposed for the corresponding rate controlling process : climb by pipe diffusion [29], jog formation during subboundary destruction [30], recombination of junction reactions [31][32]. Cross slip has also been claimed to be a possible mechanism by Dorn himself [28] but also other authors [33][34].

The precise determination of the activation parameters of the latter pro-

cess woul
necessary
crept sam
dislocati
priate al
tion forc
cessary a

A
(contract
de de la

[1] Take
[2] Poir
    Eyr
[3] Lac
[4] Sch
[5] Hirs
[6] Amel
[7] Orlo
[8] Mysh
    (197
    Mysh
    gamo
[9] Cail
[10] Douk
[11] Gerv
[12] Darb
[13] Vand
[14] Bour
[15] Rabi
[16] Cail
[17] Cail
[18] Hend
    Hend
    Press
[19] Tabat

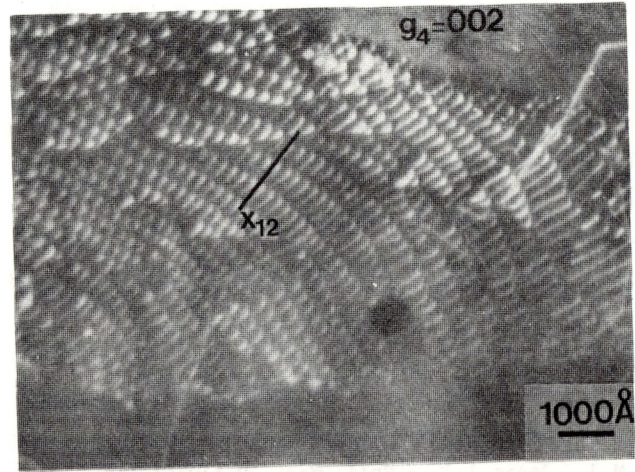

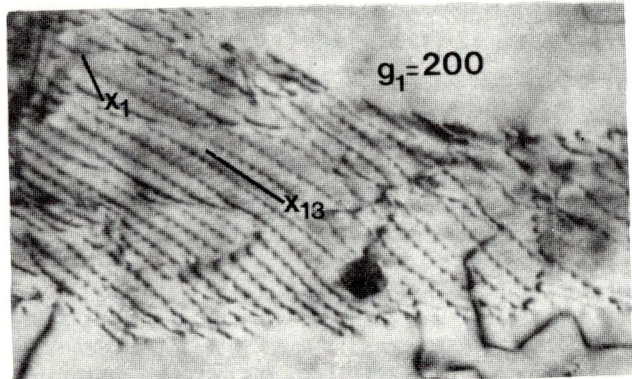

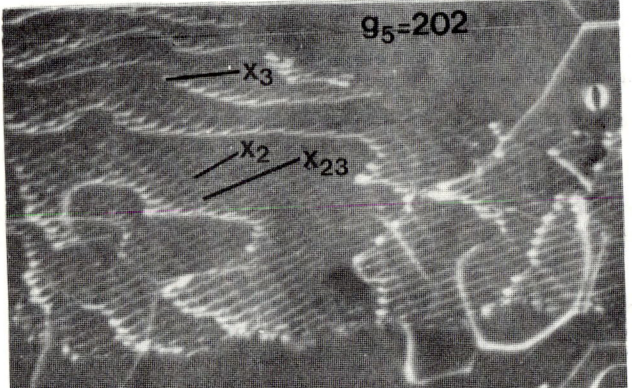

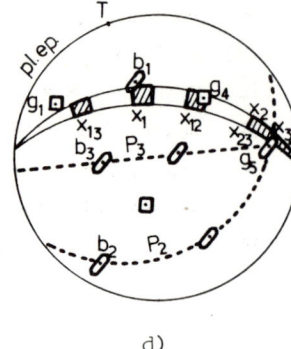

Fig. 1

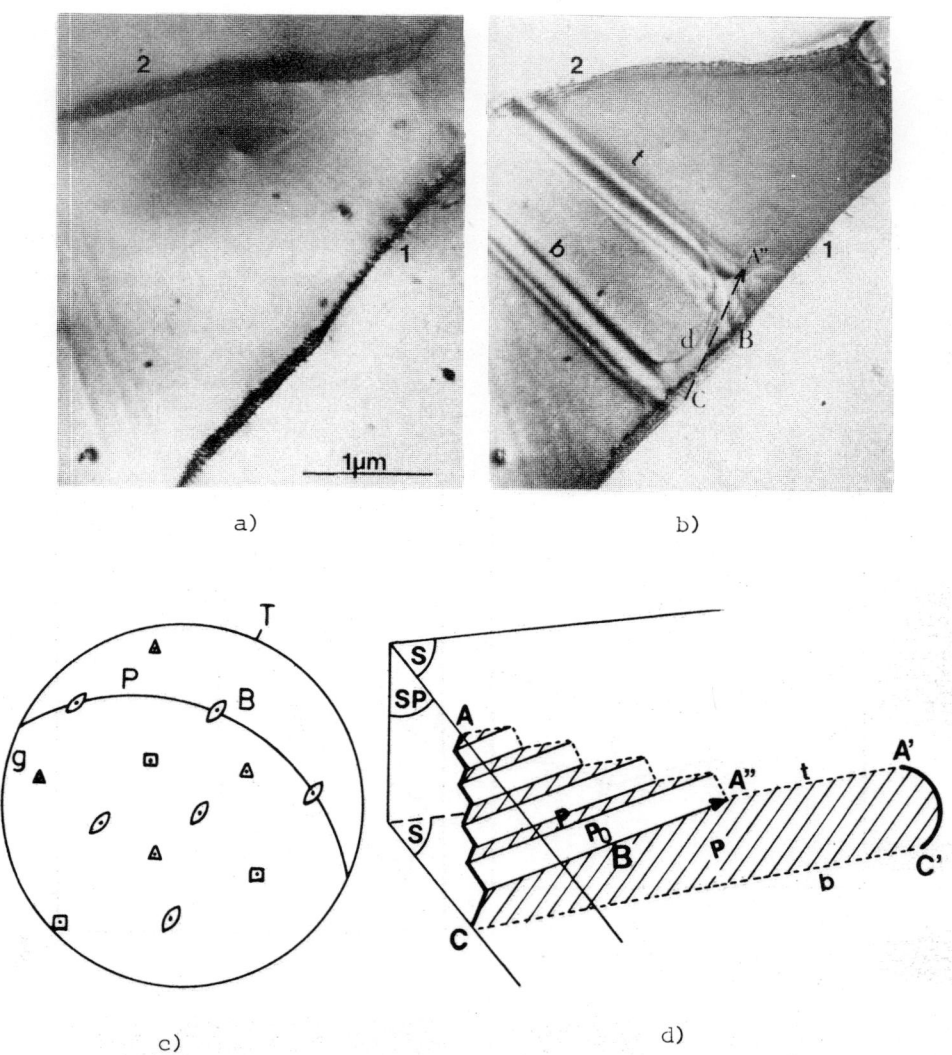

Fig. 2

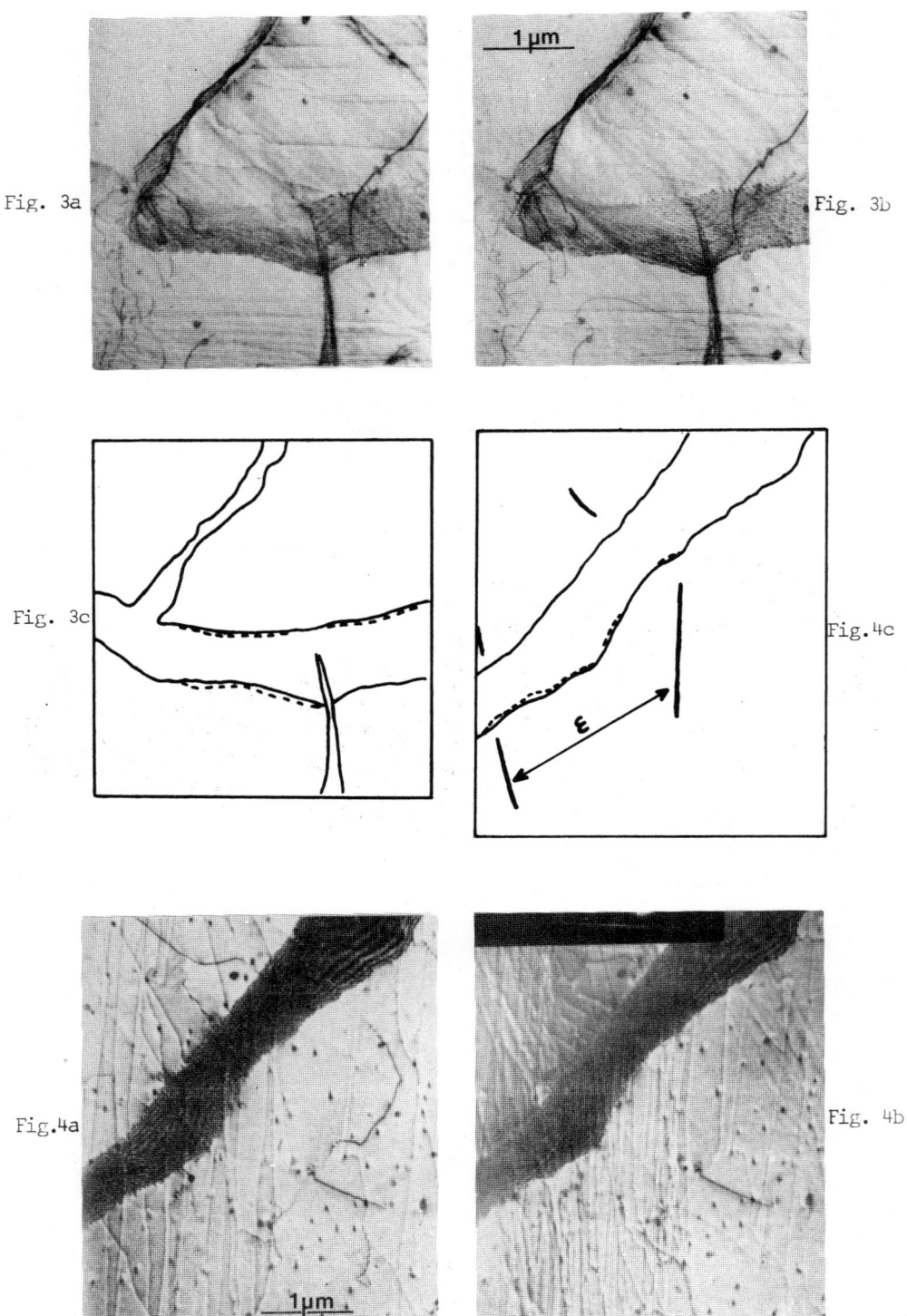

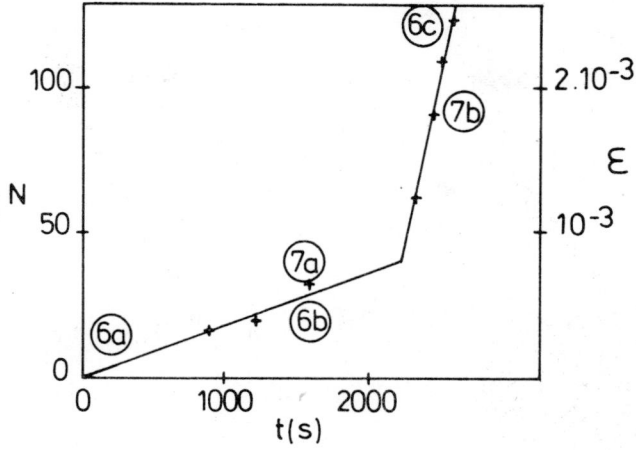

Fig. 5

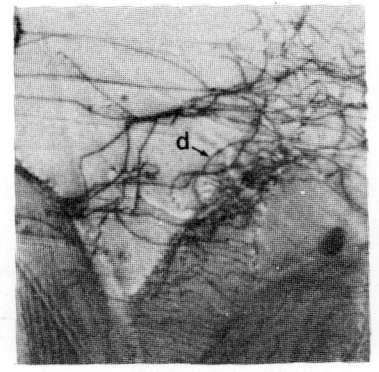

Fig. 7a

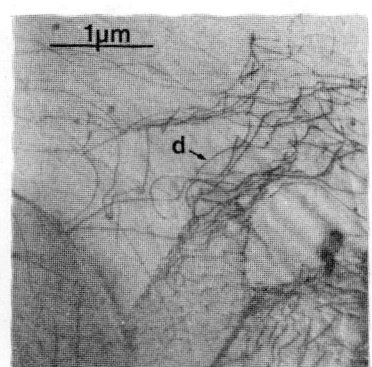

Fig. 7b

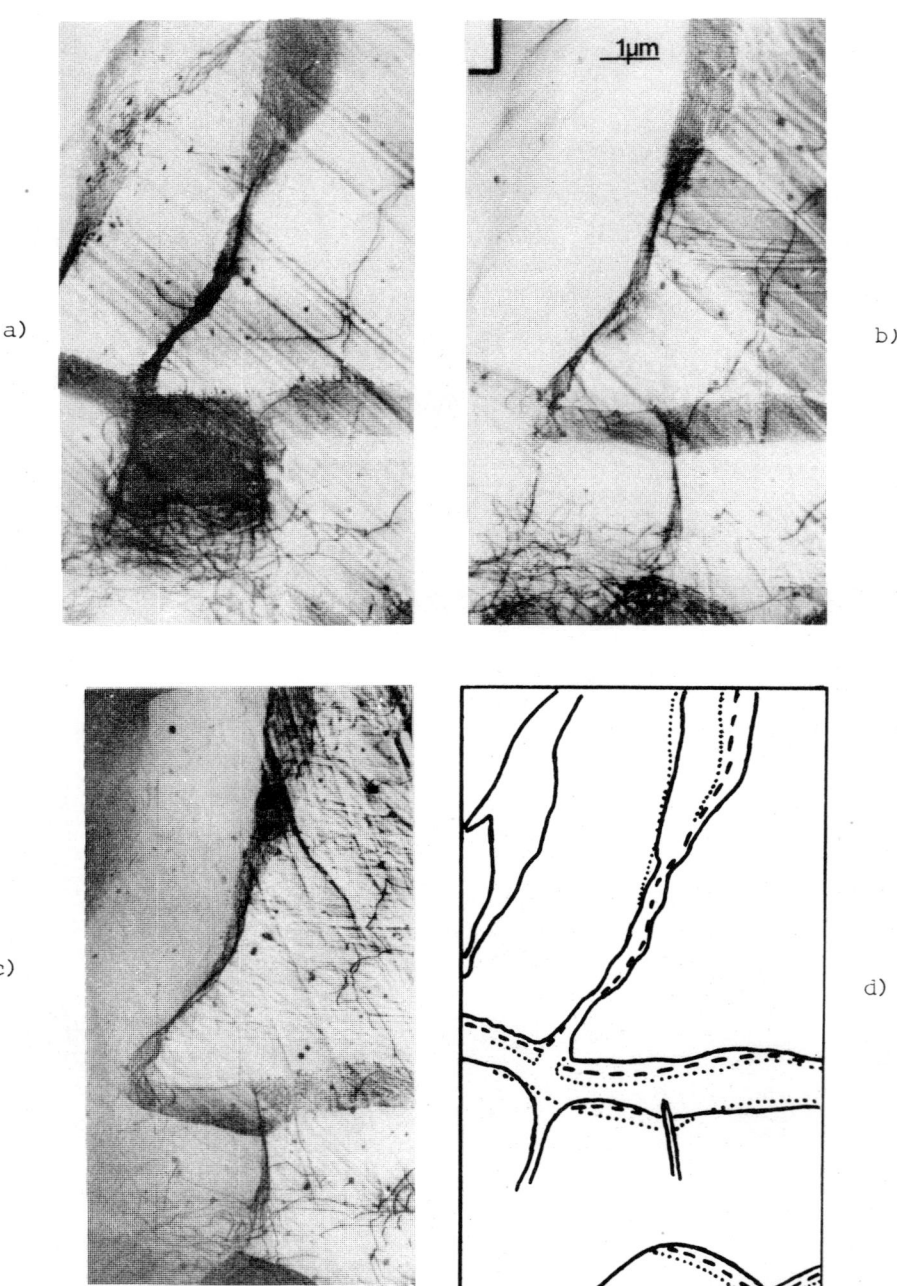

Fig. 6

Short communications presented at the symposium

Section 1: The structure and properties of dislocations
         in metals and alloys with close-packed lattices
    J. Th. M. De Hosson
Dislocations in the Ll_2 ordered structure of Cu_2NiZn
    G. Vanderschaeve, B. Escaig
Zigzag propagation of deformation microtwins in ordered
Ni_3V alloy
    H. Neuhäuser, F. Schmidt-Hohagen, E. Finkelmann
On the superposition of solid solution and strain hardening
in Cu-Zn alloys
    V. V. Demirskii, S. N. Komnik
The effect of stacking fault energy on low-temperature twinning
in copper-base alloys
    M. Saxlová
Effect of compositional modulations on strength of f.c.c. alloys
    B. Legrand, R. Le Hazif
Relationship between the electronic structure and the glide
in the hexagonal close packed metals
    S. Naka, A. Lasalmonie
The importance of the core structure of $\vec{a}$-type dislocations
in the plastic deformation of α-titanium
    V. N. Kovaleva, V. A. Moskalenko
Stacking fault energy on dislocation motion in titanium alloys
at low temperatures
    P. Lukáč, I. Stulíková, Z. Trojanová
Mobility of dislocations in hexagonal slip systems
    V. P. Soldatov, L. N. Zagoruiko
Interaction of basic dislocations with forest dislocations
in zinc leading to accelerated creep

Section 2: The structure and properties of dislocations
         in metals and alloys with a bcc lattice
    Y. Umakoshi, M. Yamaguchi, V. Vitek
Atomistic studies of the motion of $\langle 111 \rangle$ screw dislocations
in B2 ordered alloys
    G. Schoeck
The topology of screw dislocations in b.c.c. metals

E. Kuramoto, Y. Aono, T. Tsutsumi
On the energy distribution around a screw dislocation core
in model b.c.c. lattice

H.-J. Kaufmann, P. P. Pal-Val
Low-temperature ultrasound absorption in weakly deformed
molybdenum single crystals of high purity

A. Luft, H.-J. Kaufmann
Deformation behaviour and dislocation structure of molybdenum
single crystals at liquid helium temperatures

M. Bucki, J. Buchar, S. Kadečková
Dislocation structure of Fe-3.5%Si single crystal loaded
at high strain rates

E. V. Ottenberg, G. S. Burkhanov, E. M. Savitsky
Structure and mechanical properties of solid state grown
molybdenum single crystals

M. Yamaguchi, Y. Umakoshi, T. Yamane
High temperature deformation of Ni_2AlTi single crystals
with the $L2_1$ structure

E. Lunarska, V. Novák, N. Zárubová, S. Kadečková
Effect of hydrogen on work hardening and slip line pattern
in iron single crystals

G. S. Burkhanov, V. M. Kirillova, N. Mukhamedshina, M. Bucki
The study of impurity and dislocation structure of tungsten
single crystals

Section 3: The structure and properties of defects
          in non-metallic materials

V. Z. Bengus, T. P. Kovalenko, E. D. Tabachnikova
Defect structure study of KCl and LiF single crystals
at 0-stage of work-hardening

T. Suzuki
Dislocation tunneling in alkali-halides of NaCl-type

F. Appel, U. Messerschmidt
Dislocation cutting processes in ionic crystals investigated
by in-situ deformation in the HVEM and by surface decoration

U. Messerschmidt, H. Schmid, F. Appel
The shape of bowed dislocation segments in MgO crystals
loaded in high-voltage electron microscope

F. Vávra, Z. Ševčík
Temperature dependence of slip in AgCl crystals

A. B. Lebedev, S. B. Kustov, B. K. Kardashev
Amplitude-dependent internal friction during plastic deformation process

A. V. Leonteva, V. A. Romanusha, L. V. Stepanchuk
Defect behaviour pecularities near brittle-plastic transitions in crystals of a zero-group

M. Pardavi-Horváth, Á. Cziráki, I. Fellegvári, B. Keszei
Crystalline and magnetic defects in epitaxial garnet layers

M. Glogarová, J. Pavel, L. Lejček
Regular defect structure in chiral smectic C liquid crystals and its behaviour in electric field

Section 4: The structure and properties of grain boundaries

R. Z. Valiev, V. Yu. Gertsman, O. A. Kaibyshev
The interaction of grain boundaries with lattice dislocations

P. P. Pal-Val, V. Paidar, S. Kadečková
The effect of the twin boundary on the slip in Fe-5.8%Si bicrystals

Y. Estrin, K. Lücke
Vacancies in the wake of a moving grain boundary

K. Masuda, R. Yamamoto, M. Doyama, M. Hashimoto, Y. Ishida
Studies of tilt grain boundaries in cubic transition metals: atomic and electronic structures

K. Marukawa
Lattice expansion across twin boundaries in a body centered cubic metal

J. Gemperlová, A. Gemperle, V. Paidar
Lattice relaxation on antiphase boundaries in ordered Fe-Si alloys

Section 5: Collective behaviour and interaction of defects

A. E. Romanov
Elastic properties of disclination defects

D. Caillard
Weak beam in situ experiments on creep in Al at intermediate temperatures

F. Monchoux
Heterogeneous deformation of Cu-Ge alloys by collective movements of dislocations

V. Navrátil, V. Stejskalová
Discontinuous creep of Cd-Zn and Cd-Sn alloys

N. Clément, A. Coujou
In situ observation of a static aging experiment (propagation and intersection of moving pile ups)

A. Coujou, N. Clément, A. Beneteau, P. Coulomb
Interpretation of microtwinning serrations from in-situ observations in a HVEM

A. Orlová
Some applications of the dislocation link length distribution

M. Hamerský, P. Lukáč, Z. Trojanová
Lattice defects and stress relaxation

V. Novák
Stress relaxations in cyclically deformed Fe and Fe-Si alloys single crystals

ACKNOWLEDGEMENTS

The symposium on the Structure and Properties of Crystal Defects would not have been possible without the full support of the Institute of Physics and the Czechoslovak Academy of Sciences. In particular, the opportunity of holding the symposium in the conference centre of the Czechoslovak Academy of Sciences at Liblice castle is highly appreciated. In addition, the sponsorship of the Physical Section of the Union of Czechoslovak Mathematicians and Physicists, and the assistance of the Faculty of Mathematics and Physics, Charles University, Prague, in publishing part A of the symposium proceedings are gratefully acknowledged. Thanks are due to all who contributed to the organization of the symposium in particular to my colleagues from the symposium organizing committee and to Mrs. Stará and Mrs. Zichová.

V. Paidar
Symposium Secretary